The Evidence-Based Guide to ANTIDEPRESSANT MEDICATIONS

THE EVIDENCE-BASED GUIDE TO ANTIDEPRESSANT MEDICATIONS

Edited by

Anthony J. Rothschild, M.D.

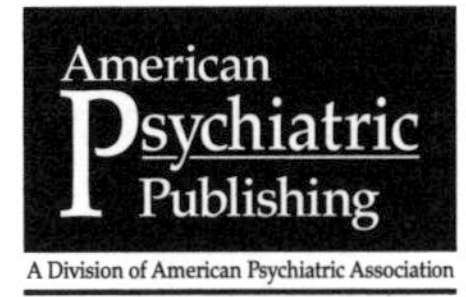

Washington, DC
London, England

Note: The authors have worked to ensure that all information in this book is accurate at the time of publication and consistent with general psychiatric and medical standards, and that information concerning drug dosages, schedules, and routes of administration is accurate at the time of publication and consistent with standards set by the U.S. Food and Drug Administration and the general medical community. As medical research and practice continue to advance, however, therapeutic standards may change. Moreover, specific situations may require a specific therapeutic response not included in this book. For these reasons and because human and mechanical errors sometimes occur, we recommend that readers follow the advice of physicians directly involved in their care or the care of a member of their family.

Manufactured in the United States of America on acid-free paper
15 14 13 12 11 5 4 3 2 1
First Edition

Typeset in Adobe's Cushing and Optima

American Psychiatric Publishing,
a Division of American Psychiatric Association
1000 Wilson Boulevard
Arlington, VA 22209–3901
www.appi.org

Library of Congress Cataloging-in-Publication Data
The evidence-based guide to antidepressant medications / edited by
Anthony J. Rothschild. — 1st ed.
p. ; cm.
Includes bibliographical references and index.
ISBN 978-1-58562-405-8 (pbk. : alk. paper)
I. Rothschild, Anthony J. II. American Psychiatric Association.
[DNLM: 1. Mental Disorders—drug therapy. 2. Antidepressive Agents—therapeutic use. 3. Evidence-Based Medicine—methods. WM 402]
LC classification not asssigned
616.85′27061—dc23

2011032536

British Library Cataloguing in Publication Data
A CIP record is available from the British Library.

To Judy, Rachel, and Amanda; to my mother, Edith Rothschild, and the memory of my father, Ernest Rothschild; and to the memory of my in-laws, Maye and Arnold Shindul.

The book is also dedicated to Betty Brudnick and in memory of Irving Brudnick, without whose generous support this book would not have been possible.

Contents

Contributors

Mary S. Ahn, M.D.
Assistant Professor, Division of Child and Adolescent Psychiatry, University of Massachusetts Medical School, Worcester, Massachusetts

Nancy Byatt, D.O., M.B.A.
Assistant Professor of Psychiatry, UMass Medical School; Attending Psychiatrist, Psychosomatic Medicine/Emergency Mental Health/Women's Mental Health, UMass Memorial Medical Center, Worcester, Massachusetts

Kristina M. Deligiannidis, M.D.
Assistant Professor of Psychiatry and Obstetrics and Gynecology, Medical Director, Depression Specialty Clinic; Psychiatrist, Women's Mental Health Specialty Clinic; Center for Psychopharmacologic Research and Treatment, University of Massachusetts Medical School/UMass Memorial Medical Center, Worcester, Massachusetts

Deepak Cyril D'Souza, M.B.B.S., M.D.
Associate Professor of Psychiatry, Yale University School of Medicine, West Haven, Connecticut

Jean A. Frazier, M.D.
Vice Chair and Director, Division of Child and Adolescent Psychiatry, Robert M. and Shirley S. Siff Endowed Chair, Professor of Psychiatry and Pediatrics, University of Massachusetts Medical School, Worcester, Massachusetts

Stacey B. Gramann, D.O., M.P.H.
Psychosomatic Medicine Fellow, Oregon Health and Science University, Portland, Oregon

Cassandra Hobgood, M.D.
Staff Psychiatrist, Baystate Medical Center, Springfield, Massachusetts; Assistant Professor of Psychiatry, Tufts University School of Medicine, Boston, Massachusetts

Michael D. Jibson, M.D., Ph.D.
Clinical Professor of Psychiatry and Director of Residency Education, Department of Psychiatry, University of Michigan Health System, Ann Arbor, Michigan

Ryan J. Kimmel, M.D.
Acting Assistant Professor, Department of Psychiatry and Behavioral Sciences, University of Washington School of Medicine; Medical Director, UWMC Inpatient Psychiatry, University of Washington Medical Center, Seattle, Washington

Benjamin Liptzin, M.D.
Chairman, Department of Psychiatry, Baystate Health, Springfield, Massachusetts; Professor and Deputy Chair of Psychiatry, Tufts University School of Medicine, Boston, Massachusetts

Avram H. Mack, M.D., F.A.P.A.
Associate Professor of Clinical Psychiatry, Georgetown University Medical Center, Washington, D.C.

Rajiv Radhakrishnan, M.B.B.S., M.D.
Postdoctoral Associate, Department of Psychiatry, Yale University School of Medicine, VA Connecticut Healthcare System, West Haven, Connecticut

Anthony J. Rothschild, M.D.
Irving S. and Betty Brudnick Endowed Chair and Professor of Psychiatry, University of Massachusetts Medical School, Worcester, Massachusetts

Peter P. Roy-Byrne, M.D.
Professor, Department of Psychiatry and Behavioral Sciences, University of Washington School of Medicine; Director, Harborview Center for Healthcare Improvement for Addictions, Mental Illness and Medically Vulnerable Populations (CHAMMP)

Judith Shindul-Rothschild, Ph.D., R.N.P.C.
Associate Professor, Fellow, National Academy of Practice, Boston College, William F. Connell School of Nursing, Chestnut Hill, Massachusetts

Kenneth R. Silk, M.D.
Professor of Psychiatry, Department of Psychiatry, University of Michigan Health System, Ann Arbor, Michigan

Lauren Yakutis, B.A.
Research Coordinator, Child and Adolescent Neurodevelopment Initiative, Department of Psychiatry, Division of Child and Adolescent Psychiatry, Worcester, Massachusetts

Disclosure of Competing Interests

The following contributors to this book have indicated a financial interest in or other affiliation with a commercial supporter, a manufacturer of a commercial product, a provider of a commercial service, a nongovernmental organization, and/or a government agency, as listed below:

Nancy Byatt, D.O., M.B.A.—*Grant support:* Meyers Primary Care Institute.

Kristina M. Deligiannidis, M.D.—*Grant/research support:* Forest Research Institute; Worcester Foundation for Biomedical Research.

Deepak Cyril D'Souza, M.B.B.S., M.D.—*Research funding (through Yale University School of Medicine):* Abbott Labs, Astra Zeneca, Cephalon; Eli Lilly, Merck, Organon/Schering Plough, Pfizer.

Jean A. Frazier, M.D.—*Research funding or participation in clinical trials:* Bristol-Myers Squibb, GlaxoSmithKline, Janssen, Johnson & Johnson, Neuropharm, Otsuka American Pharmaceutical, Pfizer.

Michael D. Jibson, M.D., Ph.D.—*Speaker's bureau (quetiapine):* AstraZeneca.

Anthony J. Rothschild, M.D.—*Research funds:* Cyberonics, St. Jude Medical, National Institute of Mental Health, Takeda; *Consultant:* AstraZeneca, Eli Lilly, GlaxoSmithKline, Pfizer; *Royalties:* Rothschild Scale for Antidepressant Tachyphylaxis (RSAT); *Clinical Manual for Diagnosis and Treatment of Psychotic Depression* (American Psychiatric Publishing, 2009); *The Evidence-Based Guide to Antipsychotic Medications* (American Psychiatric Publishing, 2010).

The following contributors to this book indicated that they have no competing interests or affiliations to declare:

Mary S. Ahn, M.D.
Stacey B. Gramann, D.O., M.P.H.
Cassandra Hobgood, M.D.
Ryan J. Kimmel, M.D.
Benjamin Liptzin, M.D.
Avram H. Mack, M.D., F.A.P.A.
Rajiv Radhakrishnan, M.B.B.S., M.D.
Peter P. Roy-Byrne, M.D.
Judith Shindul-Rothschild, Ph.D., R.N.P.C.
Kenneth R. Silk, M.D.
Lauren Yakutis, B.A.

Acknowledgments

I have many people to thank for their encouragement, advice, and support in preparing this book. My family has been patient and understanding of my need to spend time on this project. Irving and Betty Brudnick were instrumental by their endowment of the Irving S. and Betty Brudnick Endowed Chair at the University of Massachusetts Medical School, a position that has allowed me the time to focus on projects such as this evidence-based guide. I am eternally grateful for the late Irving Brudnick's wisdom and support, and I miss his guidance greatly. At American Psychiatric Publishing, Robert Hales, Editor-in-Chief; John McDuffie, Editorial Director; and Greg Kuny, Managing Editor deserve a great deal of credit for their unwavering confidence in me as an author and for their support throughout the development and production of this evidence-based guide. My assistant, Karen Lambert, provided invaluable help in the typing of the manuscript, figures, and tables. I am also appreciative of the support and encouragement of colleagues and trainees at the University of Massachusetts Medical School and UMass Memorial Healthcare. Finally, this book could not have been written without the many patients and families with whom I have had the privilege of working.

Disclaimer

Specific treatment regimens for a particular patient remain the responsibility of the treating clinician, who has access to all of the patient's relevant clinical information, can make a complete assessment of the patient using the information in this textbook as appropriate, and can provide the most informed medical advice. The information provided in this textbook is educational in nature and for general use only, and should not be seen as medical advice concerning a specific patient or the rendering of professional services. The clinician should review the latest manufacturer's package information for any medications or devices discussed in this book before prescribing for use. Information provided may include a description of the uses of therapeutic and biological products that have not been approved by the U.S. Food and Drug Administration. Medical practice, research, and pharmacological advances will occur, and therefore changes in the information and therapies in this book are expected to occur.

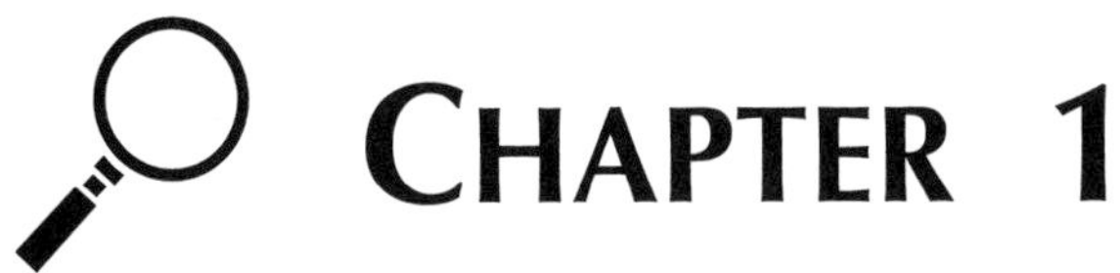

CHAPTER 1

Introduction

Anthony J. Rothschild, M.D.

ANTIDEPRESSANTS revolutionized the practice of psychiatry after their discovery in 1954. Today, they are among the most widely prescribed medications in the world. In 1954, Bloch et al. reported that patients with tuberculosis receiving iproniazid reported an improvement in mood. In 1963, Zeller reported that iproniazid was a potent inhibitor of monoamine oxidase enzymes both in vitro and in vivo and could reverse the effects of reserpine, which was known to be associated with depression as a side effect. Other monoamine oxidase inhibitors (MAOIs) replaced iproniazid, which had significant liver toxicity. Although these medications were significantly less hepatotoxic, their use declined with the introduction of the tricyclic antidepressants (TCAs) because of concerns regarding drug-drug and food-drug interactions (Blackwell et al. 1967).

In 1958, Roland Kuhn, a Swiss psychiatrist, was studying imipramine, a three-ring compound similar in structure to the phenothiazines, as a potential treatment for schizophrenia. Although it was not effective in alleviating psychotic symptoms, it did improve depressive symptoms in a subset of patients. A simple substitution of a nitrogen atom for a sulfur atom in the central ring resulted in antidepressant effects. Numerous TCAs were developed after imipramine, and this class of antidepressants was the most widely used until the development of the selective serotonin reuptake inhibitors (SSRIs).

The discovery of the TCAs and the MAOIs led to the formulation of the monoamine theory of depression (Bunney and Davis 1965; Schildkraut 1965).

As the role of monoamines in depression was investigated further, several problems with the hypothesis emerged. The hypothesis could not explain why the clinical response to antidepressants requires 1–4 weeks of treatment even though MAO inhibition and norepinephrine or serotonin reuptake blockade occur within hours of the initial treatment (Iversen and MacKay 1979; Stahl 1984). The hypothesis could also not explain why amphetamines and cocaine are not effective antidepressants (Overall 1962; Post et al. 1974; Sugrue 1983). Clearly, other mechanisms are involved. Nevertheless, the monoamine hypothesis of depression, although overly simplistic given the advances in science since 1965, is still one of the best explanations as to why antidepressants are effective treatments and has not yet been replaced with a new scientific paradigm that can explain how antidepressants work.

Although the original monoamine hypothesis of depression focused on norepinephrine, Van Praag and Leijnse (1963a, 1963b), Coppen (1967), and Maas (1975) extended the hypothesis to include serotonin. Maas (1975) suggested that some depressed patients have a more noradrenergic-based depression, whereas others have a serotonergic-based depression. Pharmaceutical research in the United States and Europe then focused on the development of medications that blocked the serotonin reuptake site without the receptor-binding profile of the TCAs, which accounted for many of the TCA's side effects. This research led to the synthesis of zimelidine, the first marketed SSRI in Europe (Huitfeldt and Montgomery 1983; Montgomery et al. 1981a, 1981b), and fluoxetine, the first SSRI marketed in the United States (Fuller et al. 1991).

Since the introduction of fluoxetine in the United States in 1987, the treatment of depression has changed dramatically. Prior to fluoxetine, only some psychiatrists, known as *psychopharmacologists,* prescribed antidepressants, mainly because of the complexity of prescribing TCAs and MAOIs. Today, in part due to the newer antidepressants, which have fewer side effects and less toxicity in overdose, many non–mental health professionals feel comfortable prescribing antidepressants. Antidepressants are prescribed for many patients in addition to those who have major depressive disorder, including patients with bipolar disorder, generalized anxiety disorder, panic disorder, posttraumatic stress disorder, obsessive-compulsive disorder, social anxiety disorder, specific phobias, psychotic depression, schizophrenia, personality disorders, substance abuse disorders, and medical illnesses. In addition, antidepressants are increasingly being prescribed by clinicians for so-called off-label use—that is, to treat illnesses for which the medications do not have U.S. Food and Drug Administration (FDA) approval.

These increased uses for antidepressants have led to the need for this evidence-based guide to antidepressant medications. The authors of each chapter in this guide present the FDA-approved and off-label uses of the antidepressant medications and the evidence base that supports (or does not support) each of their uses. The authors also discuss the use of antidepressants in several special populations including children and adolescents, geriatric patients, and pregnant and lactating women. The final chapter is on the nursing care of patients who are taking antidepressants. All of the chapter authors have synthesized a large amount of medical literature to create a comprehensive yet understandable, concise, and reader-friendly guide for the practicing clinician.

In Chapter 2, Dr. Rothschild discusses the use of antidepressants in major depressive disorder, bipolar depression, psychotic depression, and treatment-resistant depression. The chapter reviews the efficacy and side effects of TCAs, MAOIs, SSRIs, serotonin-norepinephrine reuptake inhibitors, bupropion, mirtazapine, nefazodone, trazodone, and vilazodone. The author has sorted through the vast and complex literature of antidepressants and distills the information for the practicing clinician with helpful, practical advice. Augmentation strategies and the issue of antidepressants and suicidality are also discussed.

In Chapter 3, Drs. Kimmel and Roy-Byrne discuss the use of antidepressants for anxiety disorders, including generalized anxiety disorder, panic disorder, posttraumatic stress disorder, obsessive-compulsive disorder, social anxiety disorder, and specific phobia. The authors discuss the acute management of these disorders, as well as long-term follow-up and relapse prevention. The authors also compare the use of antidepressant medications to psychological therapies and combined medication and psychological therapies.

In Chapter 4, Drs. Radhakrishnan and D'Souza review the evidence base for the use of antidepressants in schizophrenia and schizoaffective disorder. The chapter begins with an overview of the overlap among depressive symptoms, negative symptoms, and extrapyramidal side effects in patients with schizophrenia. The use of antidepressants to treat postpsychotic depression is discussed. Because antidepressants, when used to treat patients with schizophrenia, are often added to antipsychotic medications, the authors discuss drug-drug interactions that can occur when the medications are prescribed simultaneously. Finally, the authors discuss several other uses of antidepressants in patients with schizophrenia, including bupropion for smoking cessation, fluvoxamine and clomipramine for antipsychotic-induced obsessive-compulsive disorder, bupropion for antipsychotic-induced sexual dysfunction, and amitriptyline for clozapine-induced sialorrhoea and nocturia.

In Chapter 5, Drs. Silk and Jibson review the range of mood disturbances found in patients with personality disorders, both across and within specific personality disorders. The authors also review the range of other symptoms among patients with personality disorder that have responded to antidepressant medications in patients without personality disorder. The authors discuss the use of antidepressant medication in the personality disorders in general, as well as in specific personality disorders, including borderline personality disorder, schizotypal personality disorder, and avoidant personality. They also address the use of antidepressants in obsessive-compulsive personality disorder and other personality disorders.

In Chapter 6, Dr. Mack discusses the use of antidepressants in substance-related disorders. The use of antidepressants in this population is complicated by the lack of FDA indications and limited data. Dr. Mack outlines the many clinical situations in which antidepressants can be used to treat patients with substance abuse. The author discusses the use of antidepressants for the treatment of dependence, abuse, intoxication, or withdrawal; the use of antidepressants to treat diagnoses or nonspecific conditions associated with substance use disorders; and the use of antidepressants to treat substance-induced psychiatric disorders, such as alcohol-induced mood disorder. Dr. Mack also discusses the use of bupropion for nicotine dependence, SSRIs for comorbid alcohol dependence and depression, and other agents for cocaine depression.

In Chapter 7, Dr. Ahn, Ms. Yakutis, and Dr. Frazier review the use of antidepressant medications in children and adolescents. This chapter includes a review of the developmental considerations necessary to keep in mind when prescribing antidepressant medications for children and adolescents and a discussion of the background and challenges of conducting psychotropic medication trials in young people. In addition, indications for various antidepressants are reviewed. The authors outline the published controlled studies of antidepressants in children and adolescents, giving special attention to safety.

In Chapter 8, Drs. Liptzin and Hobgood review the use of antidepressant medications in geriatric patients. After discussing the general principles of medication management in the older patient, the authors review age-specific side effects of antidepressant medications and the evidence base for use of antidepressants in elderly people. They give practical advice on the use of specific antidepressants in the geriatric population. The chapter has specific sections on the use of antidepressants in depressed elderly patients with dementia, stroke, and Parkinson's disease.

In Chapter 9, Drs. Gramann and Byatt review the use of antidepressant medications in medically ill patients. After reviewing special considerations for the use of antidepressants in this population, including drug-drug interactions, pharmacokinetics, sexual side effects, akathisia, hyponatremia, and the serotonin syndrome, the authors discuss the use of antidepressants in specific medical conditions, including cardiovascular disease, pulmonary disease, gastrointestinal disease, renal disease, endocrine disease, cancer, neurological illness, chronic pain, human immunodeficiency virus infection, steroid-induced psychiatric symptoms, and burns and hospital-based trauma.

In Chapter 10, Dr. Deligiannidis discusses the use of antidepressants during pregnancy and lactation. After reviewing the risks to the baby and mother of untreated depression and anxiety during pregnancy, the author provides a thoughtful discussion, based on published research, of the risks and benefits of antidepressant use during pregnancy and lactation. Finally, Dr. Deligiannidis provides practical clinical management approaches for the pregnant and postpartum patient and for women who are breast-feeding.

In Chapter 11, Dr. Shindul-Rothschild reviews the wide range of practice settings and specialties in which patients prescribed antidepressants are provided nursing care. The chapter delineates best practices in prescribing antidepressants for advanced practice nurses and nurse practitioners in primary care, pediatric offices, rural health, and long-term-care facilities, with a focus on providing evidence-based, patient-focused care across the lifespan. The author also reviews empirically based nursing interventions to assess serious adverse effects and enhance treatment adherence for culturally diverse populations who are taking prescribed antidepressants.

This book is a condensed yet comprehensive overview of the current knowledge and evidence base regarding the use of antidepressant medications. Each chapter contains a number of useful tables and/or figures pertaining to the topic being discussed. Finally, at the end of each chapter, important clinical pearls of information are summarized in the Key Clinical Concepts.

This book is designed for the busy clinician, and I hope it will prove useful to psychiatrists, family and general practitioners, internists, neurologists, nurses, psychologists, social workers, and advanced students.

References

Blackwell B, Marley E, Price J, et al: Hypertensive interactions between monoamine oxidase inhibitors and foodstuffs. Br J Psychiatry 113:349–365, 1967

Bloch RG, Doonief AS, Buchberg AS, et al: The clinical effect of isoniazid and iproniazid in the treatment of pulmonary tuberculosis. Ann Intern Med 40:881–900, 1954

Bunney WE Jr, Davis JM: Norepinephrine in depressive reactions: a review. Arch Gen Psychiatry 13:483–494, 1965

Coppen A: The biochemistry of affective disorders. Br J Psychiatry 113:1237–1264, 1967

Fuller RW, Wong DT, Robertson DW: Fluoxetine, a selective inhibitor of serotonin uptake. Med Res Rev 11:17–34, 1991

Huitfeldt B, Montgomery SA: Comparison between zimelidine and amitriptyline of efficacy and adverse symptoms: a combined analysis of four clinical trials in depression. Acta Psychiatr Scand Suppl 308:55–69, 1983

Iversen LL, Mackay AVP: Pharmacodynamics of antidepressants and antimanic drugs, in Psychopharmacology of Affective Disorders. Edited by Paykel ES, Coppen A. Oxford, UK, Oxford University Press, 1979, pp 60–90

Kuhn R: The treatment of depressive states with G 22355 (imipramine hydrochloride). Am J Psychiatry 115:459–464, 1958

Maas JW: Biogenic amines and depression: biochemical and pharmacological separation of two types of depression. Arch Gen Psychiatry 32:1357–1361, 1975

Montgomery SA, McAuley R, Rani SJ, et al: A double-blind comparison of zimelidine and amitriptyline in endogenous depression. Acta Psychiatr Scand Suppl 290:314–327, 1981a

Montgomery SA, Rani SJ, McAuley R, et al: The antidepressant efficacy of zimelidine and maprotiline. Acta Psychiatr Scand Suppl 290:219–224, 1981b

Overall JE: Dimensions of manifest depression. J Psychiatr Res 1:239–247, 1962

Post RM, Kotin J, Goodwin FK: The effects of cocaine on depressed patients. Am J Psychiatry 131:511–517, 1974

Schildkraut JJ: The catecholamine hypothesis of affective disorders: a review of supporting evidence. Am J Psychiatry 122:509–522, 1965

Stahl SM: Regulation of neurotransmitter receptors by desipramine and other antidepressant drugs: the neurotransmitter receptor hypothesis of antidepressant action. J Clin Psychiatry 45:37–45, 1984

Sugrue M: Chronic antidepressant therapy and associated changes in central monoaminergic receptor functioning. Pharmacol Ther 21:1–33, 1983

Van Praag H, Leijnse B: Cerebral monoamines and depression: an investigation with the probenecid technique. Arch Gen Psychiatry 25:827–831, 1963a

Van Praag H, Leijnse B: The influence of some antidepressives of the hydrazine type on the glucose metabolism in depressed patients. Clin Chim Acta 8:466–475, 1963b

Zeller EA: Diamine oxidase, in The Enzymes, Vol 8, 2nd Edition. Edited by Boyer PD, Lardy H, Myrback K. London, Academic Press, 1963, pp 313–335

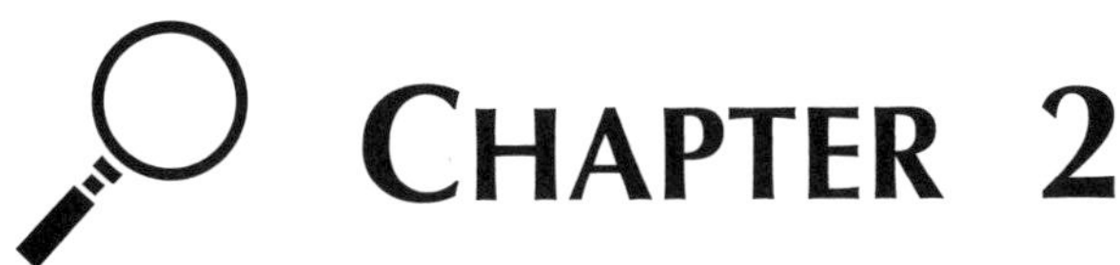

CHAPTER 2

Unipolar and Bipolar Depression

Anthony J. Rothschild, M.D.

THIS CHAPTER serves as an overview of the antidepressants available for use in clinical practice. Also in this chapter, I review the evidence base for the use of antidepressants in nonpsychotic major depressive disorder, treatment-resistant depression, major depressive disorder with psychotic features (psychotic depression, delusional depression), and bipolar disorder.

Unipolar Nonpsychotic Major Depressive Disorder

General Comments

When evaluating the response of patients treated with antidepressants, the physician should remember that the symptoms of depression resolve gradually over several weeks and that the dysphoric mood state frequently is the last symptom to improve. Consequently, although the patient may report improvement in energy levels, sleep disturbances, or somatic complaints, and the physician may observe that the patient smiles for the first time in several weeks or shows an improvement in cognitive processes, the patient's overall assessment is that he or she feels "lousy" and that the "medication is not working." Physician- or family-reported improvements in the patient's depression after the start of antidepressant therapy may be a harbinger of a full antidepressant response with continued treatment.

Although patients may experience significant improvement in the symptoms of major depression within the first week, this is uncommon. If shortly after beginning to take an antidepressant, a patient profusely thanks the physician for prescribing the medication, then the physician should consider whether the patient has a bipolar disorder and has switched to a manic episode or whether the patient is experiencing a placebo effect. If there is concern that the patient has become manic, the antidepressant should be discontinued and psychiatric consultation considered. Although predicting the occurrence of mania with antidepressant therapy is difficult, conducting a good personal and family history to detect bipolar disorder is important before the start of treatment. If a placebo effect is the more likely explanation for the patient's behavior, the patient should be encouraged to continue the prescribed medication. However, the physician should not be surprised if the patient reports 7–10 days later that the medication "has stopped working."

Antidepressant Classes

Antidepressant medications have traditionally been grouped into classes, based primarily on their mechanism of action. Despite claims from time to time over the years that one particular antidepressant or class of antidepressants has greater efficacy or a faster onset of action, no replicable findings have been able to reliably prove such claims. However, some antidepressants may indeed have greater efficacy than others for the treatment of comorbid conditions (e.g., serotonergic medications for the treatment of obsessive-compulsive disorder and other anxiety disorders; see Chapter 3, "Anxiety Disorders"). It is also unfortunately the case that two classes of effective antidepressants, the tricyclic antidepressants (TCAs) and the monoamine oxidase inhibitors (MAOIs), are underutilized (see subsections "Tricyclic and Tetracyclic Antidepressants" and "Monoamine Oxidase Inhibitors"). Antidepressants do differ in their side-effect profiles, pharmacokinetics, and potential for drug-drug interactions. The selection of a particular antidepressant for a patient will depend on factors such as history of prior medication treatment and response, patient preference, anticipated side effects, co-occurring psychiatric and general medical conditions, potential drug-drug interactions, antidepressant half-life, and cost.

The five classes of antidepressants are 1) TCAs and the tetracyclic antidepressant maprotiline; 2) MAOIs, which include isocarboxazid, phenelzine, tranylcypromine, and the transdermal formulation of selegiline; 3) selective serotonin reuptake inhibitors (SSRIs), which include citalopram, escitalopram, fluoxetine, fluvoxamine, paroxetine, and sertraline; 4) serotonin-norepinephrine reuptake inhibitors (SNRIs), which include desvenlafaxine, duloxetine, and venlafaxine; and 5) other antidepressant medications that do not fit into one of the other classes, including bupropion, mirtazapine, nefazodone, trazodone, amoxapine, and vilazodone.

The starting and usual dosages of the antidepressants are presented in Table 2–1.

Tricyclic and Tetracyclic Antidepressants

Efficacy

The TCAs include amitriptyline, desipramine, doxepin, imipramine, nortriptyline, protriptyline, and trimipramine. (Clomipramine is also a TCA and has an indication from the U.S. Food and Drug Administration [FDA] for the treatment of obsessive-compulsive disorder, as discussed in Chapter 3, "Anxiety Disorders.") Maprotiline, a tetracyclic antidepressant, is a four-ringed compound that has a mechanism of action similar to that of the TCAs. The secondary amines (e.g., nortriptyline, desipramine) have fewer of the classic TCA side effects (see following section on side effects) and are often easier for patients to take. The ability to obtain meaningful antidepressant blood levels to guide dosing is an advantage with the TCAs (see Table 2–2) and can give the clinician some guidance as to whether the dosage of the TCA is too low or too high. For example, plasma levels are particularly useful when the patient is not responding to what appears to be an adequate dosage of the TCA or has a significant number of side effects despite taking the TCA at a low dosage. For nortriptyline, a therapeutic window has been reported (Åsberg et al. 1971).

Side Effects

The side effects of TCAs can be grouped broadly into the following categories: anticholinergic, cardiovascular, central nervous system, weight gain, falls, and sexual dysfunction.

Anticholinergic side effects

All TCAs have anticholinergic side effects (e.g., dry mouth, constipation, blurry vision, urinary hesitancy, esophageal reflux). The tertiary amine TCAs (e.g., amitriptyline, imipramine) produce greater anticholinergic effects than do the secondary-amine TCAs (e.g., desipramine, nortriptyline) (Baldessarini 2006). The most common anticholinergic side effects include dry mouth, impaired ability to focus vision at close range, constipation, urinary hesita-

TABLE 2–1. Dosing of medications shown to be effective in treating major depressive disorder[a]

MEDICATION (GENERIC NAME)	STARTING DOSAGE (MG/DAY)[b]	USUAL DOSAGE (MG/DAY)[c]
Selective serotonin reuptake inhibitors[d]		
Citalopram	20	20–60[e]
Escitalopram	10	10–20
Fluoxetine	20	20–60[e]
Paroxetine	20	20–60[e]
Paroxetine, extended release	12.5	25–75
Sertraline	50	50–200[e]
Dopamine-norepinephrine reuptake inhibitor[d]		
Bupropion, immediate release	150	300–450
Bupropion, sustained release	150	300–400
Bupropion, extended release	150	300–450
Serotonin-norepinephrine reuptake inhibitors[d]		
Venlafaxine, immediate release	37.5	75–375
Venlafaxine, extended release	37.5	75–375
Desvenlafaxine	50	50[f]
Duloxetine	60	60–120
Serotonin modulators		
Nefazodone	50	150–300
Trazodone[g]	150	150–600
Vilazodone	10	40
Norepinephrine-serotonin modulator		
Mirtazapine[d]	15	15–45
Tricyclics and tetracyclics		
Amitriptyline	25–50	100–300
Doxepin	25–50	100–300
Imipramine	25–50	100–300
Desipramine	25–50	100–300
Nortriptyline	25	50–200

TABLE 2–1. Dosing of medications shown to be effective in treating major depressive disorder[a] *(continued)*

MEDICATION (GENERIC NAME)	STARTING DOSAGE (MG/DAY)[b]	USUAL DOSAGE (MG/DAY)[c]
Tricyclics and tetracyclics *(continued)*		
Trimipramine	25–50	75–300
Protriptyline	10–20	20–60
Maprotiline	75	100–225
Monoamine oxidase inhibitors (MAOIs)		
Irreversible, nonselective inhibitors		
Phenelzine	15	45–90
Tranylcypromine	10	30–60
Isocarboxazid	10–20	30–60
Irreversible, MAO-B selective inhibitor		
Selegiline transdermal[h]	6	6–12
Reversible MAO-A selective inhibitor		
Moclobemide	150	300–600

[a]For convenience, medications other than TCAs have been classified by their presumptive mechanism of action. However, the exact mechanism of action of several medications has yet to be determined or varies by dose.
[b]Lower starting doses are recommended for elderly patients and for patients with panic disorder, significant anxiety or hepatic disease, and co-occurring general medical conditions.
[c]For some of these medications (e.g., TCAs) the upper dosing limit reflects risk of toxicity or need for plasma level assessment, whereas for other medications (e.g., SSRIs), higher doses can be used safely but without evidence for overall superior efficacy.
[d]These medications are likely to be optimal medications in terms of safety, the patient's acceptance of side effects, and the quantity and quality of clinical trial data.
[e]Dose varies with diagnosis; see text for specific guidelines.
[f]Has been used at dosages up to 400 mg/day, although dosages above 50 mg/day may not provide additional benefit.
[g]This medication is not typically used for this indication.
[h]Selegiline selectively inhibits MAO-B at low doses but inhibits both MAO-A and MAO-B at the higher doses that are typically required for antidepressant activity.
Source. Adapted from American Psychiatric Association: *Practice Guideline for the Treatment of Patients with Major Depressive Disorder,* Third Edition. Washington DC, American Psychiatric Association, 2010, p. 34, Table 6.

TABLE 2–2. Approximate therapeutic serum level ranges for tricyclic and tetracyclic drugs

DRUG	SERUM LEVEL (NG/ML)
Amitriptyline[a]	100–250
Amoxapine	Unknown
Desipramine	150–300
Doxepin[a]	120–250
Imipramine[a]	150–300
Maprotiline	150–250
Nortriptyline[b]	50–150
Protriptyline	75–250
Trimipramine	Unknown

[a]Total concentration of drug and demethylated metabolic.
[b]Has a clear therapeutic window.

tion, and tachycardia. Although patients can develop some degree of tolerance to anticholinergic side effects, the symptoms may require treatment if they interfere with a person's ability to continue taking the medication. Impaired visual accommodation may be counteracted through the use of 4% pilocarpine eyedrops or bethanechol, a procholinergic medication, at dosages of 25–50 mg tid or qid. TCAs should be avoided in patients with narrow-angle glaucoma. Dry mouth may be counteracted by advising the patient to use sugarless gum or candy and ensuring adequate hydration. For severe dry mouth, bethanechol 5–10 mg sublingually can be effective. Constipation can be managed by adequate hydration and the use of bulk laxatives. Urinary hesitancy can often be alleviated by prescribing bethanechol 25–50 mg tid or qid, which is generally needed as long as the patient continues to take a TCA.

Antidepressant medications with anticholinergic side effects should be avoided in patients with cognitive impairment because these medications can impair memory and concentration and even precipitate anticholinergic delirium.

Cardiovascular side effects

In medically healthy patients with depression, TCAs produce a mild tachycardia (approximately 10 beats per minute). TCAs and maprotiline act similarly to class Ia antiarrhythmic agents, such as quinidine, and can slow cardiac conduction (Roden 2006). As a result, combinations of TCAs with other class I antiarrhythmic agents can exert additive toxic effects on cardiac conduction, and individuals with prolonged QT intervals are predisposed to develop ventricular tachycardia (Schwartz and Wolf 1978). TCAs also can decrease cardiac irritability and suppress premature contractions. Fatal cardiac arrhythmias occur primarily in the context of TCA overdose (Thanacoody and Thomas 2005).

Because of the potential for cardiac arrhythmias with TCA treatment, it is advisable for patients with significant cardiac risk factors and patients older than age 50 years to have a pretreatment electrocardiogram (ECG). Follow-up ECGs may also be indicated to identify the development of conduction changes, typically during the early phase of TCA use (Miller et al. 1998).

In addition to increasing the risk of arrhythmias, treatment with TCAs is associated with other cardiovascular effects, such as orthostatic hypotension (through α-adrenergic blockade). Orthostatic hypotension can result in dizziness, falls, or fractures—symptoms that are of particular concern for elderly patients (Joo et al. 2002). Patients who are receiving antihypertensive medications or who are dehydrated or salt depleted (e.g., from treatment with diuretics) are particularly sensitive to developing orthostatic hypotension with TCA treatment.

In the absence of a medical contraindication, patients with symptomatic orthostatic hypotension can continue to take TCAs and should be educated to maintain adequate fluid intake and not to restrict salt intake. Some evidence in studies of patients with heart disease suggests that among the TCAs, nortriptyline may be less likely to contribute to orthostatic blood pressure changes (Roose et al. 1987).

Central nervous system side effects

The central nervous system side effects of TCAs include tremor, sedation, stimulation, myoclonic twitches, seizures (particularly with maprotiline), and extrapyramidal symptoms (with amoxapine).

Tremors can be managed by reducing the TCA dosage, counseling the patient to decrease caffeine intake and cigarette smoking, or prescribing a low dosage of a β-blocker (e.g., propranolol 10 mg bid, increasing the dosage gradually to a maximum of 80 mg/day).

Myoclonus may be an indication of TCA toxicity (Garvey and Tollefson 1987). Therefore, if myoclonus is present, the physician should check the level of the TCA in the patient's blood. If the TCA level is not toxic and the patient can tolerate the myoclonus, the TCA can be continued. If the myoclonus is bothersome to the patient and the blood level is within the therapeutic range, the addition of clonazepam 0.25 mg tid can be helpful in ameliorating the symptoms of myoclonus.

A TCA-induced seizure usually does not have a prodrome and is typically a single generalized motor seizure that lasts several minutes. In nonepileptic patients, the incidence of seizures during treatment with standard dosages of TCAs is approximately 0.5% (Lowry and Dunner 1980). At one time, there was concern that maprotiline may result in a higher rate of seizures than the TCAs, but the higher rate appeared to be mainly due to prolonged treatment (>6 weeks) at high dosages (225–400 mg/day) (Dessain et al. 1986).

TCAs can produce sedation as a result of their affinity for histaminergic receptors. Therefore, I usually have patients take the TCAs as a single dose at bedtime because patients with major depressive disorder with insomnia may benefit from the sedation. If a patient is sedated the next morning, I usually advise him or her to take the TCA dose earlier in the evening. Sedation may attenuate after several weeks. In general, the secondary-amine TCAs cause less sedation than the tertiary amine TCAs (Baldessarini 2006).

Weight gain

An important side effect of TCAs is weight gain. The degree of weight gain varies across the TCAs, with amitriptyline and doxepin most frequently associated with this problem. However, patients who gain weight while taking one TCA often will continue to gain weight when switched to another TCA. The mechanism by which TCAs cause weight gain is believed to be related to their antihistaminergic properties and/or their blockade of serotonin type 2 (5-HT_2) receptors (Deshmukh and Franco 2003). The degree of weight gain is sometimes dose dependent. If a patient is having a good antidepressant response but gaining weight, the clinician and patient should discuss the risk-benefit ratio of continuing the TCA in light of the weight gain, as well as the implementation of diet and exercise programs. Weight gain will abate with cessation of TCA therapy, but the patient may still need to implement a diet and exercise regimen to lose the weight already gained.

Falls

Meta-analyses have documented an increased risk of falls for patients treated with antidepressive agents in general (Sterke et al. 2008). Use of TCAs in elderly nursing home residents has been associated with increases in falls and hip fractures (Liu et al. 1998). Although systematic reviews show a relatively small effect of orthostatic hypotension on fall risk, as discussed above in the TCA subsection "Cardiovascular Side Effects," TCAs may contribute to orthostasis in individual patients and thus increase the risk of falls (Ganz et al. 2007). Other causes of falls include bradycardia, cardiac arrhythmia, seizures, or ataxia.

Sexual dysfunction

TCAs are associated with sexual dysfunction side effects. In a placebo-controlled study of patients who took 200–300 mg of imipramine or placebo for 6 weeks, delayed orgasm was noted by 21% of the men taking imipramine and none of the men taking placebo (Harrison et al. 1986). Orgasmic delay was noted by 27% of women taking imipramine and 11% of women taking placebo (Harrison et al. 1986). Monteiro et al. (1987) reported high rates of anorgasmia in patients with obsessive-compulsive disorder treated with clomipramine.

Medication Interactions With Tricyclic Antidepressants

A number of medications that inhibit, induce, or are metabolized by hepatic microsomal enzymes can interact with TCAs (Nelson 2006). For example, medications that induce cytochrome P450 (CYP) 3A4, such as carbamazepine, barbiturates, nicotine, chloral hydrate, and phenytoin, will cause a breakdown of TCAs and a decrease in serum levels of TCAs. In contrast, antipsychotic medications (particularly the phenothiazines), the SSRIs, methylphenidate, disulfiram, and fenfluramine can inhibit metabolism via CYP2D6, resulting in reduced clearance and increased levels of TCAs. Conversely, TCAs can also alter the pharmacokinetics or pharmacodynamics of other medications; for example, TCAs can cause a lowering of valproate levels and an increase in phenothiazine plasma levels. Benzodiazepines and medications used to treat Parkinson's disease have little or no effect on TCA levels. Clinicians should keep these medication interactions in mind when TCAs are administered concomitantly with other medications.

Monoamine Oxidase Inhibitors

Efficacy

MAOIs were first discovered to be effective antidepressants when iproniazid, a medication marketed initially as a treatment for tuberculosis, was found to have antidepressant properties. Phenelzine, tranylcypromine, isocarboxazid, and transdermally delivered selegiline are MAOIs currently used to treat depression. No studies have been published comparing the newer transdermal (skin patch) formulation of selegiline to other medications; its efficacy has only been established relative to placebo (Feiger et al. 2006; Robinson et al. 2007).

MAOIs have efficacy comparable to that of other antidepressants for outpatients with major depressive disorder but are currently used primarily for patients who have not responded to trials of other antidepressants and are considered to have treatment-resistant depression (see "Treatment-Resistant Depression" later in this chapter). I prefer to use MAOIs for the treatment of depressed patients who have not had a response to previous trials of antidepressants than to use untested polypharmacy combinations of antidepressants. Although studies have shown that MAOIs are effective in depressed patients who have not responded to TCAs (Thase et al. 1995), the effectiveness of MAOIs for depressed patients who have not responded to trials with SSRIs and SNRIs is unclear (McGrath et al. 2006).

MAOIs may be particularly useful for treating patients with atypical depression, which is characterized by reactive moods; significant increases in sleep, appetite, or weight; leaden paralysis; and patterns of extreme sensitivity to interpersonal loss (often termed *rejection sensitivity*) (Thase et al. 1995). Other subsets of depression, such as depression with melancholic features and dysthymia, have also been found to be responsive to MAOI treatment.

Serum monitoring of MAOIs is not clinically indicated, and no correlations are known to exist between levels and effectiveness. One study reported a correlation between the degree of platelet MAO inhibition and response (Ravaris et al. 1976). The study, which used phenelzine, found that a higher dosage of the drug (60 mg/day) was significantly better in treating depression and anxiety than the lower dosage (30 mg/day), and only the higher dosage achieved 80% platelet MAO inhibition. However, studies with other MAOIs were not able to reproduce this effect.

Side Effects

Whereas hypertensive crises (discussed later in this section) are the most dramatic and feared side effect of MAOIs, on a day-to-day basis the most common side effects of MAOIs are orthostatic hypotension, dizziness, insomnia, daytime sedation, and daytime activation. Because MAOIs do not block acetylcholine receptors, they are associated with less dry mouth, blurry vision, constipation, and urinary hesitancy than are the TCAs.

Dizziness

Dizziness with MAOI treatment is usually secondary to orthostatic hypotension. Several strategies may be useful if dizziness occurs either alone or in combination: dosage reduction of the MAOI (with monitoring for reemergence of depressive symptoms), increased fluid intake (8 glasses of water per day), increased salt intake, use of support stockings, and the addition of a mineralocorticoid (e.g., fludrocortisone 0.3–0.8 mg/day).

Sedation and activation

Activation with MAOIs can occur either during the day or at night. Sedation during the day is frequently accompanied by activation at night with concomitant insomnia. One strategy for dealing with this side effect is to switch the time of day that patients take the MAOI. If they are taking it in the morning, the MAOI can be switched to the evening, and if they are taking it at bedtime, the MAOI can be switched to the morning. A dosage reduction (if possible) may also help to ameliorate this side effect. Some patients may require hypnotic agents to treat the insomnia.

Hypertensive crises

Use of MAOIs has often been considered risky because of the potential of developing a hypertensive crisis after ingesting high amounts of dietary tyramine. Tyramine is a potent releaser of norepinephrine and can thus elevate blood pressure. When foods high in tyramine content are ingested, the MAOI isoform MAO-A in the intestinal wall and liver safely destroys massive amounts of tyramine before it is absorbed (Gardner et al. 1996). When MAO-A is inhibited, the capacity to handle dietary tyramine is significantly reduced. A hypertensive crisis is characterized by the acute onset of severe headache, nausea, neck stiffness, palpitations, profuse perspiration, and confusion, and can possibly lead to stroke and death (Thase et al. 1995). This risk is generally alleviated by altering the diet so foods high in tyramine are avoided. Over the years, based on research and clinical experience, the list of forbidden foods (see Table 2–3) has decreased in size considerably.

Although many clinicians fear that their patients will be unable to follow the low-tyramine diet, I have had patients ranging in age from 18 to 80 who take MAOIs and follow the diet without difficulty. Before prescribing an MAOI, I review the diet with patients to see if they think they can follow it. Also, before I prescribe an MAOI, I often have patients try the diet for a week to see if they can adhere to it.

Patients taking MAOIs should be instructed that if they accidently ingest a food substance known to contain tyramine, they should go to a local emergency room. In the emergency room, antihypertensive medication (e.g., phentolamine, labetalol, sodium nitroprusside) can be administered. I also have nongeriatric patients carry two 10-mg pills of nifedipine in case of a dietary indiscretion (Schenk and Remick 1989). I advise them that if they develop symptoms of a hypertensive crisis, they should take one pill (and another dose 1 hour later if necessary) on their way to the emergency room. Use of nifedipine does increase the risk of hypotension (Grossman et al. 1996).

The clinician should be aware of two general types of potentially dangerous drug interactions with MAOIs: those that can raise blood pressure by sympathomimetic actions and those that can cause a potentially fatal serotonin syndrome. In overdose, patients may present with a combination of serotonin syndrome and hypertensive crisis. Many clinicians recommend that their patients wear bracelets stating that they are taking MAOIs in case the patients are unconscious in an emergency situation.

Combination of MAOIs with sympathomimetic medications. Potentially dangerous hypertensive reactions can occur when medications that boost adrenergic stimulation by a mechanism other than MAO inhibition are added to an MAOI. For example, decongestants can boost adrenergic activity. Decongestants to be avoided include over-the-counter phenylephrine and

TABLE 2–3. Food restrictions for patients taking monoamine oxidase inhibitors

Severe
Aged cheeses
Aged meats (pepperoni, sausage, salami)
Spoiled meats and fish
Sauerkraut
Soy sauce
Fava or broad bean pods
Banana peels
All beers on tap
Use in moderation (2 glasses or less a day)
Red wine (4-oz glasses)
White wine (4-oz glasses)
Bottled or canned beers
Mild to none
Avocados
Banana pulp
Bouillon
Chocolate
Fresh cheeses (cottage cheese, cream cheese, processed cheese slices)
Fresh or processed meat

Source. Adapted from Amsterdam 2006; Shulman and Walker 2001.

oxymetazoline, both relatively selective α_1-adrenergic agonists, and pseudoephedrine. An additional ingredient found in cold medicines is the cough suppressant and opiate derivative dextromethorphan, which should be avoided not because it is a sympathomimetic agent but because it is a weak serotonin reuptake inhibitor (see the following subsection on combining MAOIs with serotonergic medications). Any medications that block norepinephrine reuptake, including stimulants and antidepressants, attention-deficit/hyperactivity drugs (e.g., atomoxetine), appetite suppressants (e.g., sibutramine and other sympathomimetics), and the analgesic tramadol should generally be avoided in combination with an MAOI.

Combination of MAOIs with serotonergic medications. Another potentially dangerous reaction can occur when medications that inhibit serotonin reuptake are combined with those that inhibit MAO. This combination can result in the so-called serotonin syndrome, characterized by abdominal pain, diarrhea, flushing, sweating, hyperthermia, lethargy, mental status changes, tremor and myoclonus, rhabdomyolysis, renal failure, cardiovascular shock, and possibly death.

Usually, the serotonin syndrome caused by an MAOI together with a serotonin reuptake inhibitor results when the prescriber does not recognize that a patient taking an MAOI is also taking a drug, such as an analgesic, appetite suppressant, or antihistamine, that has serotonin reuptake inhibiting properties. These medications would include any SSRI or SNRI, and clomipramine, a serotonergic TCA. Opioids that block 5-HT reuptake, including meperidine, methadone, propoxyphene, dextromethorphan, and tramadol, especially at high dosages, must also be avoided in the presence of an MAOI. Consequently, when patients are being switched from an SSRI other than fluoxetine or an SNRI to an MAOI, a waiting period of at least 2 weeks is needed between the discontinuation of one medication and the initiation of the other. When the medication is being changed from fluoxetine to an MAOI, a waiting period of at least 5 weeks is needed before the MAOI is started. Injection of meperidine given concomitantly with an MAOI may be the most frequent drug combination causing serious complications and even death (Fuller and Snoddy 1975). Analgesics, including opiates, that are safe to administer with an MAOI are those lacking serotonin reuptake–inhibiting properties, such as aspirin, acetaminophen, nonsteroidal anti-inflammatory drugs, codeine, oxycodone, fentanyl, buprenorphine, and morphine. Treatment of serotonin syndrome includes discontinuation of all serotonergic agents and subsequent supportive care.

MAOIs and cough and cold medications. Patients taking an MAOI can take cough and cold medication, but they should avoid oral phenylephrine to minimize the risk of a hypertensive reaction. Patients taking an MAOI should also avoid ingredients in cough and cold preparations that inhibit serotonin reuptake, such as dextromethorphan and some antihistamines (e.g., chlorpheniramine, brompheniramine). Other antihistamines and cough suppressants, including codeine, are generally acceptable to be administered with MAOIs.

Sexual side effects

In general, the sexual side effects seen with MAOI therapy include anorgasmia, decreased libido, and erectile or ejaculatory dysfunction. Sexual side effects may diminish over time or with reductions in MAOI dosages. In a placebo-controlled study of patients who took between 60 and 90 mg of phenelzine or placebo for 6 weeks, delayed orgasm was noted by 30% of the men taking phenelzine and none of the men taking placebo (Harrison et al. 1986). Orgasmic delay was noted by 36% of women taking phenelzine and 11% of women taking placebo (Harrison et al. 1986).

Neurological side effects

Besides insomnia and sedation (discussed previously in this "Side Effects" section), other neurological side effects that can occur with MAOI treatment include headaches, myoclonic jerks, paresthesias, and, rarely, peripheral neuropathy.

Selective Serotonin Reuptake Inhibitors

Efficacy

SSRIs remain the most widely prescribed class of antidepressants. Currently available SSRIs include fluoxetine, sertraline, paroxetine, fluvoxamine, citalopram, and escitalopram. (Fluvoxamine, however, does not have an FDA indication for depression.) Numerous studies support the superiority of SSRIs compared with placebo for the treatment of major depressive disorder, and more than 10 systematic reviews and meta-analyses have found that SSRIs have efficacy comparable to that of other antidepressants, including the TCAs (Cipriani et al. 2005a; Geddes et al. 2000). Although an occasional study indicates that a particular SSRI is more effective than another, the majority of studies show no differences in efficacy among individual SSRIs (Cipriani et al. 2005a; Gartlehner et al. 2008). Also, no significant evidence suggests the superiority of any other class of antidepressants over SSRIs (Barbui et al. 2000; Cipriani et al. 2005a; Gartlehner et al. 2008; Geddes et al. 2000).

Side Effects

Although the various SSRIs have similar side effects, individual SSRIs may differ in the degree to which they are associated with a particular side effect. The SSRIs do differ in their pharmacokinetics (half-lives) and the degree to which they inhibit the CYP isoenzyme system affecting the metabolism of concomitant medications the patient may be taking.

Common transient side effects

SSRIs are associated with nausea, vomiting, diarrhea, and headache (Edwards and Anderson 1999). These adverse events are generally dose dependent and tend to dissipate over the first few weeks of treatment. Compared with the other SSRIs, sertraline is more frequently associated with loose stools and diarrhea. SSRIs have also been reported to help prevent and treat migraine headaches (Doughty and Lyle 1995).

Most patients taking SSRIs do not experience either insomnia or somnolence. If a patient reports somnolence after starting an SSRI, I usually recommend taking the dose at bedtime. If a patient is experiencing insomnia, I recommend taking the dose in the morning if he or she has been taking the SSRI in the evening or at bedtime. Because insomnia is a common symptom of depression, it is important to ascertain the patient's baseline level of insomnia before the patient starts taking an SSRI or any antidepressant. Insomnia can be treated by using sleep hygiene techniques or by adding a sedative-hypnotic medication or trazodone.

Sexual side effects

Because sexual dysfunction (particularly decreased libido) can be secondary to the depressive illness, a medical problem, a medication, or problems in a relationship, the clinician should obtain a baseline history of any sexual dysfunction before prescribing an antidepressant (Rothschild 2000). Although sexual side effects can occur with any antidepressant medication, sexual dysfunction appears to occur at higher rates in patients taking SSRIs than in those taking other classes of antidepressants. In a large study, Montejo-González et al. (1997) reported rates of sexual dysfunction (defined as decrease in libido, delay of orgasm or ejaculation, anorgasmia or no ejaculation, or impotence) in patients who were taking various SSRIs: paroxetine (64.71%), fluvoxamine (58.94%), sertraline (56.4%), and fluoxetine (54.38%). No statistically significant differences were found among the individual SSRIs in the rates of sexual dysfunction.

If the sexual dysfunction is deemed to be a side effect of the SSRI, a number of factors need to be considered in the risk-benefit analysis of how to proceed. If the patient has not responded to the antidepressant, then a switch to a different medication is advisable. If the patient has had an antidepressant response to the first antidepressant ever taken, then a switch to a different antidepressant can be implemented. However, if the patient has previously taken several antidepressants without a response and is now responding to an antidepressant (but has sexual dysfunction side effects), a number of strategies can be employed that will hopefully allow the patient to continue taking the antidepressant. Unfortunately, with the exception of sildenafil augmentation (Fava et al. 2006; Nurnberg et al. 2008), most of these strategies have not been studied systematically in a double-blind randomized controlled trial. However, it is clear that waiting for the patient to accommodate to sexual dysfunction side effects is usually not effective (Rothschild 2000). Strategies to implement if sexual dysfunction occurs include lowering the dosage of the SSRI, timing sexual activity to when the antidepressant blood level is at its nadir, taking drug holidays, switching to a different antidepressant, or augmentation with "antidotes" such as amantadine, buspirone, bupropion, cyproheptadine, psychostimulants, sildenafil, tadalafil, or yohimbine (Fava et al. 2006; Nurnberg et al. 2008; Rothschild 1995, 2000; Segraves et al. 2007).

Effects on weight

Most patients who take SSRIs do not experience substantial weight changes. At one time, acute treatment with fluoxetine was thought to be associated with weight loss, but over time people regained any weight that had been lost (Michelson et al. 1999). It is always important to remember that some patients have lost a considerable amount of weight due to the depressive illness and can be expected to regain the lost weight as they improve. Other patients, however, will gain weight secondary to SSRI treatment (Papakostas 2007). Overall, the SSRIs are associated with weight gain to a much lesser degree than the TCAs or MAOIs.

Serotonin syndrome

Serotonin syndrome rarely occurs with SSRI monotherapy, but it can occur if more than one serotonergic medication is taken. The symptoms of serotonin syndrome include tremor, diaphoresis, abdominal pain, diarrhea, flushing, rigidity, myoclonus, mental status changes, and autonomic dysfunction, which can progress to hyperthermia, rhabdomyolysis, coma, and death. The keys to treatment of serotonin syndrome are discontinuation of the serotonergic medications and provision of supportive care.

Serotonin syndrome can occur when a patient is taking more than one serotonergic medication, including any combination of SSRIs, MAOIs, tramadol, high-dose triptans, linezolid (an antibiotic), and over-the-counter preparations (e.g., St. John's wort, L-tryptophan). Clinicians need to remember that once a medication is stopped, time may be needed for it to completely leave the body or for its pharmacological effects to dissipate. Therefore, when an SSRI is being changed to an MAOI or vice versa, the patient should stop taking the first medication at least 2 weeks before taking the second, or 5 weeks when switching from fluoxetine. Concerns regarding serotonin syndrome also apply to patients taking more than one SSRI simultaneously (the efficacy of which has never been demonstrated).

Drug-drug interactions

All SSRIs are metabolized extensively in the liver by the CYP microsomal enzyme system. However, the extent to which various SSRIs in their usual therapeutic dosages inhibit different isoenzymes of the CYP system differs. Interaction with other drugs is higher for fluoxetine, fluvoxamine, and paroxetine than for sertraline, citalopram, and escitalopram (Sandson et al. 2005).

CYP2D6 is the most well characterized of these isoenzymes and is important in the metabolism of a number of commonly prescribed medications, including TCAs, antiarrhythmics (quinidine), haloperidol, some benzodiazepines, codeine, and dextromethorphan, the ingredient found in several over-the-counter medications (e.g., Dristan, Comtrex, Tylenol Cold and Flu, Robitussin DM, and Benylin DM). Inhibitory effects on the CYP isoenzymes may slow the metabolism or inhibit the clearance of affected drugs, resulting in higher plasma concentrations. Thus, the clinician may need to lower the dosage of affected drugs when therapy is initiated or start with a lower dosage of the affected drug when it is added to an ongoing regimen with fluoxetine, fluvoxamine, or paroxetine. Likewise, when withdrawing the antidepressant from therapy, the clinician may need to increase the dosage of the coadministered drug. For example, when SSRIs that strongly inhibit the CYP2D6 isoenzyme (e.g., fluoxetine, fluvoxamine, paroxetine) are administered concomitantly with tamoxifen, the metabolism of tamoxifen to its active metabolite is reduced (Desmarais and Looper 2009), resulting in a potential decrease in its efficacy in preventing breast cancer relapse (Kelly et al. 2010).

Other side effects

Extrapyramidal side effects, including akathisia, dystonia, parkinsonism, and tardive dyskinesia, are not commonly associated with SSRI use, although some reports in the literature suggest that these side effects can occur (Gerber and Lynd 1998). Other uncommon side effects reported include bruxism, restlessness, agitation, and anxiety. If akathisia occurs in a patient with depression, a β-blocker or benzodiazepine can be used to reduce symptoms.

Discontinuation of SSRIs

Generally, as with all antidepressants, the recommended practice is to taper SSRIs rather than to stop them abruptly. This is less of an issue with fluoxetine, due to the long half-life of its active metabolite, norfluoxetine. Discontinuation side effects are predictable and manageable and consist of transient effects, including flulike experiences such as nausea, headache, light-headedness, chills, and body aches, and neurological symptoms such as paresthesias, insomnia, and "electric shock–like" phenomena. These symptoms, which tend to be mild and seldom require treatment, can occur within 2–3 days of stopping treatment with SSRIs (except fluoxetine) and abate with no intervention within 6–10 days.

Discontinuation side effects can be alleviated or prevented by tapering or by reinstituting low dosages of the SSRI for a few days if symptoms appear after abrupt discontinuation.

Serotonin-Norepinephrine Reuptake Inhibitors

Efficacy

The SNRIs currently available are venlafaxine, desvenlafaxine (the principal metabolite of venlafaxine), and duloxetine. Each of these medications has been shown to be effective when compared with placebo (Gartlehner et al. 2008; Thase et al. 2009). At low dosages, venlafaxine is an SSRI; significant norepinephrine reuptake does not occur until the dosage is 225 mg/day or greater. In contrast, duloxetine has significant serotonin and norepinephrine reuptake effects at the starting dosage of 60 mg/day.

Whether SNRIs offer an efficacy advantage over SSRIs is the subject of debate. Some analyses of pooled data sets have suggested a small advantage for SNRIs over SSRIs, particularly for patients who have not responded to previous trials of SSRIs or those with more severe depression (Bauer et al. 2009; Papakostas et al. 2008a; Thase et al. 2007c). However, other meta-analyses have shown equivalent efficacy for SSRIs and SNRIs (Gartlehner et al. 2008). In individual studies, venlafaxine and duloxetine are generally as effective as SSRIs (Keller et al. 2007a, 2007b; Thase et al. 2007c). Venlafaxine's efficacy is also comparable to that of the TCAs (Agency for Healthcare Policy Research 1999; Bauer et al. 2009).[1]

Side Effects

The most common side effects of the SNRIs (venlafaxine, desvenlafaxine, and duloxetine) are similar to those seen with the SSRIs, including nausea and vomiting and sexual dysfunction, although the SNRIs may have a greater propensity to induce nausea. The rates of sexual dysfunction with SNRI treatment are similar to those with the SSRIs. As with the SSRIs, the side effects with SNRIs (except sexual dysfunction) can attenuate with continued medication use. Because of their noradrenergic effects, the SNRIs are also associated with side effects such as increased pulse rate, dilated pupils, dry mouth, excessive sweating, constipation, and increased blood pressure. The risk of increased blood pressure is greatest at venlafaxine dosages of >150 mg/day (Thase 1998). As with all antidepressants, tapering the dosage of the SNRI is preferable to abrupt cessation, to avoid any discontinuation side effects. This is particularly true for venlafaxine (Fava et al. 1997) and may also be true for desvenlafaxine. As discussed previously in the section on MAOI side effects,

---

[1]Duloxetine and desmethylvenlafaxine have not been compared with TCAs.

SNRIs and MAOIs should not be prescribed simultaneously because of the risk of the serotonin syndrome.

Other Antidepressant Medications

Trazodone

Trazodone is an effective antidepressant (Cunningham et al. 1994) but is very sedating and can produce acute dizziness and fainting when taken on an empty stomach (particularly in high dosages). In combination with nonsedating antidepressants, such as the SSRIs, the sedative properties of trazodone are sometimes useful to treat insomnia associated with depression. Trazodone also has been used successfully to treat antidepressant-associated insomnia (Nierenberg et al. 1994).

The most common side effects associated with trazodone include sedation and postural hypotension (particularly among elderly patients). Trazodone has also been associated with priapism and erectile dysfunction in men (Thompson et al. 1990).

Bupropion

The mechanism of action of bupropion is not entirely clear, although it appears to have norepinephrine and dopamine reuptake inhibitor effects and little to no effect on serotonin (Fava et al. 2005). Bupropion has been shown in double-blind studies to have efficacy comparable to that of the TCAs (Feighner et al. 1986). There are three formulations of bupropion: immediate release, sustained release, and extended release.

Bupropion's lack of effects on serotonergic transmission has both advantages and disadvantages. An advantage is a significantly decreased rate of sexual side effects when compared with SSRIs (Segraves et al. 2000). A disadvantage is that bupropion is not likely to be efficacious in comorbid conditions that are helped by increasing serotonergic transmission, such as anxiety, obsessive-compulsive disorder, and eating disorders. In fact, bupropion may be less well tolerated than other antidepressants among patients with significant anxiety and is contraindicated in patients with anorexia nervosa or bulimia nervosa (see next paragraph).

Bupropion has a low incidence of anticholinergic side effects (Lineberry et al. 1990), orthostatic hypotension (Farid et al. 1983), and effects on cardiac conduction (Wenger et al. 1983). Neurological side effects with bupropion include headaches, tremors, and seizures (Fava et al. 2005). The risk of seizures is minimized by avoiding high dosages (e.g., using no more than 450 mg/day), avoiding rapid titration, using divided dosing schedules for the immediate-release and sustained-release formulations, and avoiding use of bupropion in patients with risk factors for seizures. Bupropion should not be used in patients with anorexia nervosa or bulimia nervosa because of an elevated risk of seizures (American Psychiatric Association 2006). The risk of seizures may also be increased by concomitant use of inhibitors of CYP2D6 (e.g., paroxetine, fluoxetine) because of the resulting increase in bupropion blood levels. Other side effects of bupropion include agitation, jitteriness, mild cognitive dysfunction, insomnia, and gastrointestinal disturbances. Patients typically experience minimal weight gain or even weight loss when taking bupropion (Li et al. 2005). Because of its weak dopaminergic effects, bupropion should be used cautiously in patients with psychotic disorders, including psychotic depression. Bupropion has also been approved by the FDA as a treatment for smoking cessation (American Psychiatric Association 2007); therefore, it may be particularly useful in depressed patients who wish to stop smoking (and do not have concomitant anxiety).

Nefazodone

Nefazodone is chemically related to trazodone and is a potent antagonist of the 5-HT_2 receptor and is also a weak SSRI. The use of nefazodone in clinical practice has decreased dramatically over the past 10 years, mainly because of concerns regarding liver toxicity (see next paragraph). In fact, Bristol-Myers Squibb, the original manufacturer of Serzone (brand of nefazodone), discontinued the sale of Serzone in the United States and Canada in 2004. However, several generic formulations of nefazodone are still available.

In comparison to the SSRIs, nefazodone has comparable efficacy and overall tolerability (Papakostas et al. 2007). Common side effects of nefazodone include dry mouth, nausea, constipation, orthostatic hypotension, and sedation (Schatzberg et al. 2002). Nefazodone has not been associated with priapism. Compared with the SSRIs, nefazodone has a lower incidence of treatment-emergent sexual dysfunction (Ferguson et al. 2001). Nefazodone has also been associated with rare but potentially fatal liver failure (DeSanty and Amabile 2007). In one report, 88% of the cases of liver toxicity occurred during the first 6 months of nefazodone therapy (Stewart 2002). Nefazodone should be avoided in patients with active liver disease or elevated serum transaminases.

Nefazodone is a potent inhibitor of the CYP3A4 isoenzyme system and can raise the blood levels of medications metabolized by this isoenzyme system, such as aripiprazole, benzodiazepines, digoxin, and some antihistamines.

Mirtazapine

Mirtazapine is chemically related to mianserin, an antidepressant used in Europe but not in the United States. Although mirtazapine has a tetracyclic structure, its mechanism of action is quite different from that of the TCAs, and it is not a reuptake blocker of any monoamine transmitter. Through antagonism of α_2-adrenergic receptors, mirtazapine acts to release norepinephrine. The increased noradrenergic tone promotes a rapid increase in synaptic serotonin levels as a result of stimulation of α_1-adrenergic receptors on serotonin cell bodies (Artigas et al. 2002). Mirtazapine is also an antagonist of 5-HT_2 and 5-HT_3 receptors.

Mirtazapine has efficacy comparable to that of the SSRIs (Papakostas et al. 2008b). The most common side effects of mirtazapine include dry mouth, sedation, somnolence, and weight gain. Although weight gain is a problem for many patients taking mirtazapine, this is a particularly good antidepressant to prescribe for depressed patients with insomnia who have lost considerable weight. Because somnolence is common, mirtazapine is usually given at bedtime. Somnolence is more pronounced at lower dosages than at higher dosages because at low dosages the antihistaminergic effects predominate relative to noradrenergic or serotonergic effects. Thus, a starting dosage of 30 mg/day is often tolerated as well as a dosage of 7.5 mg/day. Except for weight gain, the side effects of mirtazapine frequently attenuate with time. Sexual dysfunction side effects associated with mirtazapine may be less than those observed with the SSRIs (Koutouvidis et al. 1999).

Vilazodone

Vilazodone is a dual-acting serotonergic antidepressant approved by the FDA in 2011 for the treatment of depression. Vilazodone combines the effects of an SSRI with 5-HT_{1A} receptor partial agonist activity. Vilazodone showed significant antidepressant efficacy compared with placebo, with a statistically significant onset of effect at 1 week (Rickels et al. 2009). The most common side effects were diarrhea, nausea, and somnolence (Rickels et al. 2009). In addition, no significant difference was found between placebo and vilazodone in terms of sexual dysfunction as measured by the Arizona Sexual Experiences Scale (Rickels et al. 2009). The effects of vilazodone could conceivably be duplicated by prescribing the combination of an SSRI and buspirone, a partial 5-HT_{1A} agonist.

Continuation and Maintenance Treatment

Continuation phase pharmacotherapy is strongly recommended following successful acute phase antidepressant therapy, with a recommended duration of continuation therapy of approximately 4–9 months (assuming good and consistent control of depression symptoms). Because studies indicate that relapse rates are greater if antidepressant treatment is discontinued or reduced in dosage or intensity following recovery (Papakostas et al. 2007), treatment should generally continue with the same medication at the same dosage. If a relapse does occur during the continuation phase, an initial step can be to increase the dosage of medication (Schmidt et al. 2002).

Patients who have had three or more prior major depressive episodes should receive maintenance treatment (American Psychiatric Association 2010). Studies indicate that the number of lifetime major depressive episodes is significantly associated with the probability of recurrence, such that the risk of recurrence increases by 16% with each successive episode (Solomon et al. 2000). Additional risk factors for the recurrence of a major depressive episode include "persistence of subthreshold depressive symptoms; prior history of multiple episodes of major depressive disorder; severity of initial and any subsequent episodes; earlier age at onset; presence of an additional nonaffective psychiatric diagnosis; presence of a chronic general medical disorder; family history of psychiatric illness, particularly mood disorder; ongoing psychosocial stressors or impairment; negative cognitive style; and persistent sleep disturbances" (American Psychiatric Association 2010, p. 58).

Results from more than 30 trials of pharmacotherapy in the maintenance phase have generally demonstrated the effectiveness of antidepressant medication for relapse prevention (Agency for Healthcare Policy Research 1999; Hansen et al. 2008; Keller 2006). In general, the treatment that was effective in the acute and continuation phases should be used in the maintenance phase with the same medication and at the same dosage (Frank et al. 1993).

Unfortunately, in some patients the antidepressant appears to lose its effectiveness during maintenance despite being prescribed at the same dosage to which the patient responded during the acute treatment phase. An observational investigation of participants in the National Institute of Mental Health Collaborative Depression Study found that 25% of participants had a loss of antidepressant response (Solomon et al. 2005). Rates of recurrence in clinical trials assessing maintenance pharmacotherapy have been found to vary considerably, ranging from 9% to 57% (Byrne and Rothschild 1998). Some evidence suggests that the likelihood of the loss of antidepressant response varies across antidepressant class. Specifically, patients receiving maintenance treatment with SSRIs have been found to be at an increased risk for recurrence of depression. In a retrospective, naturalistic analysis of patients with major depressive disorder, those receiving antidepressants that modulate serotonin and norepinephrine neurotransmission (i.e., venlafaxine or TCAs) had significantly lower rates (3.7%) of the recurrence of depression than did those being treated with SSRIs (14.1%; $P=0.01$) (Posternak and Zimmerman 2005).

Byrne and Rothschild (1998) hypothesized that the phenomenon of tachyphylaxis is distinct from that of an initial or recurrent major depressive episode. *Tachyphylaxis* is defined as symptoms of apathy or decreased motivation (commonly known as "the blahs"), fatigue, dullness in cognitive function, sleep disturbance, weight gain, and sexual dysfunction (Rothschild 2008). Defining tachyphylaxis as a clinical phenomenon that is distinct from a full recurrence has significant clinical utility. It may serve as an early marker for an impending recurrence, indicating the need for a change in clinical intervention to prevent a worsening of the patient's status, and may ultimately serve as a phenotype for studies seeking to identify genetic markers for recurrence. Other names for this phenomenon include *acquired drug tolerance, antidepressant tolerance, antidepressant "poop-out,"* and *breakthrough depression* (Byrne and Rothschild 1998; Solomon et al. 2005). Regardless of the label applied and its perceived causes, tachyphylaxis is a clinically significant phenomenon that deleteriously impacts the care of depressed patients. In a study that explored this new definition of antidepressant tachyphylaxis or "poop-out," no differences were found between fluoxetine and venlafaxine in rates of tachyphylaxis over a 2-year period (Rothschild et al. 2009). However, the occurrence of tachyphylaxis was a harbinger or predictor of the later development of a full relapse into an episode of major depression (Rothschild et al. 2009).

Treatment-Resistant Depression

Every clinician's practice includes patients with so-called treatment-resistant depression (TRD). Although there is no universally accepted definition of TRD, results from the U.S. National Institute of Mental Health's (NIMH's) Sequenced Treatment Alternatives to Relieve Depression (STAR*D) study indicate that after the failure of two treatment trials, the chances of remission decrease significantly (Rush et al. 2004).

Although psychiatrists have a plethora of antidepressants available to treat patients, and many more than when I finished my psychiatric training in 1983, it seems as if many more patients have TRD now than 30 years ago when fewer antidepressants were in the therapeutic armamentarium. Why is that? Although there are several possible explanations, I cannot begin to count the number of times in the past 15 years a patient has been referred to me with so-called TRD, having had numerous trials of antidepressants, yet when I take the history, I discover that the patient has *never* had a trial of a TCA or MAOI. Unfortunately, a generation of psychiatrists appears to have graduated from psychiatry residency training programs having never prescribed an MAOI. It is unfortunately also becoming increasingly common for graduates not to have prescribed a TCA during their training. A 1997 survey of the Michigan Psychiatric Association reported that 12% of practicing psychiatrists had never prescribed an MAOI, whereas another 27% had not prescribed an MAOI in the prior 3 years (Balon et al. 1999). Only 2% of respondents reported frequent use of MAOIs (Balon et al. 1999), compared with reports of approximately 25% a decade earlier (Clary et al. 1990). Although no similar survey has been done since 1997, my impression is that the use of MAOIs to treat depression has continued to decline. When beginning work with patients who are considered to have TRD, the clinician should ask the following questions: 1) Have they ever had an adequate trial of a TCA? 2) Have they ever had an adequate trial of an MAOI? Electroconvulsive therapy (ECT) remains an effective therapy for patients with treatment-resistant symptoms (Pagnin et al. 2004). However, the results of clinical trials differ regarding whether patients with medication-resistant symptoms have responses to ECT that are comparable to those of patients without documented medication resistance (Rasmussen et al. 2007).

The pharmacological treatments of TRD can be grouped into two main strategies: switching antidepressants or combining medications. In the first strategy, treatment is switched within and between classes of compounds. The benefits of switching include avoidance of polypharmacy (Glezer et al. 2009), a narrower range of treatment-emergent adverse events, and lower costs. An inherent disadvantage of any switching strategy is that partial treatment responses resulting from the initial treatment may be lost by the discontinuation of the antidepressant. The advantage of combination strategies is the potential to build on achieved improvements; these strategies are generally recommended if partial response was achieved with the current treatment trial. Various non-antidepressant augmenting agents, such as lithium and thyroid hormones, are well studied, although not commonly used. There is also evidence of the efficacy and increasing use of atypical antipsychotics in combination with antidepressants (e.g., olanzapine in combination with fluoxetine or augmentation with aripiprazole or quetiapine). The disadvantages of a combination strategy include multiple medications, a broader range of treatment-emergent adverse events, and higher costs.

Switching Strategies

If a patient does not show a response to an initial antidepressant trial that is typically of sufficient dosage and duration, the patient is not likely to improve by continuation of the antidepressant, and therefore switching medications and the prevention of unnecessary polypharmacy is indicated (Alao et al. 2003; Glezer et al. 2009). Although no specific patient characteristics predict which medication to choose, results from STAR*D suggest that changing to a second-step treatment results in additional remission rates of about 25%, and further changes are associated with continued remission, albeit at lower rates (about 13%–14%) (Rush et al. 2008). Treatment can be changed to a medication from the same pharmacological class (e.g., from one SSRI to another

SSRI) or to one from a different class (e.g., from an SSRI to a TCA) (Rush et al. 2006; Thase et al. 2007b).

Augmentation Strategies

Generally, in patients who have had some response to an antidepressant, the preferable action is to continue the antidepressant to maintain the gains that have been made and to augment with another medication (Pridmore and Turnier-Shea 2004). Of the many possible augmenting agents from which the clinician can choose, lithium and thyroid hormone have the longest history and record of efficacy (Carvalho et al. 2007).

Lithium is the most extensively studied augmentation strategy (Cipriani et al. 2006; Crossley and Bauer 2007) and may also reduce the long-term risk of suicide (Cipriani et al. 2005b). Lithium was first introduced by de Montigny et al. (1981) as an augmenting agent used with TCA treatment of nonresponders. To date, 11 placebo-controlled studies have been reported, 8 of which found lithium augmentation to be more effective than placebo (Shelton et al. 2010). In 9 of these placebo-controlled trials, initial treatment with a TCA was augmented with lithium, whereas in 2 studies, initial SSRI treatment was augmented with lithium (Shelton et al. 2010). The response rates in the placebo-controlled studies augmenting antidepressive efficacy of TCAs with lithium varied widely, from 12.5% to 100% (Shelton et al. 2010). Lithium augmentation of SSRI treatment produced response rates from 50% to 60% (Shelton et al. 2010). The interval before full response to adjunctive lithium is in the range of several days to 6 weeks. The blood level of lithium required to enhance the effects of antidepressants is not known. If effective and well tolerated, lithium should be continued at least for the duration of acute treatment and perhaps beyond the acute phase for purposes of relapse prevention.

The addition of thyroid hormone (triiodothyronine [T_3], liothyronine), even in euthyroid patients, may increase the effectiveness of antidepressant medication treatment when used as an augmentation agent (Aronson et al. 1996) or in combination with an antidepressant from the outset of therapy (Cooper-Kazaz et al. 2007). The dosage typically used for this purpose is 25 μg/day of triiodothyronine, which is increased to 50 μg/day if the response is inadequate after about a week. The duration of treatment required has not been well studied.

In the STAR*D study, the investigators compared the efficacy of lithium augmentation with that of liothyronine augmentation in patients with TRD who had not achieved remission in two preceding treatment trials. Both groups showed only modest remission rates (lithium 15.9% vs. liothyronine 24.7%), which were not statistically significantly different (Nierenberg et al. 2006).

Although the addition of bupropion to an SSRI is a frequent strategy used in clinical practice, only a few studies support this practice. In one study, combined treatment with bupropion and an SSRI resulted in better outcomes than either therapy alone (Lam et al. 2004). This combination is generally well tolerated, although bupropion, a moderately potent inhibitor of CYP2D6, increases blood levels of several SSRIs (Kennedy et al. 2002).

Another commonly used strategy in clinical practice is the combination of mirtazapine and an SSRI or venlafaxine. Generally, mirtazapine 15–30 mg at bedtime is added to the incompletely effective antidepressant, and the dosage of mirtazapine is titrated up to 45 mg/day on the basis of response and tolerability (Carpenter et al. 2002).

Many clinicians find that augmentation of antidepressants with low dosages of stimulants such as methylphenidate or dextroamphetamine may help ameliorate otherwise suboptimally responsive depression (Ravindran et al. 2008), although not all clinical trials have shown benefits from this strategy (Patkar et al. 2006).

In recent years, the off-label use of atypical antipsychotic medications for the treatment of nonpsychotic depression has been increasing. At the present time, both aripiprazole and quetiapine have an FDA indication as an addition to antidepressant treatment for use in treating nonpsychotic major depressive disorder. At the present time, olanzapine combined with fluoxetine has an FDA indication for the acute treatment of TRD (defined as two failed attempts of adequate dosage and duration with other antidepressants in the current episode).

In deciding to use an atypical antipsychotic medication for nonpsychotic depression, the clinician needs to take into account the potential benefits and risks of this class of medications (Rothschild 2010). The long-term efficacy, tolerability, and safety of atypical antipsychotic medications for the treatment of nonpsychotic major depressive disorder remain to be determined. Generally, in clinical practice, lower dosages of antipsychotic medication are used for antidepressant augmentation than for treatment of psychosis. For example, the combination of olanzapine and fluoxetine (Shelton et al. 2001; Thase et al. 2007a) is typically initiated at 6 mg/day of olanzapine and 25 mg/day of fluoxetine, and the dosage is titrated upward as tolerated to a maximum of 18 mg/day of olanzapine and 75 mg/day of fluoxetine. Aripiprazole is typically initiated at 2.5–5 mg/day, and the dosage is titrated upward as tolerated to a maximum of 30 mg/day (Berman et al. 2007). With quetiapine, dosages of 150–300 mg/day are recommended for augmentation of antidepressants in unipolar major depression, with benefits for depressive symptoms found in some (Doree et al. 2007; McIntyre et al. 2007) but not all (Garakani et al. 2008) clinical trials.

Unipolar Major Depression With Psychotic Features

Psychotic depression (major depression with psychotic features, delusional depression) is a serious illness during which a person suffers from the dangerous combination of depressed mood and psychosis, with the psychosis commonly manifesting itself as nihilistic, "bad things are about to happen"–type delusions (Rothschild 2009). In samples of patients with major depression, a European study observed that 18.5% of them also had symptoms that fulfilled criteria for major depressive episode with psychotic features (Ohayon and Schatzberg 2002), and in a study in the United States (Johnson et al. 1991), 14.7% of the patients who met the criteria for major depression had a history of psychotic features. In outpatient studies of adolescents with major depression, the prevalence of psychotic symptoms was reported to be 18% (Ryan et al. 1987). In people older than 60 years, the prevalence of psychotic depression in the community is between 14 and 30 per 1,000 (Baldwin and Jolley 1986; Blazer 1994). In a Finnish community sample of people over the age of 60, the rate of psychotic depression was found to be 12 per 1,000 in women and 6 per 1,000 in men (Kivela and Pahkala 1989).

Currently, no drugs, devices, or treatments, including any antipsychotic medication, have been approved by the FDA specifically for the treatment of major depression with psychotic features. In *Practice Guideline for the Treatment of Patients With Major Depressive Disorder,* Third Edition, the American Psychiatric Association (2010) Work Group recommends, with substantial clinical confidence, the combination of an antipsychotic and an antidepressant or ECT for the pharmacological treatment of psychotic depression. Despite these recommendations, recent data suggest that only 5% of patients with psychotic depression receive an adequate combination of an antidepressant and an antipsychotic (Andreescu et al. 2007). These findings indicate a persisting low rate of adequate dosage and duration of treatment (particularly the use of an antipsychotic medication) of psychotic depression and little change from a study published a decade earlier, which also reported inadequate dosage and duration of medication treatment prescribed to patients with psychotic depression (Mulsant et al. 1997).

Effectiveness of Antidepressant Monotherapy

Amoxapine, a dibenzoxazepine-derivative TCA, is converted by the liver to 8-hydroxyamoxapine, which has considerable dopamine receptor binding properties, and is associated with extrapyramidal side effects including tardive dyskinesia. Because of this, amoxapine is rarely used anymore for the treatment of major depressive disorder, although it may have a role in the treatment of psychotic depression (Rothschild 2009). However, even when amoxapine is used for the treatment of psychotic depression, the amount of antidepressant and antipsychotic in the patient's body is controlled by the patient's liver.

In the 1990s, an Italian research group published a series of studies that reported marked improvement of inpatients with psychotic depression using SSRI monotherapy including fluvoxamine, paroxetine, and sertraline (Zanardi et al. 1996, 1998, 2000). In these studies, the response rates to SSRI monotherapy were comparable to the response rate observed in other studies with ECT or with a combination of TCA and antipsychotic. These response rates were remarkably high given the relatively short duration of treatment (i.e., ≤6 weeks). These studies have been criticized because of the lack of a placebo control, concerns regarding the diagnostic inclusion criteria, and the validity of the scales used for evaluation of response (Rothschild and Phillips 1999). The results have not been replicated by another research group. An 8-week open-label study using sertraline monotherapy (mean dosage=177 mg/day) for psychotic depression failed to replicate these findings (Simpson et al. 2005).

Only two randomized clinical trials have compared antidepressant monotherapy with an antidepressant-antipsychotic combination (Mulsant et al. 2001; Spiker et al. 1985). Spiker et al. (1985) found that the antidepressant-antipsychotic combination was superior to antidepressant monotherapy. In contrast, Mulsant et al. (2001), in a study of older patients (mean age=72 years) with psychotic depression, observed no difference between antidepressant monotherapy and the combination of antidepressant and antipsychotic. In fact, the response was mediocre for both groups. The Mulsant et al. study was a double-blind trial comparing the tolerability and the efficacy of nortriptyline plus perphenazine versus nortriptyline plus placebo in a group of older inpatients who presented with a major depressive episode with psychotic features. Fifty-two patients (mean age=72 years) were included in the trial, and open-label nortriptyline was started and the dosage titrated to yield a therapeutic plasma level (target=100 ng/mL; range=50–150 ng/mL). After 2 weeks, patients who had not responded were randomly assigned to receive perphenazine ($n=17$) or placebo ($n=19$) in addition to the nortriptyline. The dosage was titrated up to a maximum of 24 mg/day (mean dosage=18.9 mg/day) until either patients showed therapeutic response or extrapyramidal side effects were detected. After patients had received nortriptyline for at least 4 weeks combined with either perphenazine or placebo for at least 2 weeks (median= 9 weeks), no statistical differences were observed on the Hamilton Rating Scale for Depression (Ham-D) or the Psychoticism subscale of the Brief Psychiatric Rating Scale (BPRS). Rates of response to nortriptyline plus perphenazine (50%) and nortriptyline monotherapy (44%) did not statistically differ among the 30 treatment completers ($P=0.99$).

A meta-analysis of these two studies (Wijkstra et al. 2006) did not show a statistically significant difference between a TCA-antipsychotic combination and a TCA alone (relative risk [RR]=1.44; 95% CI=0.86–2.41; P=0.16), leading the authors to conclude that either antidepressant monotherapy or an antidepressant-antipsychotic combination was an appropriate pharmacotherapy option for psychotic depression. I disagree with this conclusion. The Spiker et al. (1985) study clearly found a statistically significant efficacy advantage of the combination of amitriptyline and perphenazine over amitriptyline monotherapy. When data from the Mulsant et al. (2001) study—which had a different study design from that of the Spiker study and mediocre results on both nortriptyline monotherapy and the combination of nortriptyline and perphenazine—are added to the Spiker data, the finding of the Spiker study is obscured.

In a post hoc analysis (Birkenhager et al. 2008) of two randomized controlled clinical trials of imipramine monotherapy with plasma level–targeted dosing and response defined as a ≥50% decrease in Ham-D score, 55% of patients with mood-congruent psychotic depression responded compared with 39% of depressed patients without psychotic features (P=0.09). Rates of remisison (defined as a 50% decrease in Ham-D score and a final Ham-D score ≤7) were not different between psychotic (25%) and nonpsychotic (24%) depressed patients (P=0.94).

Over the years, there have been case reports of an association between TCA or SSRI monotherapy and an exacerbation of psychotic symptoms in patients with unipolar psychotic depression (Narayan et al. 1995; Nelson et al. 1979). In an analysis of 20 studies of psychotic depression, Kantrowitz and Tampi (2008) reported that 15 of 177 subjects (8.5%) undergoing antidepressant monotherapy (8 of whom were taking TCAs) had an exacerbation of psychosis, whereas only 2 of 129 subjects (1.6%) undergoing either antipsychotic or combination treatment had an exacerbation of psychosis. Thus, TCA monotherapy was statistically significantly more likely (P=0.007) to be temporally associated with an exacerbation of psychosis than was antipsychotic monotherapy or the combination of an antidepressant and an antipsychotic.

Taken together, the studies of antidepressant monotherapy provide little evidence that antidepressants by themselves are as efficacious as the combination of antidepressant plus antipsychotic. Furthermore, antidepressant monotherapy may carry some risk of exacerbating the psychotic symptoms in psychotic depression.

Choice of Antidepressant

Which antidepressant should be used (in combination with an antipsychotic medication) for the treatment of major depression with psychotic features? Although in theory any of the antidepressant medications could be used, only four antidepressant-antipsychotic combinations have been studied in randomized controlled clinical trials of patients with psychotic depression and have been shown to be effective (see Table 2–4). Because other combinations of antidepressants and antipsychotics have not been studied, I recommend using these particular pairs of antidepressants and antipsychotics until evidence indicates that other combinations are effective. If a patient does not respond to trials of one or two of these combinations, the clinician should seriously consider ECT.

Bipolar Disorder

The use of antidepressants to treat the depressed phase of bipolar disorder has been the subject of considerable debate over the years. The controversy has focused on whether antidepressants are efficacious for the treatment of the depressed phase of bipolar disorder and on the concern that antidepressants, particularly TCAs, may destabilize mood by inducing an affective switch to mania or hypomania (Sidor and MacQueen 2011). Warnings against the administration of antidepressants to patients with bipolar depression are reflected in current U.S. treatment guidelines, such as the American Psychiatric Association's (2002) practice guideline. On the other hand, European treatment guidelines, such as the British Association for Psychopharmacology guidelines, are less cautious in recommending antidepressants for bipolar disorder (Goodwin and Young 2003). The debate is further complicated by the fact that in bipolar disorder, switch from depression into hypomania or mania commonly occurs as a natural course of the illness.

In recent years, the approval by the FDA of pharmacological treatments such as an olanzapine-fluoxetine combination (Symbyax) and quetiapine for the acute treatment of the depressed phase of bipolar disorder has made the resolution of the controversy less crucial.[2] Nevertheless, some patients with bipolar disorder will not respond to or tolerate the FDA-approved treatments for the depressed phase of bipolar disorder, resulting in the clinician's considering the use of antidepressants. Indeed, approximately 50% of patients with bipolar disorder are prescribed an antidepressant (Goldberg et al. 2009). Thus, the clinician needs to assess the current evidence base for the use of antidepressants in the depressed phase of bipolar disorder.

In 2004, Gijsman et al. published a systematic review and meta-analysis of 12 randomized controlled trials of antidepressant use in the acute treatment of bipolar depression. Their analysis strongly supported an average positive efficacy for antidepressants versus placebo for the depressed phase of

---

[2]Lamotrigine, aripiprazole, and long-acting risperidone (Risperdal Consta) are indicated for the maintenance treatment of bipolar I disorder.

TABLE 2–4. Combinations of antidepressant and antipsychotic medications with demonstrated efficacy in psychotic depression in randomized controlled clinical trials

STUDY	SAMPLE SIZE	ANTIDEPRESSANT	ANTIPSYCHOTIC
Meyers et al. 2009	259	Sertraline	Olanzapine
Rothschild et al. 2004[a]	249	Fluoxetine	Olanzapine
Wjikstra et al. 2008	122	Venlafaxine	Quetiapine
Spiker et al. 1985	51	Amitriptyline	Perphenazine

[a]Only study with a placebo control group.
Source. Adapted from Rothschild AJ: *Clinical Manual for Diagnosis and Treatment of Psychotic Depression.* Washington DC, American Psychiatric Publishing, 2009, p. 94. Copyright © 2009 American Psychiatric Publishing. Used with permission.

bipolar disorder in trials lasting up to 10 weeks. The size of the antidepressant effect was comparable to that in unipolar depression (Geddes et al. 2003), suggesting that antidepressants may be of comparable efficacy in unipolar and bipolar depression. The rates of switching to mania in the short time spans of 4–10 weeks covered by these studies were low and did not support the belief that switching is a common early complication of treatment with antidepressants. However, as Gijsman et al. pointed out, the numbers of patients switching into mania were small, and larger studies, especially those with longer follow-up and systematic monitoring of manic symptoms, could change this conclusion. However, the authors argued that the use of antidepressants in the short term was supported by their meta-analysis.

The Gijsman et al. (2004) analysis supported the previous findings of nonrandomized studies in bipolar disorder and comparative studies in unipolar patients that had suggested a higher risk of switching to mania for patients taking TCAs (Bottlender et al. 1998; Peet 1995). The study also suggested that TCAs cause more switching to mania and that TCAs are not more, and may even be less, effective than other classes of antidepressants. The authors speculated that antidepressant response and a switch into mania may not be correlated and thus may make TCAs less suitable for bipolar patients in general. Finally, Gijsman et al.'s analysis was unable to show a difference between an antidepressant used as monotherapy and a combined antidepressant and mood stabilizer.

In the NIMH-funded Systematic Treatment Enhancement Program for Bipolar Disorder (STEP-BD), subjects with bipolar depression were randomly assigned to receive up to 26 weeks of treatment with a mood stabilizer plus adjunctive antidepressant therapy (paroxetine or bupropion) or a mood stabilizer plus a matching placebo, in a double-blind, placebo-controlled study under conditions generalizable to routine clinical care (Sachs et al. 2007). Forty-two of the 179 subjects (23.5%) receiving a mood stabilizer plus adjunctive antidepressant therapy had a durable recovery, as did 51 of the 187 subjects (27.3%) receiving a mood stabilizer plus a matching placebo (P= 0.40) (Sachs et al. 2007). The authors concluded that the use of adjunctive, standard antidepressant medication, as compared with the use of mood stabilizers, was not associated with increased efficacy or with increased risk of treatment-emergent affective switch (see below) (Sachs et al. 2007).

A recent meta-analysis of 15 double-blind randomized controlled clinical trials (4–16 weeks) did not find that the use of antidepressant medications to treat the depressed phase of bipolar disorder was associated with a statistically significant increase in efficacy compared with placebo or other pharmacological treatments (Sidor and MacQueen 2011). Sidor and MacQueen, in their meta-analysis, included three new placebo-controlled studies (including the STEP-BD study discussed above) published since the Gijsman et al. (2004) meta-analysis and also excluded two studies that Gijsman et al. used in their meta-analysis.

Antidepressants and the Potential for Risk of Switch Into Mania

Two meta-analyses, as well as the STEP-BD study, suggest that SSRIs and bupropion do not increase the risk of switch into mania when used to treat the depressed phase of bipolar disorder (Gijsman et al. 2004; Sachs et al. 2007; Sidor and MacQueen 2011). Although bupropion is no more efficacious in the treatment of the depressed phase of bipolar disorder than other treatments (McIntyre et al. 2002; Sachs et al. 2007; Sidor and MacQueen 2011), expert guidelines often give bupropion a prominent role in the treatment of the depressed phase of bipolar disorder because of the belief that it is less likely to be associated with switching the patient into the manic phase (Keck et al. 2004; Sachs et al. 2000), despite reports of switching occurring in patients with a history of antidepressant-associated switching (Fogelson et al. 1992). However, the number of studies that evaluated potential for affective switching during bupropion treatment is small. Apart from some open studies, only two studies (Post et al. 2006; Sachs et al. 1994) have examined the use of bupropion for the treatment of the depressed phase of bipolar disorder. In the smaller study of 10 desipramine-treated patients and 9 bupropion-treated patients (Sachs et al. 1994), bupropion was less statistically significantly likely to induce mood elevation than was desipramine. However, in a larger study, a double-blind comparison of bupropion, sertraline, and venlafaxine, a significantly higher rate of switch from depression to mania or hypomania was observed among subjects receiving venlafaxine than among those receiving bupropion or sertraline (Leverich et al. 2006; Post et al. 2006). A retrospective study failed to replicate this study, finding no difference in the incidence of switching into mania among bupropion (36%), SSRIs (30%), and venlafaxine (31%) in rapid-cycling bipolar patients, although monotherapy with second-generation antidepressants was associated with treatment-emergent mania (Gao et al. 2008).

In the STEP-BD study, neither paroxetine nor bupropion was associated with an increased rate of treatment-emergent affective switch (Sachs et al. 2007). No significant difference in the rates of prospectively observed treatment-emergent mania, hypomania, or mixed episodes was found between the patients receiving a mood stabilizer plus an antidepressant (10.1%) and those receiving a mood stabilizer plus placebo (10.7%) (Sachs et al. 2007). Among subjects reporting treatment-emergent affective switch associated with one or more previous courses of treatment with antidepressants, switch rates did not differ significantly between the group receiving a mood stabilizer plus an antidepressant and the group receiving a mood stabilizer plus placebo (10.2% and 17.9%, respectively; P=0.22) (Sachs et al. 2007). Among the subjects receiving a mood stabilizer plus an antidepressant, no significant differences were found in the rate of any primary or secondary outcome between subjects receiving bupropion and those receiving paroxetine.

In a meta-analysis that included the studies by Post et al. (2006) and Sachs et al. (1994), Sidor and MacQueen (2011) reported that bupropion was associated with a significantly reduced risk for affective switch compared with other antidepressants, particularly TCAs and SNRIs (RR=0.34; 95% CI= 0.13–0.88). The switch rate was 5% for bupropion, 7% for SSRIs, 15% for SNRIs, and 43% for TCAs (Sidor and MacQueen 2011). However, the study by Sachs et al. (1994) used a modest dose of bupropion compared with a maximally tolerated dose of desipramine, which may have inflated the switch rates in the TCA group (Sidor and MacQueen 2011). Furthermore, in the Post et al. (2006) study, some subjects were unblinded. Of note, in the Post et al. study, no difference in switch rates occurred between bupropion and venlafaxine in patients with non-rapid-cycling bipolar disorder.

Finally, in a critical review of the randomized controlled studies in the literature that took the methodological limitations into account, Licht et al. (2008) could not find any conclusive unbiased evidence supporting the notion that antidepressants can induce switching or accelerate cycling. Unfortunately, no systematic data are available that help the clinician decide whether to continue or discontinue an antidepressant when hypomanic or manic symptoms develop in a patient treated with an antidepressant.

Practical Conclusions for Clinical Practice

The belief that antidepressants (even in combination with mood stabilizers) induce switches, rapid cycling, or both in patients with bipolar disorder is not sufficiently justified by the scientific evidence in the medical literature and may, unfortunately, create unnecessary anxiety among clinicians, patients, and their relatives. The available evidence does suggest, however, that antidepressant medications have little efficacy in the acute treatment of the depressed phase of bipolar disorder. This is particularly important in light of the fact that other medications, including the olanzapine-fluoxetine combination and quetiapine, have shown strong evidence for efficacy in the acute treatment of depression in patients with bipolar I disorder. Furthermore, despite a lack of systematic studies, almost all experts would agree that the prescription of antidepressants in the absence of a mood stabilizer is not recommended for patients with bipolar I disorder. Finally, if a patient develops mania or a mixed state in the aftermath of depression (or later) while taking an antidepressant, stopping the antidepressant (or reducing the dosage) is clinically advisable in most cases.

Special Topics

Do Antidepressants Work?

Clinicians have successfully used antidepressants to treat patients suffering from depression for 50 years. In 2008, Kirsch et al. published a meta-analysis of the data held by the FDA from 35 randomized placebo-controlled trials of four newer antidepressants in the acute treatment of major depression. The authors claimed that although antidepressants are statistically superior to placebo, the magnitude of the drug-placebo difference is small, and that these differences were only clinically relevant in patients with severe depression. Surprisingly, the paper received considerable attention in the popular press, including radio and front-page newspaper coverage. The focus on questions about whether antidepressants really worked needlessly upset patients and their families. What has not received equal coverage in the popular media is that many experts in the field have argued that the analysis by Kirsch and colleagues is seriously flawed (Bech 2009; Broich 2009; Hegerl and Mergl 2010; Horder et al. 2010). Furthermore, the efficacy of antidepressants is documented by the experience of clinicians worldwide and the millions of patients who have benefited from taking them.

Do Antidepressants "Cause" Suicide?

Recurring questions are whether treatment with the SSRIs and other antidepressants can induce suicidal ideation and whether they make existing suicidal ideation worse. Although the reliable scientific evidence indicates that SSRIs and other antidepressants do not cause suicide (as discussed in the following subsections), the FDA has required that all antidepressants contain a black box warning that they are associated with "suicidality" in children, adolescents, and young adults up to age 24 years. Clinicians should be aware of two important points: 1) The FDA's black box warning does not indicate that antidepressants increase the risk of suicide in anyone, or that they increase the risk of suicidal thinking or behavior in patients ages 25 and older. 2) Although the FDA used the concept of "suicidality" as a proxy for completed suicide, they are not the same thing. The term *suicidality* has been criticized as grossly overestimating the risk of suicide (Klein 2006) and as not being as clinically useful as more specific terminology such as *ideation, behavior, attempts,* and *suicide* (Meyer et al. 2010).

Ecological Studies About Antidepressants and Suicide

Ecological studies provide confirmatory evidence that antidepressants do not cause suicide. A substantial body of evidence suggests that increases in the use of antidepressants have been accompanied by decreases in suicide rates in various countries (Grunebaum et al. 2004; Hall et al. 2003; Isacsson et al. 2009; 2010a, 2010b). Also, Bramness et al. (2007) reported an association between a decrease in suicide rates in Norway and its counties from 1980 to 2004 and increased sales of nontricyclic antidepressants. U.S. government statistics indicate that since the advent of SSRIs, the age-adjusted suicide rate dropped approximately 13.5% between 1985 and 1999 while antidepressant prescription rates increased over fourfold, with the increase mostly due to SSRIs (Grunebaum et al. 2004). In a study examining the association between antidepressant medication prescriptions and suicide rate at the county level across the United States broken down by age, sex, income, and race for the period 1996–1998 (Gibbons et al. 2005), prescriptions for SSRIs and newer non-SSRI antidepressants (e.g., nefazodone, mirtazapine, bupropion, venlafaxine) were associated with lower suicide rates (both within and between counties). On the contrary, as detailed in an article by Gibbons et al. (2007), there is good reason to believe that the FDA's warnings, beginning with the 2003 FDA Talk Paper concerning the use of Paxil to treat pediatric depression (U.S. Food and Drug Administration 2003), have had the effect of deterring or frightening both pediatric and young adult patients (and their physicians) away from treatment and that, as a consequence, there has been a reversal of the historic downward trend in pediatric and young adult suicides associated with increasing use of antidepressants in these populations.

Thus, rather than revealing an increased risk of suicide with SSRI treatment, the available evidence suggests that suicide rates have dropped in parallel with the increased use of SSRIs. In contrast, a positive association between TCA prescriptions and suicide rate has been observed (Gibbons et al. 2005). A study of computerized health plan records of 65,103 patients with 82,285 episodes of antidepressant treatment between January 1, 1992, and June 30, 2003, failed to demonstrate a significant increase in risk of suicide or serious suicide attempts after starting treatment with newer antidepressant drugs (Simon et al. 2006). In fact, the risk of death by suicide was not significantly higher in the month after starting medication than in subsequent months. Not surprisingly, the risk of suicide attempt was highest in the month before starting antidepressant treatment and declined progressively after starting medication. Finally, in a study in patients age 65 and older, the use of SSRIs was not associated with an increased risk of suicide (Rahme et al. 2008).

Population-based, ecological studies do not, by themselves, prove causation with respect to increasing antidepressant rates and falling suicide rates. They do, however, provide confirmatory information that is consistent with the hypothesis that SSRIs do not cause suicide, and in fact are protective against suicide, as would be expected from a medication that effectively treats depression, which itself is a major cause of suicide.

Food and Drug Administration Analyses

After repeated reviews of available data, the FDA has not found a causal relationship between antidepressant treatment and suicidality in adults (Hammad 2003; U.S. Food and Drug Administration 2003, 2004). In an analysis of the FDA database of 207 trials including a total of 40,028 patients, Hammad et al. (2006) concluded that neither the use of placebo nor the use of antidepressants in short-term randomized controlled clinical trials was associated with an increased risk of completed suicide among patients with major depressive disorder or various anxiety disorders.

In 2006, the FDA analyzed data from studies involving nine antidepressant medications in 251 randomized trials. Dr. Thomas Laughren, director of the FDA's Division of Psychiatry Products, wrote a memorandum outlining the FDA's findings and attached the FDA Clinical Review with analyses of the data (Laughren 2006). Laughren noted that there does not appear to be an increased risk of completed suicide in patients taking antidepressants. The FDA analysis of all SSRIs compared with placebo did not find an increased risk of completed suicide for patients taking SSRIs (odds ratio [OR]=0.86; 95% CI=

0.12–6.30; not significant) (FDA Clinical Review, Table 30). The data were analyzed for the primary endpoint (suicidality); a protective effect was found for antidepressants compared to placebo in adults ages 25–64 (OR= 0.79; 95% CI=0.64–0.98; *P*=0.03) and in adults ages 65 and older (OR=0.37; 95% CI= 0.18–0.76; *P*=0.007) (FDA Clinical Review, Table 17), and no increased risk of suicidality was found for people age 24 and younger (OR=1.62; 95% CI= 0.97–2.71; *P*=0.07).

Other Studies

Gibbons et al. (2007) analyzed data on 226,866 veterans who received a diagnosis of depression in 2003 or 2004, had at least 6 months of follow-up, and had no history of depression from 2000 to 2002. Suicide attempt rates overall, as well as before and after initiation of antidepressant therapy, were compared for patients who received SSRIs, new-generation non–serotonergic-specific (non-SSRI) antidepressants (bupropion, mirtazapine, nefazodone, and venlafaxine), TCAs, or no antidepressant. The data indicated that suicide attempt rates were lower among patients who were treated with antidepressants than among those who were not, with a statistically significant odds ratio for SSRIs and TCAs. For SSRIs versus no antidepressant, this effect was significant in all adult age groups. Suicide attempt rates were also higher prior to treatment than after the start of treatment, with a significant relative risk for SSRIs and for non-SSRIs. For SSRIs, this effect was seen in all adult age groups and was significant in all but the age 18–25 group. These findings suggest that SSRI treatment has a protective effect in all adult age groups and do not support the hypothesis that SSRI treatment places patients at greater risk of suicide.

Further evidence that antidepressants do not cause suicide was reported by Simon and Savarino (2007), who used outpatient claims from a prepaid health plan and identified new episodes of depression treatment beginning with an antidepressant prescription in primary care (*N*=70,368), an antidepressant prescription from a psychiatrist (*N*=7,297), or an initial psychotherapy visit (*N*=54,123). Outpatient and inpatient claims were used to identify suicide attempts or possible suicide attempts during the 90 days before and 180 days after the start of treatment. The pattern of attempts over time was the same in all three groups: highest in the month before starting treatment, next highest in the month after starting treatment, and declining thereafter. The pattern of suicide attempts before and after starting antidepressant treatment is not specific to medication. Differences between treatments and changes over time probably reflect referral patterns and the expected improvement in suicidal ideation after the start of treatment.

Finally, in a meta-analysis of eight large-scale observational studies that compared the risk of suicide among patients with depression who received

SSRIs and those with no exposure to antidepressants, Barbui et al. (2009) reported that SSRIs had a beneficial effect in the group ages 18–24 years.

Professional Organizations

The American College of Neuropsychopharmacology (1993, 2004) and the American Psychiatric Association (2003) have expressed the view that there is no causal link between SSRIs and suicidality. Moreover, despite the black box warning, experts in the field generally accept that a cause-effect relationship between SSRIs and suicidality in children and adolescents has not been established.

KEY CLINICAL CONCEPTS

- Despite some claims that antidepressants are not effective, an extremely large evidence base supports antidepressants as efficacious treatments for depression.
- A sufficient number of well-studied antidepressants with different mechanisms of action have been approved by the FDA, so that clinicians can prescribe several monotherapy trials of different antidepressants before using polypharmacy.
- For partial responders to antidepressants, augmentation with lithium carbonate, thyroid hormone, atypical antipsychotic medications (aripiprazole, olanzapine, quetiapine), and other medications may be useful.
- For patients with major depression with psychotic features, antidepressants should be combined with antipsychotic medications.
- Although the risk of switch into mania when antidepressants are prescribed to patients with bipolar disorder may have been overestimated, evidence does suggest that antidepressants may not be effective in treating the depressed phase of bipolar disorder.
- No reliable scientific evidence indicates that antidepressants cause people to commit suicide.

References

Agency for Healthcare Policy Research: Evidence Report on Treatment of Depression—Newer Pharmacotherapies. San Antonio Evidence-Based Practice Center. Washington, DC, Agency for Healthcare Policy Research, Evidence-Based Practice Centers, 1999

Alao AO, Malhotra K, Pies R, et al: Pharmacological strategies in treatment-resistant depression. West Afr J Med Sep; 22: 211–218, 2003

American College of Neuropsychopharmacology: Suicidal behavior and psychotropic medication. Accepted as a consensus statement by the ACNP Council, March 2, 1992. Neuropsychopharmacology 8:177–183, 1993

American College of Neuropsychopharmacology: Executive summary: preliminary report of the Task Force on SSRIs and suicidal behavior in youth. Brentwood, TN, American College of Neuropsychopharmacology, January 21, 2004

American Psychiatric Association: Practice guideline for the treatment of patients with bipolar disorder (revision). Am J Psychiatry 159 (suppl 4):1–50, 2002

American Psychiatric Association: Guideline for the Assessment and Treatment of Patients With Suicidal Behaviors. Washington, DC, American Psychiatric Association, 2003

American Psychiatric Association: Practice guideline for the treatment of patients with eating disorders, third edition. Am J Psychiatry 163(suppl):4–54, 2006

American Psychiatric Association: Practice guideline for the treatment of patients with substance use disorders, second edition. Am J Psychiatry 164(suppl):5–123, 2007

American Psychiatric Association: Practice Guideline for the Treatment of Patients With Major Depressive Disorder, Third Edition. 2010. Available at: www.psychiatryonline.com/pracGuide/pracGuidehome.aspx

Amsterdam J: Monoamine oxidase inhibitor therapy in severe and resistant depression. Psychiatr Ann 36:606–613, 2006

Andreescu C, Mulsant BH, Peasley-Micklus C, et al: Persisting low use of antipsychotics in the treatment of major depressive disorder with psychotic features. J Clin Psychiatry 68:194–200, 2007

Aronson R, Offman HJ, Joffe RT, et al: Triiodothyronine augmentation in the treatment of refractory depression: a meta-analysis. Arch Gen Psychiatry 53:842–848, 1996

Artigas F, Nutt DJ, Shelton R: Mechanism of action of antidepressants. Psychopharmacol Bull 36 (suppl 2):123–132, 2002

Åsberg M, Crönholm B, Sjöqvist F, et al: Relationship between plasma level and therapeutic effect of nortriptyline. BMJ 3:331–334, 1971

Baldessarini RJ: Drug therapy of depression and anxiety disorders, in Goodman and Gilman's The Pharmacological Basis of Therapeutics. Edited by Brunton LL, Lazo JS, Parker KL. New York, McGraw-Hill, 2006, pp 429–460

Baldwin RC, Jolley DJ: The prognosis of depression in old age. Br J Psychiatry 149:574–583, 1986

Balon R, Mufti R, Arfken C: A survey of prescribing practices for monoamine oxidase inhibitors. Psychiatr Serv 50:945–947, 1999

Barbui C, Hotopf M, Freemantle N, et al: Selective serotonin reuptake inhibitors versus tricyclic and heterocyclic antidepressants: comparison of drug adherence. Cochrane Database Syst Rev CD002791, 2000

Barbui C, Esposito E, Cipriani A: Selective serotonin reuptake inhibitors and risk of suicide: a systematic review of observational studies. CMAJ 180:291–297, 2009

Bauer M, Tharmanathan P, Volz HP, et al: The effect of venlafaxine compared with other antidepressants and placebo in the treatment of major depression: a meta-analysis. Eur Arch Psychiatry Clin Neurosci 259:172–185, 2009

Bech P: Is the antidepressive effect of second-generation antidepressants a myth? Psychol Med 40:181–186, 2009

Berman RM, Marcus RN, Swanink R, et al: The efficacy and safety of aripiprazole as adjunctive therapy in major depressive disorder: a multicenter, randomized, double-blind, placebo-controlled study. J Clin Psychiatry 68:843–853, 2007

Birkenhager TK, van den Broek WW, Mulder PG, et al: Efficacy of imipramine in psychotic versus nonpsychotic depression. J Clin Psychopharmacol 28:166–170, 2008

Blazer D: Epidemiology of late-life depression, in Diagnosis and Treatment of Depression in Late Life. Edited by Schneider L, Reynolds C, Lebowitz B, et al. Washington, DC, American Psychiatric Press, 1994, pp 9–20

Bottlender R, Rudolf D, Strauss A, et al: Antidepressant associated maniform states in acute treatment of patients with bipolar-I depression. Eur Arch Psychiatr Clin Neurosci 248:296–300, 1998

Bramness JG, Walby FA, Tverdal A: The sales of antidepressants and suicide rates in Norway and its counties 1980–2004. J Affect Disord 102:1–9, 2007

Broich K: Committee for Medicinal Products for Human Use (CHMP) assessment on efficacy of antidepressants. Eur Neuropsychopharmacol 19:305–308, 2009

Byrne SE, Rothschild AJ: Loss of antidepressant efficacy during maintenance therapy: possible mechanisms and treatments. J Clin Psychiatry 59:279–288, 1998

Carpenter LL, Yasmin S, Price LH: A double-blind, placebo-controlled study of antidepressant augmentation with mirtazapine. Biol Psychiatry 51:183–188, 2002

Carvalho AF, Cavalcante JL, Castelo MS, et al: Augmentation strategies for treatment-resistant depression: a literature review. J Clin Pharm Ther 32:415–428, 2007

Clary C, Mandos LA, Schweizer E: Results of a brief survey on the prescribing practices for monoamine oxidase inhibitor antidepressants. J Clin Psychiatry 51:226–231, 1990

Cipriani A, Brambilla P, Furukawa TA, et al: Fluoxetine versus other types of pharmacotherapy for depression. Cochrane Database of Systematic Reviews 2005a, Issue 4. Art. No.: CD004185. DOI: 10.1002/14651858.CD004185.pub2.

Cipriani A, Pretty H, Hawton K, et al: Lithium in the prevention of suicidal behavior and all-cause mortality in patients with mood disorders: a systematic review of randomized trials. Am J Psychiatry 162:1805–1819, 2005b

Cipriani A, Smith KA, Burgess SSA, et al: Lithium versus antidepressants in the long-term treatment of unipolar affective disorder. Cochrane Database of Systematic Reviews 2006, Issue 4. Art. No.: CD003492. DOI: 10.1002/14651858.CD003492.pub2.

Cooper-Kazaz R, Apter JT, Cohen R, et al: Combined treatment with sertraline and liothyronine in major depression: a randomized, double-blind, placebo-controlled trial. Arch Gen Psychiatry 64:679–688, 2007

Crossley NA, Bauer M: Acceleration and augmentation of antidepressants with lithium for depressive disorders: two meta-analyses of randomized, placebo controlled trials. J Clin Psychiatry 68:935–940, 2007

Cunningham LA, Borison RL, Carman JS, et al: A comparison of venlafaxine, trazodone, and placebo in major depression. J Clin Psychopharmacol 14:99–106, 1994

de Montigny C, Grunberg F, Mayer A, et al: Lithium induces rapid relief of depression in tricyclic antidepressant drug non-responders. Br J Psychiatry 138:252–256, 1981

DeSanty KP, Amabile CM: Antidepressant-induced liver injury. Ann Pharmacother 41:1201–1211, 2007

Deshmukh R, Franco K: Managing weight gain as a side effect of antidepressant therapy. Cleve Clin J Med 70:614, 616, 618, passim, 2003

Desmarais JE, Looper KJ: Interactions between tamoxifen and antidepressants via cytochrome P450 2D6. J Clin Psychiatry 70:1688–1697, 2009

Dessain EC, Schatzberg AF, Woods BT, et al: Maprotiline treatment in depression: a perspective on seizures. Arch Gen Psychiatry 43:86–90, 1986

Doree JP, Des Rosiers J, Lew V, et al: Quetiapine augmentation of treatment-resistant depression: a comparison with lithium. Curr Med Res Opin 23:333–341, 2007

Doughty MJ, Lyle WM: Medications used to prevent migraine headaches and their potential ocular adverse effects. Optom Vis Sci 72:879–891, 1995

Edwards JG, Anderson I: Systematic review and guide to selection of selective serotonin reuptake inhibitors. Drugs 58:1207–1209, 1999

Farid FF, Wenger TL, Tsai SY, et al: Use of bupropion in patients who exhibit orthostatic hypotension on tricyclic antidepressants. J Clin Psychiatry 44:170–173, 1983

Fava M, Mulroy R, Alpert J, et al: Emergence of adverse events following discontinuation of treatment with extended-release venlafaxine. Am J Psychiatry 154:1760–1762, 1997

Fava M, Rush AJ, Thase ME, et al: 15 years of clinical experience with bupropion HCl: from bupropion to bupropion SR to bupropion XL. Prim Care Companion J Clin Psychiatry 7:106–113, 2005

Fava M, Nurnberg HG, Seidman SN, et al: Efficacy and safety of sildenafil in men with serotonergic antidepressant–associated erectile dysfunction: results from a randomized, double-blind, placebo-controlled trial. J Clin Psychiatry 67:240–246, 2006

Feiger AD, Rickels K, Rynn MA, et al: Selegiline transdermal system for the treatment of major depressive disorder: an 8-week, double-blind, placebo-controlled, flexible-dose titration trial. J Clin Psychiatry 67:1354–1361, 2006

Feighner JP, Hendrickson G, Miller L, et al: Double-blind comparison of doxepin versus bupropion in outpatients with a major depressive disorder. J Clin Psychopharmacol 6:27–32, 1986

Ferguson JM, Shrivastava RK, Stahl SM, et al: Reemergence of sexual dysfunction in patients with major depressive disorder: double-blind comparison of nefazodone and sertraline. J Clin Psychiatry 62:24–29, 2001

Fogelson DI, Bystritsky A, Pasnau R: Bupropion in the treatment of bipolar disorders: the same old story? J Clin Psychiatry 53:443–446, 1992

Frank E, Kupfer DJ, Perel JM, et al: Comparison of full-dose versus half-dose pharmacotherapy in the maintenance treatment of recurrent depression. J Affect Disord 27:139–145, 1993

Fuller RW, Snoddy HD: Inhibition of serotonin uptake and the toxic interaction between meperidine and monoamine oxidase inhibitors. Toxicol Appl Pharmacol 32:129–134, 1975

Ganz DA, Bao Y, Shekelle PG, et al: Will my patient fall? JAMA 297:77–86, 2007

Gao K, Kemp DE, Banocy SJ, et al: Treatment emergent mania/hypomania during antidepressant monotherapy in patients with rapid cycling bipolar disorder. Bipolar Disord 10:907–915, 2008

Garakani A, Martinez JM, Marcus S, et al: A randomized, double-blind, and placebo-controlled trial of quetiapine augmentation of fluoxetine in major depressive disorder. Int Clin Psychopharmacol 23:269–275, 2008

Gardner DM, Shulman KI, Walker SE, et al: The making of a user friendly MAOI diet. J Clin Psychiatry 57:99–104, 1996

Gartlehner G, Gaynes BN, Hansen RA, et al: Comparative benefits and harms of second-generation antidepressants: background paper for the American College of Physicians. Ann Intern Med 149:734–750, 2008

Garvey MJ, Tollefson GD: Occurrence of myoclonus in patients treated with cyclic antidepressants. Arch Gen Psychiatry 44:269–272, 1987

Geddes J, Freemantle N, Mason J, et al: SSRIs versus other antidepressants for depressive disorder. Cochrane Database Syst Rev CD001851, 2000

Geddes J, Butler R, Hatcher S: Depressive disorders. Clin Evid 9:1034–1057, 2003

Gerber PE, Lynd LD: Selective serotonin-reuptake inhibitor-induced movement disorders. Ann Pharmacother 32:692–698, 1998

Gibbons RD, Hur K, Bhaumik DK, et al: The relationship between antidepressant medication use and rate of suicide. Arch Gen Psychiatry 62:165–172, 2005

Gibbons RD, Brown CH, Hur K, et al: Relationship between antidepressants and suicide attempts: an analysis of the Veterans Health Administration Data Sets. Am J Psychiatry 164:1044–1049, 2007

Gijsman H, Geddes J, Rendell J, et al: Antidepressants for bipolar depression: a systematic review of randomized, controlled trials. Am J Psychiatry 161:1537–1547, 2004

Glezer A, Byatt N, Cook R Jr, et al: Polypharmacy prevalence rates in the treatment of unipolar depression in an outpatient clinic. J Affect Disord 117:18–23, 2009

Goldberg JF, Brooks JO 3rd, Kurita K, et al: Depressive illness burden associated with complex polypharmacy in patients with bipolar disorder: findings from the STEP-BD. J Clin Psychiatry 70:155–162, 2009

Goodwin GM, Young AH: The British Association for Psychopharmacology guidelines for treatment of bipolar disorder: a summary. J Psychopharmacol 17 (suppl 4):3–6, 2003

Grossman E, Messerli FH, Grodzicki T, et al: Should a moratorium be placed on sublingual nifedipine capsules given for hypertensive emergencies and pseudoemergencies? JAMA 276:1328–1331, 1996

Grunebaum MF, Ellis SP, Li S, et al: Antidepressants and suicide risk in the United States, 1985–1999. J Clin Psychiatry 65:1456–1462, 2004

Hall WD, Mant A, Mitchell PB, et al: Association between antidepressant prescribing and suicide in Australia, 1991–2000: trend analysis. BMJ 326:1008–1011, 2003

Hammad TA: Incidence of suicide in randomized controlled trials of patients with major depressive disorder. Pharmacoepidemiol Drug Saf 12:S156, 2003

Hammad TA, Laughren TP, Racoosin JA: Suicide rates in short-term randomized controlled trials of newer antidepressants. J Clin Psychopharmacology 26:203–207, 2006

Hansen R, Gaynes B, Thieda P, et al: Meta-analysis of major depressive disorder relapse and recurrence with second-generation antidepressants. Psychiatr Serv 59:1121–1130, 2008

Harrison WM, Rabkin JG, Ehrhardt AA, et al: Effects of antidepressant medication on sexual function: a controlled study. J Clin Psychopharmacol 6:144–149, 1986
Hegerl U, Mergl R: The clinical significance of antidepressant treatment effects cannot be derived from placebo-verum response differences. J Psychopharmacol 24:445–448, 2010
Horder J, Matthews P, Waldmann R: Placebo, Prozac, and PLoS: significant lessons for psychopharmacology. J Psychopharmacol June 22, 2010 [Epub ahead of print]
Isacsson G, Holmgren A, Osby U, et al: Decrease in suicide among the individuals treated with antidepressants: a controlled study of antidepressants in suicide, Sweden 1995–2005. Acta Psychiatr Scand 129:37–44, 2009
Isacsson G, Reutfors J, Papadopoulos FC, et al: Antidepressant medication prevents suicide in depression. Acta Psychiatr Scand 122:454–460, 2010a
Isacsson G, Rich CL, Jureidini J, et al: The increased use of antidepressants has contributed to the worldwide reduction in suicide rates. Br J Psychiatry 196:429–433, 2010b
Johnson J, Horwath E, Weissman MM: The validity of major depression with psychotic features based on a community sample. Arch Gen Psychiatry 48:1075–1081, 1991
Joo JH, Lenze EJ, Mulsant BH, et al: Risk factors for falls during treatment of late-life depression. J Clin Psychiatry 63:936–994, 2002
Kantrowitz JT, Tampi RR: Risk of psychosis exacerbation by tricyclic antidepressants in unipolar major depressive disorder with psychotic features. J Affect Disord 106:279–284, 2008
Keck PE, Perlis RH, Otto MW, et al: The Expert Consensus Guideline Series: Treatment of Bipolar Disorder 2004. Postgraduate Medicine Special Report 1–116, 2004
Keller MB: Long-term treatment of patients with recurrent unipolar major depression: evidence to clinical practice. CNS Spectr 11 (12, suppl 15):4–5, 2006
Keller MB, Trivedi MH, Thase ME, et al: The Prevention of Recurrent Episodes of Depression with Venlafaxine for Two Years (PREVENT) study: outcomes from acute and continuation phases. Biol Psychiatry 62:1371–1379, 2007a
Keller MB, Trivedi MH, Thase ME, et al: The Prevention of Recurrent Episodes of Depression with Venlafaxine for Two Years (PREVENT) study: outcomes from the 2-year and combined maintenance phases. J Clin Psychiatry 68:1246–1256, 2007b
Kelly CM, Juurlink DN, Gomes T, et al: Selective serotonin reuptake inhibitors and breast cancer mortality in women receiving tamoxifen: a population based cohort study. BMJ 340:c693, 2010 [doi: 10.1136/bmj.c693]
Kennedy SH, McCann SM, Masellis M, et al: Combining bupropion SR with venlafaxine, paroxetine, or fluoxetine: a preliminary report on pharmacokinetic, therapeutic, and sexual dysfunction effects. J Clin Psychiatry 63:181–186, 2002
Kirsch I, Deacon BJ, Huedo-Medina TB, et al: Initial severity and antidepressant benefits: a meta-analysis of data submitted to the Food and Drug Administration. PLoS Med 5(2):e45, 2008
Kivela SL, Pahkala K: Delusional depression in the elderly: a community study. J Gerontol 22:236–241, 1989
Klein DF: The flawed basis for FDA post-marketing safety decisions: the example of anti-depressants and children. Neuropsychopharmacology 31:689–699, 2006
Koutouvidis N, Pratikakis M, Fotiadou A: The use of mirtazapine in a group of 11 patients following poor compliance to selective serotonin reuptake inhibitor treatment due to sexual dysfunction. Int Clin Psychopharmacol 14:253–255, 1999

Lam RW, Hossie H, Solomons K, et al: Citalopram and bupropion-SR: combining versus switching in patients with treatment-resistant depression. J Clin Psychiatry 65:337–340, 2004

Laughren T: Memorandum: Department of Health and Human Services Public Health Service, Food and Drug Administration, Center for Drug Evaluation and Research: Overview for December 13 Meeting of Psychopharmacologic Drugs Advisory Committee (PDAC). November 16, 2006. Available at: www.fda.gov/ohrms/dockets/ac/06/briefing/2006-4272b1-01-FDA.pdf. Accessed April 29, 2011.

Leverich GS, Altshuler LL, Frye MA, et al: Risk of switch in mood polarity to hypomania or mania in patients with bipolar depression during acute and continuation trials of venlafaxine, sertraline, and bupropion as adjuncts to mood stabilizers. Am J Psychiatry 163:232–239, 2006

Li Z, Maglione M, Tu W, et al: Meta-analysis: pharmacologic treatment of obesity. Ann Intern Med 142:532–546, 2005

Licht RW, Gijsman H, Nolen WA, et al: Are antidepressants safe in the treatment of bipolar depression? A critical evaluation of their potential risk to induce switch into mania or cycle acceleration. Acta Psychiatr Scand 118:337–346, 2008

Lineberry CG, Johnston A, Raymond RN, et al: A fixed-dose (300 mg) efficacy study of bupropion and placebo in depressed outpatients. J Clin Psychiatry 51:194–199, 1990

Liu B, Anderson G, Mittman N, et al: Use of selective serotonin reuptake inhibitors or tricyclic antidepressants and risk of hip fractures in elderly people. Lancet 351:1303–1307, 1998

Lowry MR, Dunner FJ: Seizures during tricyclic therapy. Am J Psychiatry 137:1461–1462, 1980

McGrath PJ, Stewart JW, Fava M, et al: Tranylcypromine versus venlafaxine plus mirtazapine following three failed antidepressant medication trials for depression: a STAR*D report. Am J Psychiatry 163:1531–1541, 2006

McIntyre A, Gendron A, McIntyre A: Quetiapine adjunct to selective serotonin reuptake inhibitors or venlafaxine in patients with major depression, comorbid anxiety, and residual depressive symptoms: a randomized, placebo-controlled pilot study. Depress Anxiety 24:487–494, 2007

McIntyre RS, Mancini DA, McCann S, et al: Topiramate versus bupropion bipolar disorder: a preliminary single-blind study. Bipolar Disord 4:207–213, 2002

Meyer RE, Salzman C, Youngstrom EA, et al: Suicidality and risk of suicide—definition, drug safety concerns, and a necessary target for drug development: a brief report. J Clin Psychiatry 71:1040–1046, 2010

Meyers BS, Flint AJ, Rothschild AJ, et al: A double-blind randomized controlled trial of olanzapine plus sertraline vs. olanzapine plus placebo for psychotic depression: the study of pharmacotherapy of psychotic depression (STOP-PD). Arch Gen Psychiatry 66:838–847, 2009

Michelson D, Amsterdam JD, Quitkin FM, et al: Changes in weight during a 1-year trial of fluoxetine. Am J Psychiatry 156:1170–1176, 1999

Miller MD, Curtiss EI, Marino L, et al: Long-term ECG changes in depressed elderly patients treated with nortriptyline: a double-blind, randomized, placebo-controlled evaluation. Am J Geriatr Psychiatry 6:59–66, 1998

Monteiro WO, Noshirvani HF, Marks IM, et al: Anorgasmia from clomipramine in obsessive-compulsive disorder: a controlled trial. Br J Psychiatry 151:107–112, 1987

Montejo-González AL, Llorca G, Izquierdo JA, et al: SSRI-induced sexual dysfunction: fluoxetine, paroxetine, sertraline, and fluvoxamine in a prospective, multicenter, and descriptive clinical study of 344 patients. J Sex Marital Ther 23:176–194, 1997

Mulsant BH, Haskett RF, Prudic J, et al: Low use of neuroleptic drugs in the treatment of psychotic major depression. Am J Psychiatry 154:559–561, 1997

Mulsant BH, Sweet RA, Rosen J, et al: A randomized double-blind comparison of nortriptyline plus perphenazine vs. nortriptyline plus placebo in the treatment of psychotic depression in late life. J Clin Psychiatry 62:597–604, 2001

Narayan M, Meckler L, Nelson JC: Fluoxetine-induced delusions in psychotic depression (letter). J Clin Psychiatry 56:329, 1995

Nelson JC: Tricyclic and tetracyclic drugs, in Essentials of Clinical Psychopharmacology, 2nd Edition. Edited by Schatzberg AF, Nemeroff CB. Washington, DC, American Psychiatric Publishing, 2006, pp 5–29

Nelson JC, Bowers MB, Sweeney DR: Exacerbation of psychosis by tricyclic antidepressants in delusional depression. Am J Psychiatry 136:574–576, 1979

Nierenberg AA, Alder LA, Peselow E, et al: Trazodone for antidepressant-associated insomnia. Am J Psychiatry 151:1069–1072, 1994

Nierenberg AA, Fava M, Trivedi MH, et al: A comparison of lithium and T(3) augmentation following two failed medication treatments for depression: a STAR*D report. Am J Psychiatry 163:1519–1530, 2006

Nurnberg HG, Hensley PL, Heiman JR, et al: Sildenafil treatment of women with antidepressant-associated sexual dysfunction: a randomized controlled trial. JAMA 300:395–404, 2008

Ohayon MM, Schatzberg AF: Prevalence of depressive episodes with psychotic features in the general population. Am J Psychiatry 159:1855–1861, 2002

Pagnin D, de Queiroz V, Pini S, et al: Efficacy of ECT in depression: a meta-analytic review. J ECT 20:13–20, 2004

Papakostas GI: Limitations of contemporary antidepressants: tolerability. J Clin Psychiatry 68 (suppl 10):11–17, 2007

Papakostas GI, Fava M: A meta-analysis of clinical trials comparing the serotonin (5HT)-2 receptor antagonists trazodone and nefazodone with selective serotonin reuptake inhibitors for the treatment of major depressive disorder. Eur Psychiatry 22:444–447, 2007

Papakostas GI, Perlis RH, Seifert C, et al: Antidepressant dose reduction and the risk of relapse in major depressive disorder. Psychother Psychosom 76:266–270, 2007

Papakostas GI, Fava M, Thase ME: Treatment of SSRI-resistant depression: a meta-analysis comparing within- versus across-class switches. Biol Psychiatry 63:699–704, 2008a

Papakostas GI, Homberger CH, Fava M: A meta-analysis of clinical trials comparing mirtazapine with selective serotonin reuptake inhibitors for the treatment of major depressive disorder. J Psychopharmacol 22:843–848, 2008b

Patkar AA, Masand PS, Pae CU, et al: A randomized, double-blind, placebo-controlled trial of augmentation with an extended release formulation of methylphenidate in outpatients with treatment resistant depression. J Clin Psychopharmacol 26:653–656, 2006

Peet M: Induction of mania with selective serotonin re-uptake inhibitors and tricyclic antidepressants. Br J Psychiatry 164:549–550, 1995

Post RM, Altshuler LL, Leverich GS, et al: Mood switch in bipolar depression: comparison of adjunctive venlafaxine, bupropion and sertraline. Br J Psychiatry 189:124–131, 2006

Posternak MA, Zimmerman M: Dual reuptake inhibitors incur lower rates of tachyphylaxis than selective serotonin reuptake inhibitors: a retrospective study. J Clin Psychiatry 66:705–707, 2005

Pridmore S, Turnier-Shea Y: Medication options in the treatment of treatment-resistant depression. Aust N Z J Psychiatry 38:219–225, 2004

Rahme E, Dasgupta K, Turecki G, et al: Risks of suicide and poisoning among elderly patients prescribed selective serotonin reuptake inhibitors: a retrospective cohort study. J Clin Psychiatry 69:349–357, 2008

Rasmussen KG, Mueller M, Knapp RG, et al: Antidepressant medication treatment failure does not predict lower remission with ECT for major depressive disorder: a report from the consortium for research in electroconvulsive therapy. J Clin Psychiatry 68:1701–1706, 2007

Ravaris C, Nies A, Robinson D, et al: A multiple dose, controlled study of phenelzine in depression-anxiety states. Arch Gen Psychiatry 33:347–350, 1976

Ravindran AV, Kennedy SH, O'Donovan MC, et al: Osmotic-release oral system methylphenidate augmentation of antidepressant monotherapy in major depressive disorder: results of a double-blind, randomized, placebo-controlled trial. J Clin Psychiatry 69:87–94, 2008

Rickels K, Athanasiou M, Robinson DS, et al: Evidence for efficacy and tolerability of vilazodone in the treatment of major depressive disorder: a randomized, double-blind, placebo-controlled trial. J Clin Psychiatry 70:326–333, 2009

Robinson DS, Gilmor ML, Yang Y, et al: Treatment effects of selegiline transdermal system on symptoms of major depressive disorder: a meta-analysis of short-term, placebo-controlled, efficacy trials. Psychopharmacol Bull 40:15–28, 2007

Roden DM: Antiarrhythmic drugs, in Goodman and Gilman's The Pharmacological Basis of Therapeutics. Edited by Brunton LL, Lazo JS, Parker KL. New York, McGraw-Hill, 2006, pp 899–932

Roose SP, Glassman AH, Giardina EG, et al: Tricyclic antidepressants in depressed patients with cardiac conduction disease. Arch Gen Psychiatry 44:273–275, 1987

Rothschild AJ: SSRI-induced sexual dysfunction: efficacy of a drug holiday. Am J Psychiatry 152:1514–1516, 1995

Rothschild AJ: Sexual side effects of antidepressants. J Clin Psychiatry 61 (suppl 11):28–36, 2000

Rothschild AJ: The Rothschild Scale for Antidepressant Tachyphylaxis: reliability and validity. Compr Psychiatry 49:508–513, 2008

Rothschild AJ (ed): Clinical Manual for the Diagnosis and Treatment of Psychotic Depression. Washington, DC, American Psychiatric Press, 2009

Rothschild AJ (ed): The Evidenced-Based Guide to Antipsychotic Medications. Washington, DC, American Psychiatric Press, 2010

Rothschild AJ, Phillips KA: Selective serotonin reuptake inhibitors and delusional depression. Am J Psychiatry 156:977–978, 1999

Rothschild AJ, Williamson DJ, Tohen MF, et al: Olanzapine-fluoxetine combination for major depression with psychotic features. J Clin Psychopharmacol 24:365–373, 2004

Rothschild AJ, Dunlop BW, Dunner DL, et al: Assessing rates and predictors of tachyphylaxis during the Prevention of Recurrent Episodes of Depression with Venlafaxine ER for Two Years (PREVENT) study. Psychopharmacol Bull 42:5–20, 2009

Rush AJ, Fava M, Wisniewski SR, et al: Sequenced treatment alternatives to relieve depression (STAR*D): rationale and design. Control Clin Trials 25:119–142, 2004
Rush AJ, Trivedi MH, Wisniewski SR, et al: Bupropion-SR, sertraline, or venlafaxine-XR after failure of SSRIs for depression. N Engl J Med 354:1231–1242, 2006
Rush AJ, Wisniewski SR, Warden D, et al: Selecting among second-step antidepressant medication monotherapies: predictive value of clinical, demographic, or first-step treatment features. Arch Gen Psychiatry 65:870–880, 2008
Ryan ND, Puig-Antich J, Ambrosini P, et al: The clinical picture of major depression in children and adolescents. Arch Gen Psychiatry 44:854–861, 1987
Sachs GS, Lafer B, Stoll AL, et al: A double-blind trial of bupropion versus desipramine for bipolar depression. J Clin Psychiatry 55:391–393, 1994
Sachs GS, Printz DJ, Kahn DA, et al: The expert consensus guideline series: medication treatment of bipolar disorder 2000. Postgraduate Medicine Special Report 1–104, 2000
Sachs GS, Nierenberg AA, Calabrese JR, et al: Effectiveness of adjunctive antidepressant treatment for bipolar depression. N Engl J Med 356:1711–1722, 2007
Sandson NB, Armstrong SC, Cozza KL: An overview of psychotropic drug-drug interactions. Psychosomatics 46:464–494, 2005
Schatzberg AF, Prather MR, Keller MB, et al: Clinical use of nefazodone in major depression: a 6-year perspective. J Clin Psychiatry 63 (suppl 1):18–31, 2002
Schenk CH, Remick RA: Sublingual nifedipine in the treatment of hypertensive crisis associated with monoamine oxidase inhibitors. Ann Emerg Med 18:114–115, 1989
Schmidt ME, Fava M, Zhang S, et al: Treatment approaches to major depressive disorder relapse, part 1: dose increase. Psychother Psychosom 71:190–194, 2002
Schwartz PJ, Wolf S: QT interval prolongation as predictor of sudden death in patients with myocardial infarction. Circulation 57:1074–1077, 1978
Segraves RT, Kavoussi R, Hughes AR, et al: Evaluation of sexual functioning in depressed outpatients: a double-blind comparison of sustained-release bupropion and sertraline treatment. J Clin Psychopharmacol 20:122–128, 2000
Segraves RT, Lee J, Stevenson R, et al: Tadalafil for treatment of erectile dysfunction in men on antidepressants. J Clin Psychopharmacol 27:62–66, 2007
Shelton RC, Tollefson GD, Tohen M, et al: A novel augmentation strategy for treating resistant major depression. Am J Psychiatry 158:131–134, 2001
Shelton RC, Osuntokun O, Heinloth AN, et al: Therapeutic options for treatment-resistant depression. CNS Drugs 24:131–161, 2010
Shulman K, Walker S: A reevaluation of dietary restrictions for irreversible monoamine oxidase inhibitors. Psychiatr Ann 31:378–384, 2001
Sidor M, MacQueen G: Antidepressants for the acute treatment of bipolar depression: a systematic review and meta-analysis. J Clin Psychiatry 72:156–167, 2011
Simon GE, Savarino J: Suicide attempts among patients starting depression treatment with medications or psychotherapy. Am J Psychiatry 164:1029–1034, 2007
Simon GE, Savarino J, Operskalski B, et al: Suicide risk during antidepressant treatment. Am J Psychiatry 163:41–47, 2006
Simpson GM, El Sheshai A, Loza N, et al: An 8-week open-label trial of a 6-day course of mifepristone for the treatment of psychotic depression. J Clin Psychiatry 66:598–602, 2005
Solomon DA, Keller MB, Leon AC, et al: Multiple recurrences of major depressive disorder. Am J Psychiatry 157:229–233, 2000

Solomon DA, Leon AC, Mueller TI, et al: Tachyphylaxis in unipolar major depressive disorder. J Clin Psychiatry 66:283–290, 2005

Spiker DG, Weiss JC, Dealy RS, et al: The pharmacological treatment of delusional depression. Am J Psychiatry 142:430–436, 1985

Sterke CS, Verhagen AP, van Beeck EF, et al: The influence of drug use on fall incidents among nursing home residents: a systematic review. Int Psychogeriatr 20:890–910, 2008

Stewart DE: Hepatic adverse reactions associated with nefazodone. Can J Psychiatry 47:375–377, 2002

Thanacoody HK, Thomas SH: Tricyclic antidepressant poisoning: cardiovascular toxicity. Toxicol Rev 24:205–214, 2005

Thase ME: Effects of venlafaxine on blood pressure: a meta-analysis of original data from 3744 depressed patients. J Clin Psychiatry 59:502–508, 1998

Thase ME, Trivedi MH, Rush AJ: MAOIs in the contemporary treatment of depression. Neuropsychopharmacology 12:185–219, 1995

Thase ME, Corya SA, Osuntokun O, et al: A randomized, double-blind comparison of olanzapine/fluoxetine combination, olanzapine, and fluoxetine in treatment-resistant major depressive disorder. J Clin Psychiatry 68:224–236, 2007a

Thase ME, Friedman ES, Biggs MM, et al: Cognitive therapy versus medication in augmentation and switch strategies as second-step treatments: a STAR*D report. Am J Psychiatry 164:739–752, 2007b

Thase ME, Pritchett YL, Ossanna MJ, et al: Efficacy of duloxetine and selective serotonin reuptake inhibitors: comparisons as assessed by remission rates in patients with major depressive disorder. J Clin Psychopharmacol 27:672–676, 2007c

Thase ME, Kornstein SG, Germain JM, et al: An integrated analysis of the efficacy of desvenlafaxine compared with placebo in patients with major depressive disorder. CNS Spectr 14:144–154, 2009

Thompson JW Jr, Ware MR, Blashfield RK: Psychotropic medication and priapism: a comprehensive review. J Clin Psychiatry 51:430–433, 1990

U.S. Food and Drug Administration: FDA statement regarding the anti-depressant Paxil for pediatric population. FDA Talk Paper, June 19, 2003. Available at: www.ahrp.org/infomail/0603/19a.php. Accessed April 29, 2011.

U.S. Food and Drug Administration: Public health advisory: Worsening depression and suicidality in patients being treated with antidepressants. March 22, 2004. Available at: www.fda.gov/Drugs/DrugSafety/PostmarketDrugSafetyInformationforPatientsandProviders/DrugSafetyInformationforHealthcareProfessionals/PublicHealthAdvisories/ucm161696.htm. Accessed April 29, 2011.

Wenger TL, Cohn JB, Bustrack J: Comparison of the effects of bupropion and amitriptyline on cardiac conduction in depressed patients. J Clin Psychiatry 44:174–175, 1983

Wijkstra J, Lljmer J, Balk FJ, et al: Pharmacological treatment for unipolar psychotic depression. Br J Psychiatry 188:410–415, 2006

Wijkstra J, Burger H, van den Broek WW, et al: Treatment of unipolar psychotic depression: a randomized, double-blind study comparing imipramine, venlafaxine, and venlafaxine plus quetiapine. Acta Psychiatr Scand 121:190–200, 2010

Zanardi R, Franchini L, Gasperini M, et al: Double-blind controlled trial of sertraline versus paroxetine in the treatment of delusional depression. Am J Psychiatry 153:1631–1633, 1996

Zanardi R, Franchini L, Gasperini M, et al: Faster onset of action of fluvoxamine in combination with pindolol in the treatment of delusional depression: a controlled study. J Clin Psychopharmacol 18:441–446, 1998

Zanardi R, Franchini L, Serritti A, et al: Venlafaxine versus fluvoxamine in the treatment of delusional depression: a pilot double-blind controlled study. J Clin Psychiatry 61:26–29, 2000

CHAPTER 3

Anxiety Disorders

Ryan J. Kimmel, M.D.
Peter P. Roy-Byrne, M.D.

PANIC ATTACKS, "generalized" or free-floating anxiety, and context-dependent fears (phobias) are modern syndromes that when historically formulated as "neurotic anxiety," were felt to be poorly responsive to pharmacotherapy. Pioneering studies of antidepressants in patients with anxiety that were conducted by Donald Klein in the 1960s (Klein 1964) led to a belief that antidepressants were specifically effective only for anxiety marked by panic attacks and phobias. Other early data (reported in the "Obsessive-Compulsive Disorder" section below) suggested that the serotonergic antidepressant clomipramine was specifically effective for obsessive-compulsive disorder (OCD). After anxiety disorders were reformulated for DSM-III (American Psychiatric Association 1980), additional studies concluded that antidepressants—at the time, only tricyclic antidepressants (TCAs) and monoamine oxidase inhibitors (MAOIs)—were also effective for nonpanic, nonphobic (i.e., generalized) anxiety. At the same time, the category of anxiety disorders was expanded to include OCD and posttraumatic stress disorder (PTSD), in addition to panic disorder, generalized anxiety disorder, and the phobic disorders (agoraphobia and social phobia). With the advent of selective serotonin reuptake inhibitors (SSRIs), it became clear that these agents were effective for OCD and PTSD.

Antidepressants now constitute the mainstay of pharmacological treatment for a broad swath of anxiety disorders and, because of their efficacy for comorbid depression, are increasingly replacing benzodiazepines as the first-line option for anxiety treatment. Research in recent decades also has clearly established the potent efficacy of cognitive-behavioral therapy (CBT) for all of the anxiety disorders. Thankfully, debate about which modality is superior is dying down. Many comparative studies show that antidepressants and CBT have roughly comparable efficacy, at least in the short term. The exception is in treating OCD, for which CBT appears to have a distinct advantage. Outstanding questions now focus on whether combination treatment offers an advantage over single-modality treatment, whether there is differential treatment modality efficacy over the longer term, and how best to accommodate patient preferences for specific modalities.

In this chapter, we review extant data on the efficacy of antidepressants for the major anxiety disorders, with a focus on randomized, double-blind, placebo-controlled trials. Our strategy is to highlight more recent studies, as well as the larger seminal studies, and to remark on meta-analytic summaries for the majority of earlier studies. Although we also note some of the open-trial efficacy for medications that have not been studied in a controlled trial, experience over the years has shown that many open-trial reports fail to be confirmed in subsequent double-blind studies. Hence, such evidence should be viewed skeptically.

Unfortunately, the majority of evidence focuses on short-term outcomes. These medications, however, are often used very long term, often for years and sometimes for decades. Although some longer-term studies have been published, most of these do not extend beyond 6–12 months. Hence, there is still much to learn.

Panic Disorder

The diagnosis of panic disorder (PD) requires both panic attacks (discrete periods of fear and somatic symptoms peaking in 10 minutes) and a month of fear or changed behavior (e.g., phobic avoidance, excessive medical diagnostic tests, emergency room visits) due to anticipation of another attack. The somatic symptoms include palpitations, sweating, trembling, shortness of breath, chest pain, sense of choking, nausea, dizziness, paresthesias, and chills or hot flashes. PD is further divided into two subtypes: PD with agoraphobia (i.e., a fear and avoidance of places or situations from which escape is difficult or embarrassing) and PD without agoraphobia (American Psychiatric Association 2000). Although 15% of people may have a panic attack in their lifetime (Eaton et al. 1994), the lifetime prevalence of PD was reported to be 4.1% in a survey by Kessler et al. (2005a). Peak age at onset is the late teens and early twenties. There have been numerous genetic linkage and genetic association studies of patients with PD, and several dozen specific genes are currently being explored; however, no definitive and replicable findings have been reported yet (Hamilton 2009). PD has a high rate of comorbidity with major depressive disorder (Hettema et al. 2003).

A wide variety of medication classes has been employed for PD (Kumar and Malone 2008). In the largest meta-analysis, however, Mitte (2005) found no difference in effect size between medication classes.

Acute Management

SSRIs

The SSRIs paroxetine, sertraline, and fluoxetine have been approved by the U.S. Food and Drug Administration (FDA) for PD. All three of these medications are supported by numerous placebo-controlled trials. Kumar and Malone (2008) assimilated 36 reviews and calculated a number needed to treat (NNT) of 5–8 for acute phase treatment.

Despite not having specific FDA approval for PD, the three other SSRIs do have placebo-controlled evidence to support their use. Fluvoxamine's benefit has been replicated most frequently and is reviewed by Irons (2005). Citalopram showed benefit in two studies (Leinonen et al. 2000; Lepola et al. 1998). Escitalopram's use is supported by placebo-controlled studies (Davidson et al. 2004a; Stahl et al. 2003), and an additional study demonstrated improvement in measurements of quality of life in patients with PD treated with escitalopram (Bandelow et al. 2007).

The issue of dosing SSRIs in PD is not fully resolved. In the aforementioned meta-analysis, Mitte (2005) found no connection between fixed and variable dosing. A recent trial (Simon et al. 2009) sought to address this issue with a 6-week open-label study of sertraline up to 100 mg/day or escitalopram up to 15 mg/day, followed by a 6-week randomized controlled trial (RCT) for patients with continued panic symptoms, with half receiving either sertraline up to 200 mg/day or escitalopram up to 30 mg/day. The increased dosages of these SSRIs did not result in a significant increase in efficacy, although it remains appropriate practice to maximize the dosage in patients not responding to treatment.

SNRIs

The serotonin-norepinephrine reuptake inhibitor (SNRI) venlafaxine ER (extended release) has FDA approval for PD. The first placebo-controlled trial of venlafaxine dates back to 1996 (Pollack et al. 1996). A trial by Pollack et al. (2007) contains the most significant data in favor of the use of venlafaxine ER for PD. In the most recent placebo-controlled trial (Liebowitz et al. 2009), however, venlafaxine at a mean dosage of 188.3 mg/day in completers failed to rise to the level of statistical significance for the primary outcome measure (percentage of panic-free patients). The other placebo-controlled venlafaxine trial also failed to yield significantly more panic-free patients but did demonstrate attenuated panic frequency and a reduction in the anticipatory fear and avoidance symptoms (Bradwejn et al. 2005).

Neither duloxetine nor desvenlafaxine has been the subject of a placebo-controlled trial for PD.

TCAs

The TCAs imipramine and clomipramine have, combined, been the subject of more than a dozen RCTs in patients with PD. The most recent meta-analysis of their efficacy found an effect size identical to that of the SSRIs (Mitte 2005). However, even in an analysis of PD study completers who tolerated sertraline and imipramine well, the favorable side-effect profile of the SSRI was evident (Mavissakalian 2003). Two head-to-head placebo-controlled trials between TCAs have been reported. In the first, clomipramine was found to be superior to imipramine (Modigh et al. 1992). The second was a double-blind crossover trial in which clomipramine and desipramine were compared (Sasson et al. 1999). Both medications significantly reduced panic attack frequency, although clomipramine had some advantages over desipramine according to several of the other outcomes used in the study. In another RCT, desipramine failed to significantly beat placebo (Lydiard et al. 1993). The data suggest that predominant serotonergic mechanisms, wherein clomipramine is superior to other TCAs, may be advantageous for panic. Evidence that response to treatment continues to increase between the short (3-month) and medium (6-month) term was present from the earliest imipramine studies (Zitrin et al. 1983).

MAOIs

No placebo-controlled trials of the MAOI phenelzine have been published since the modern definition of PD was added in DSM-III. However, in the pre–DSM-III era, five RCTs of patients with panic attacks, anxiety, and phobias showed robust and sustained antipanic, antiphobic, and antianxiety effects for phenelzine (Mountjoy et al. 1977; Sheehan et al. 1980; C. Solyom et al. 1981, L. Solyom et al. 1973; Tyrer et al. 1973).

Recently, in a double-blind comparison of tranylcypromine 30 mg/day versus 60 mg/day in 36 patients, at the higher dosage, there was a significant reduction in frequency of panic attacks among patients with comorbid PD and social anxiety disorder (Nardi et al. 2010). This finding is consistent with evidence that maximal antianxiety effects with MAOIs require higher dosages, on the order of a minimum of 60 mg/day of phenelzine or 40 mg/day of tranylcypromine.

Evaluation of moclobemide, at various dosages, is ongoing in Europe, but this reversible, selective MAOI is not available in the United States.

Mirtazapine

Mirtazapine has not been the subject of double-blinded, placebo-controlled trials for PD. Although two open-label trials showed a reduction in panic attacks (Boshuisen et al. 2001; Sarchiapone et al. 2003), neither employed the more rigorous outcome of percentage of panic-free patients that is used in some trials.

Bupropion

An older trial with a small sample size did not find bupropion to be effective for PD (Sheehan et al. 1983). However, a more recent open trial of 20 patients suggested some efficacy (Simon et al. 2003).

Maintenance and Relapse Prevention

In their meta-analysis of relapse prevention, Donovan et al. (2010) examined six studies related to PD and found that the data argued in favor of antidepressant use. In those six studies, patients who initially responded to the antidepressant and then were randomized to placebo experienced relapse 8%–50% of the time. In contrast, patients whose antidepressant was continued relapsed 3%–22% of the time. These data yielded an odds ratio of 0.35 (95% CI, 0.23–0.51) in favor of antidepressant treatment.

Naturalistic studies show a 30%–90% relapse rate at 6–12 months after medication discontinuation (Roy-Byrne and Cowley 1994). Our current recommendations, based on the limited controlled and naturalistic data, suggest that treatment should be continued for 1–2 years after full response is achieved.

Comparison With Psychological Treatment and Combined Treatment

A meta-analysis by Mitte (2005) suggested that medication and CBT were similarly effective for patients with PD, although CBT was favored in some analyses and outcome measures. After 6-month maintenance (Barlow et al. 2000), the combination of imipramine and CBT demonstrated greater efficacy than either intervention alone, although all three treatments were comparable in acute management. A meta-analysis that included the Barlow et al. study reached similar conclusions (Furukawa et al. 2006). In contrast, the most recent study showed that combined SSRI and CBT treatment in the acute phase was superior to either treatment alone (van Apeldoorn et al. 2010). In clinical practice, combination treatment should be considered if the patient continues to have residual symptoms after single-modality treatment.

Generalized Anxiety Disorder

A diagnosis of generalized anxiety disorder (GAD) requires excessive, impairing, hard-to-control worry on most days, along with three or more of the six following symptoms: restlessness, becoming easily fatigued, irritability, poor concentration, muscle tension, and sleep disturbance. The criteria must be met for 6 months, although recent studies show that people with shorter durations of this syndrome have equivalent impairment and associated characteristics (Ruscio et al. 2007). Lifetime prevalence was 5.7% in a study employing DSM-IV (American Psychiatric Association 1994) criteria (Kessler et al. 2005b). GAD is twice as common in women as in men, and the rate of comorbidity with other psychiatric disorders is as high as 90% (Wittchen et al. 1994). GAD is associated with significant impairment and reduced quality of life, even when researchers control for its most common comorbidity, major depressive disorder (Wittchen et al. 2000). Given the high rate of observed comorbidity between major depressive disorder and GAD, the high rate of genetic overlap in twin studies is not surprising (Kendler et al. 2007).

The evolving criteria for the diagnosis of GAD, with changes in duration of symptoms, the prominence of worry, and differentiation from other comorbid Axis I mood and anxiety diagnoses, have made it difficult to compare evidence from different eras. However, significant amounts of data are available from the DSM-IV (post-1994) era and several more modern studies that examine older medications. In a Cochrane meta-analysis on GAD that included six antidepressant trials published between 1997 and 2001, as well as one published in 1993, antidepressants were found to be effective and well tolerated, with an NNT of about 5 (Kapczinski et al. 2003).

Acute Management

SSRIs

The SSRIs paroxetine and escitalopram have FDA approval for use in GAD. All of the available placebo-controlled trials for paroxetine were pooled and examined in a large analysis totaling 1,800 patients (Rickels et al. 2006). In the acute phase, covering the first 8 weeks of treatment, paroxetine resulted in remission of GAD in 35% of patients, compared with 25% in the placebo groups, yielding an

NNT of 10. For the short-term studies, using combined criteria of a Sheehan Disability Scale score <5 and a Hamilton Anxiety Scale (Ham-A) score ≤7, paroxetine is favored with an odds ratio of 1.7–2.0, which would be equivalent to an NNT of about 10. The mean dosage was 24.3 mg/day. The short-term studies revealed the three most common paroxetine side effects to be abnormal ejaculation (24.7%), nausea (20.1%), and headache (16.9%).

Pooled data from three placebo-controlled escitalopram trials, allowing dosing up to 20 mg/day, demonstrated efficacy via Ham-A scores (Goodman et al. 2005). Moreover, pooled data from four escitalopram trials demonstrated efficacy in patients with GAD, based on results from the Quality of Life Enjoyment and Satisfaction Questionnaire (Demyttenaere et al. 2008). More recently, escitalopram 20 mg/day again demonstrated superiority over placebo (Coric et al. 2010). In a study of patients 60 years and older, however, escitalopram demonstrated a higher cumulative response rate for improvement than did placebo over 12 weeks, but just missed a significant difference using the intention-to-treat analysis (Lenze et al. 2009). These results are somewhat compromised by the high dropout rate, which limited the intent-to-treat analysis. In a double-blind, non-placebo-controlled trial pitting escitalopram against paroxetine, both demonstrated equal efficacy based on Ham-A scores (Bielski et al. 2005).

Sertraline, at a mean dosage of 149.1 mg/day, was found to be more effective than placebo in treating GAD (Brawman-Mintzer et al. 2006). Similar results were found at a mean dosage of 95.1 mg/day in another trial (Allgulander et al. 2004a). Ham-A psychic and somatic anxiety factors were significantly improved in a third trial (Dahl et al. 2005). In a double-blind study comparing sertraline and paroxetine, neither demonstrated an advantage over the other, either in efficacy or in tolerability (Ball et al. 2005).

A citalopram study of anxiety disorders in patients over age 60, wherein 30 of 34 enrolled patients had a diagnosis of GAD, demonstrated statistical significance for a 50% reduction in Ham-A scores, but not for remission (defined in this study as a Ham-A score ≤10, P=0.07) (Lenze et al. 2005).

Neither fluoxetine nor fluvoxamine has been the subject of a placebo-controlled trial for GAD in adults.

SNRIs

The SNRIs venlafaxine ER and duloxetine have FDA approval for GAD. Although dosages up to 225 mg/day are often employed in these studies, the efficacy of venlafaxine ER at 75 mg/day has been demonstrated in fixed-dose, placebo-controlled trials (Davidson et al. 1999; Montgomery et al. 2006). Response rates increase significantly between the short (3-month) and intermediate (6-month) terms (Meoni et al. 2001); this increase is likely not specific for SNRIs, but rather a property of GAD response to antidepressants in general.

Duloxetine, similarly, has recently garnered FDA approval for GAD. In a pooled analysis of placebo-controlled trials of duloxetine (60–120 mg/day) and venlafaxine ER (75–225 mg/day), both demonstrated efficacy compared with placebo. Moreover, neither SNRI demonstrated superior efficacy or tolerability compared with each other (Allgulander et al. 2008). A post hoc review of three studies argues for efficacy of duloxetine for painful physical symptoms associated with GAD (Beesdo et al. 2009).

In a meta-analysis that included five placebo-controlled venlafaxine ER trials, one paroxetine trial, and one fluoxetine trial (in which patients had comorbid GAD and depression), no statistically significant difference in effect size was found between the SSRIs and venlafaxine ER (Mitte et al. 2005). Similarly, in a meta-analysis that included three escitalopram trials, two paroxetine trials, two sertraline trials, a pediatric fluvoxamine trial, and five venlafaxine ER trials, no statistically significant differences in effect sizes were found for these classes (Hidalgo et al. 2007).

Desvenlafaxine has not been the subject of a placebo-controlled trial for GAD.

TCAs

Imipramine is the only TCA that has been studied extensively and in comparison with other pharmacological modalities for GAD (Rickels et al. 1993; Rocca et al. 1997). Results from a study by Rocca et al. (1997) suggested that imipramine had efficacy similar to that of paroxetine. The NNT for imipramine has been calculated as 4 (Kapczinski et al. 2003).

MAOIs

No RCTs of MAOIs have been reported in the literature on GAD.

Mirtazapine

Although no placebo-controlled trials of mirtazapine in GAD have been reported, a fixed-dose (30-mg), an open-label trial suggested that mirtazapine has some merit in the acute management of GAD (Gambi et al. 2005).

Nefazodone

No RCTs of nefazodone have been reported in the literature on GAD.

Bupropion

In a double-blind study involving 24 patients with GAD, comparing bupropion XL (extended release; 150–300 mg/day) with escitalopram (10–20 mg/day), both medications demonstrated comparable efficacy (Bystritsky et al. 2008). No placebo-controlled trials have been reported.

Maintenance and Relapse Prevention

A meta-analysis on relapse prevention (Donovan et al. 2010) favored antidepressant treatment, with a pooled odds ratio of 0.2, based on placebo-controlled studies of escitalopram, duloxetine, and paroxetine. Relapse rate upon switch to placebo was in the range of 35%–60%, whereas only 4%–14% of patients who continued antidepressant therapy relapsed in these 12- to 24-week studies of treatment responders.

Comparison With Psychological Treatment and Combined Treatment

Although studies have demonstrated the efficacy of CBT, as well as other psychotherapy modalities, for GAD, no controlled study has directly compared CBT with antidepressants, or combined CBT-antidepressant treatment with single-modality treatment.

Social Anxiety Disorder

The diagnosis of social anxiety disorder (SAD; formerly social phobia) requires marked fear of social or performance situations in which the person may be exposed to scrutiny by known, or unknown, individuals. The person fears that he or she will act in a manner that will invite humiliation or embarrassment in these settings. The evoked anxiety is excessive and, even when accompanied by good insight, results in avoidance and impaired functioning. Individuals may have a fear of a "specific" situation (e.g., speaking or other performance fears) or "generalized" fears of most social situations.

SAD is, by psychiatry standards, a relatively recent construct. Marks and Gelder (1966) described the syndrome under the rubric "social phobia." Social phobia was included and subsumed under specific phobias by the 1980 DSM-III. A recent review of the extant evidence for DSM-5 (Bögels et al. 2010) suggests that except for specific performance anxiety, SAD should be viewed along a spectrum, depending on the number and severity of social fears. This same review suggests that although avoidant personality disorder overlaps substantially with severe SAD, enough cases are related to the schizophrenia spectrum to warrant retention of a separate personality disorder category.

In Western countries, the lifetime prevalence of SAD is 7%–13% (Furmark 2002). The female-to-male ratio is on the order of 3:2 (Schneier et al. 1992). Patients with SAD are four times more likely to develop major depression than persons without the disorder (Kessler et al. 1994). SAD shows a moderate level of genetic heritability (Mosing et al. 2009).

Most, but not every, placebo-controlled medication trial lists the SAD subtype of the participants. Of those studies that have specified subtype, some enrolled both subtypes and others enrolled exclusively so-called generalized patients. No placebo-controlled studies have yet enrolled exclusively specific-subtype patients. No trend in efficacy can be found among studies that included both subtypes, when compared with those that enrolled exclusively generalized social anxiety.

Acute Medication Management

SSRIs

SSRIs are considered first-line treatment for SAD. Paroxetine and sertraline have FDA approval for SAD. As a class, SSRIs demonstrate statistically significant reductions in symptom severity (Lochner et al. 2004). In the acute phase, patients are two times more likely to respond to SSRIs than placebo. An updated version of an older Cochrane review (Stein et al. 2004) calculated an NNT of 4.19 (Ipser et al. 2008).

Placebo-controlled trials of paroxetine have demonstrated efficacy at dosages ranging from 20 to 60 mg/day (Allgulander 1999; Baldwin et al. 1999; Lepola et al. 2004; Stein et al. 1998). In a placebo-controlled trial done by Liebowitz et al. (2002), paroxetine 20 mg/day was statistically more efficacious than placebo but no less effective than paroxetine 60 mg/day.

Sertraline, at dosages of 50–200 mg/day, is supported by multiple placebo-controlled trials (Katzelnick et al. 1995; Liebowitz et al. 2003; Van Ameringen et al. 2001).

Although not formally approved by the FDA for SAD, fluvoxamine, at dosages of 50–300 mg/day, demonstrated similar efficacy to sertraline and paroxetine in placebo-controlled trials (Davidson et al. 2004c; Stein et al. 1999). Evidence also suggests that response to fluvoxamine increases between 3 and 6 months, mirroring effects for other anxiety disorders with other antidepressants (Stein et al. 2003b).

In a study by Lader et al. (2004), escitalopram demonstrated efficacy beginning at 5 mg/day. This study is unique in that it contains the only head-to-head comparison of SSRIs: escitalopram 20 mg/day was superior to paroxetine 20 mg/day. It is not clear whether this difference is due to the pharmacology or to the relative dosing, considering that the dose potencies are by no means equivalent (escitalopram dosing is more potent).

Fluoxetine, at dosages of 10–60 mg/day, with effect sizes similar to those of the other SSRIs, is supported by several placebo-controlled trials (Davidson et al. 2004b; Kobak et al. 2002).

The placebo-controlled data that support the use of citalopram 40 mg/day are limited to a 36-patient study, in which citalopram was compared with a neurokinin-1 antagonist and placebo (Furmark et al. 2005).

SNRIs

Venlafaxine ER, which has been well studied in SAD, has consistently been demonstrated to be superior to placebo (Allgulander et al. 2004b; Liebowitz et al. 2005b; March et al. 2007; Rickels et al. 2004). Interestingly, venlafaxine ER has also been studied in head-to-head trials with paroxetine (Allgulander et al. 2004b; Liebowitz et al. 2005a); efficacy was similar for the two medications in both studies. Mean dosages in the Liebowitz et al. study were 202 mg/day for venlafaxine and 46 mg/day for paroxetine. The overall side effect risk also was similar. Systolic blood pressure in the venlafaxine ER group rose 1 mm Hg, but the study was large enough that this small change yielded a significant *P* value. This finding is consistent with data that blood pressure elevations do not commonly occur at dosages of <225 mg/day of venlafaxine.

No placebo-controlled trials of duloxetine or desvenlafaxine in patients with SAD have been reported.

TCAs

The current consensus is that TCAs do not work for SAD. No placebo-controlled trials of TCAs in SAD have been reported. In the 1970s, results from a large open-label trial (Beaumont 1977) suggested that clomipramine may have some efficacy; however, clomipramine may not be the best representative of the TCA class because it is strongly serotonergic. Little efficacy was found in a 15-patient open-label trial of imipramine (Simpson et al. 1998a). Both of these TCA trials had high dropout rates due to side effects.

MAOIs

Although the MAOI phenelzine has some significant risk factors, including hypertensive crisis, insomnia, weight gain, and sexual dysfunction, some placebo-controlled trials support its use, at dosages up to 90 mg/day, in SAD (Blanco et al. 2010; Heimberg et al. 1998; Liebowitz et al. 1992; Versiani et al. 1992), with NNTs similar to those seen in SSRI trials.

At low dosages, selegiline is an irreversible selective MAO-B inhibitor that is available in the United States. In one limited study, selegiline showed some efficacy in SAD (Simpson et al. 1998b).

Moclobemide and brofaromine, two medications not available in the United States, bind reversibly and selectively to the A isoenzyme of monoamine oxidase. Compared with phenelzine, for example, these two medications have a lower risk of hypertensive crisis. These medications have been studied in numerous placebo-controlled trials and were found to be effective in a meta-analysis by Blanco et al. (2003).

Mirtazapine

Mirtazapine demonstrated efficacy at 30 mg/day in a placebo-controlled trial (Muehlbacher et al. 2005). Interestingly, all of the study participants were women with social phobia. As expected with mirtazapine, the most common side effects in this study were dry mouth (21%), weight gain (21%), sedation (18%), drowsiness (18%), and increased appetite (12%).

Nefazodone

In the lone placebo-controlled trial, the efficacy of nefazodone was not significantly different from that of placebo in patients with social phobia (Van Ameringen et al. 2007).

Bupropion

No placebo-controlled trials of bupropion in SAD have been reported, although successful treatment has been reported in an open-label study (Emmanuel et al. 2000).

Long-Term Follow-Up and Relapse Prevention

Most placebo-controlled studies of SAD follow patients for a maximum of 12 weeks. Donovan et al. (2010) performed a meta-analysis of four studies that followed patients up to 6 months. Of the four trials, two employed paroxetine, one used sertraline, and one used escitalopram. In these studies, 40%–60% of patients whose antidepressant was discontinued went on to relapse. The odds ratio of relapse for SSRI continued versus discontinued ranged from 0.07 to 0.28.

Comparison With Psychological Treatment and Combined Treatment

CBT is an accepted treatment modality for SAD, and studies have shown comparable efficacy when directly comparing CBT with medication. Evidence for whether combined CBT and medication has an advantage over monotherapy is mixed. In a recent study, phenelzine and CBT demonstrated greater efficacy than placebo in SAD, with the combination of the two interventions superior to either treatment alone (Blanco et al. 2010). In contrast, another study showed individual but not combined benefit with fluoxetine and CBT (Davidson et al. 2004b). These contrasting findings provide indirect support for long-standing clinical lore that MAOIs may have an advantage over SSRIs in treatment-refractory anxiety, although of course a direct comparison between the two medications would be required.

Specific Phobia

Specific phobia (formerly called "simple phobia") is an excessive fear, recognized as excessive by the patient, brought on by a specific situation or object. This class of phobias has been divided into three subtypes: animal phobias (based on a characteristic early age at onset), blood/injury phobias (based on a characteristic bradycardia and hypotensive fear response), and any other specific phobias. Kessler and colleagues estimated the 12-month prevalence to be 12.5% in the continental United States (Kessler et al. 2005b) and the lifetime prevalence in women to be double that of men (Kessler et al. 1994). A genetic contribution is likely, as demonstrated in twin studies (Kendler 2001).

Acute Management

Although the clear treatment of choice for specific phobia is systematic desensitization, a few attempts at antidepressant intervention have been reported. In an early study, a combination of psychotherapy and clomipramine was reported to have some efficacy (Waxman 1977). More recently, two placebo-controlled studies of SSRIs for this disorder have been done. In an escitalopram study, where the mean dose was 17 mg/day, the authors demonstrated a strong effect in favor of the antidepressant, but the study was too underpowered to yield statistical significance over placebo (Alamy et al. 2008). A 12-patient placebo-controlled study of paroxetine 20 mg/day, however, did show statistically significant improvement (Benjamin et al. 2000). In both studies, the main phobias were varied and included heights, flying, specific animals, confined spaces, driving, storms, and dentists.

Long-Term Follow-Up and Relapse Prevention

There have been no long-term placebo-controlled studies for antidepressants in treating specific phobia. The aforementioned paroxetine study lasted 4 weeks (Benjamin et al. 2000), and the escitalopram trial lasted 12 weeks (Alamy et al. 2008).

Obsessive-Compulsive Disorder

The diagnosis of OCD requires either uncontrollable thoughts or images (obsessions) or compulsive, repetitive acts driven by obsessions or rigid rules. The symptoms must cause significant functional impairment due to the time consumed. Using DSM-IV criteria, Kessler et al. (2005b) estimated a lifetime prevalence of 1.6% for OCD. The disorder adversely impacts multiple domains of functioning and quality of life (Hollander et al. 1996).

OCD is a heterogeneous disorder, with some patients experiencing a chronic course and others a relapsing-remitting course (Ravizza et al. 1997). The longest follow-up study (Skoog and Skoog 1999), a 40-year case-note review of 144 patients, suggested that complete remission was achieved in only 20% of OCD cases.

According to Crino et al. (2005), 79.7% of patients who met criteria for OCD using DSM-IV criteria also met criteria for another mood, anxiety, substance use, or personality disorder. In fact, 46% met criteria for OCD and three or more other disorders. The significant Axis I comorbidity seen in OCD patients also contributes to the high level of disability and low remission rate. OCD appears to have significant genetic heterogeneity (Nicolini et al. 2009), and the variability of symptoms, illness course, and comorbidities suggests a broad OCD phenotype.

Acute Management

SSRIs

SSRIs are considered a first-line treatment for OCD. Fluoxetine (up to 80 mg/day), fluvoxamine (up to 300 mg/day), sustained-release fluvoxamine (up to 300 mg/day), paroxetine (up to 50 mg/day), and sertraline (up to 200 mg/day) have FDA approval for treatment of OCD. Treating OCD with SSRIs often requires dosing at the high end of the usual antidepressant range. Moreover, trials lasting longer than 13 weeks show a trend toward improved effect size compared with shorter trials (Soomro et al. 2008), suggesting that patients may need to continue an SSRI trial for longer than 3 months before final efficacy is assessed. The Cochrane meta-analysis by Soomro et al. (2008) confirmed efficacy for the SSRI class as a whole but did not show a statistically significant difference between any of the individual agents. The NNT for SSRIs in OCD ranges from about 6 to 12.

Compared with trials of the other SSRIs in OCD, far fewer controlled trials of citalopram and escitalopram have been reported. Although trials have shown the benefit of these two medications in OCD (Montgomery et al. 2001; Stein et al. 2008), the studies are too limited to make meaningful recommendations in regard to dosing. Based on the limited data available for OCD, dosages of up to 60 mg/day of citalopram and up to 30 mg/day of escitalopram are generally suggested.

SNRIs

No placebo-controlled trials for SNRIs have been reported. The strongest case for use of venlafaxine in OCD comes from trials suggesting no statistical difference in efficacy for venlafaxine, clomipramine, and paroxetine (Albert et al. 2002; Denys et al. 2003, 2004). Venlafaxine dosing in these trials was up to 300 mg/day.

The evidence supporting duloxetine's efficacy for OCD is confined to case reports and series, with dosages of 120–180 mg/day reported (Dell'osso et al. 2008; Yeh et al. 2009).

No studies of desvenlafaxine use in OCD have been reported.

TCAs

Binding affinities for serotonin, norepinephrine, and dopamine receptors vary significantly among medications in the TCA class. Evidence from OCD medication trials suggests that antidepressants whose binding profiles include a serotonin reuptake inhibition (SRI) component are more effective than antidepressants that are primarily noradrenergic or dopaminergic. Since the first report of its efficacy in 1967 by Fernandez-Cordoba and Lopez-Ibor, clomipramine, whose significant SRI action augments its noradrenergic and dopaminergic modalities, has consistently demonstrated efficacy in treating OCD. The largest placebo-controlled report, by the Clomipramine Collaborative Study Group (1991), included two placebo-controlled studies, one with patients who had been ill for at least 1 year, and one with patients who had been ill for at least 2 years. This study involved 21 treatment centers, 520 patients, and clomipramine dosing ≤300 mg/day. For the 239 patients who had been ill for 2 years, clomipramine yielded a 38% mean reduction of symptoms, whereas placebo produced only a 3% improvement of symptoms. For the 281 patients who had been ill for at least a year, clomipramine resulted in a 44% reduction in symptoms, compared with 5% for placebo. The NNT was calculated at 2.5.

Much OCD work has compared clomipramine with SSRIs, in terms of both efficacy and tolerability. Although head-to-head trials of clomipramine against fluoxetine, fluvoxamine, and sertraline have suggested that these medications are equally efficacious, a series of meta-analyses suggests that clomipramine slightly outperforms SSRIs (Ackerman and Greenland 2002; Greist et al. 1995; Piccinelli et al. 1995).

Desipramine, on the other hand, has very little SRI action and has less efficacy than, for example, sertraline in head-to-head trials in patients with OCD (Hoehn-Saric et al. 2000).

The issue of antidepressant tolerability in OCD is complicated. Clomipramine is certainly associated with more side effects than SSRIs in large analyses. However, in one analysis of a large multicenter clomipramine trial, the presence of anticholinergic side effects predicted a better response (Ackerman et al. 1999). The connection between the presence of side effects and effect size has also been commented on by Abramowitz (1997). It is not clear if this phenomenon is biological, either as a marker of metabolism or an anticholinergic contribution to efficacy, or psychological. Blinded study participants with anticholinergic side effects may have felt reassured that they were in the active drug arm. Although anticholinergic side effects do not predict responsivity for anxiety disorders as a whole, anticholinergic medications have recently demonstrated some efficacy in depression (Drevets and Furey 2010).

MAOIs

No RCTs of MAOI use have been reported for OCD.

Mirtazapine

Mirtazapine has effects on serotonergic and noradrenergic neurotransmission via serotonin and norepinephrine receptor blockade, rather than effects on reuptake inhibition (Kent 2000). A 12-week open-label trial of mirtazapine up to 60 mg/day in 30 subjects showed a 28% improvement in scores on the Yale-Brown Obsessive Compulsive Scale. Fifteen of the responders agreed to be randomly assigned to receive placebo, and a statistically significant difference between mirtazapine and placebo was noted during an 8-week follow-up (Koran et al. 2005). Results from another study suggest that mirtazapine augmentation of citalopram may accelerate the response rate of the SSRI (Pallanti et al. 2004).

Nefazodone

No RCTs of nefazodone have been reported for OCD.

Bupropion

Although no RCTs of bupropion have been reported for OCD, an open-label trial demonstrated no efficacy (Vulink et al. 2005).

Long-Term Follow-Up and Relapse Prevention

Fineberg et al. (2007) produced a thorough review of the body of literature on long-term treatment of OCD. As these authors pointed out, OCD is a long-term illness, and chronic treatment is expected. However, in the longest placebo-controlled medication trial for acute responders, which lasted 1 year, Katz et al. (1990) found a sustained benefit to clomipramine. Thus, American Psychiatric Association (2007) guidelines, as well as guidelines from the World Council of Anxiety (Greist et al. 2003), suggest that patients who are having an adequate response be maintained on medication for 1–2 years, with slow taper considered after that time.

Comparison With Psychological Treatment and Combined Treatment

Among the psychological/behavioral treatment possibilities, exposure with response prevention has shown the greatest efficacy in OCD. Because this treatment has been found to be superior to SSRIs in large trials, the American Psychiatric Association (2007) guidelines suggest that exposure may be considered a first-line treatment for OCD. Data also suggest that more cognitive forms of behavioral treatment—that is, more classic CBT—may also be effective. Finally, findings from a study by Simpson et al. (2008) suggest that adding exposure to a treatment plan that already includes a serotonin reuptake inhibitor can further reduce symptom severity.

Posttraumatic Stress Disorder

The diagnosis of PTSD requires exposure to a traumatic event involving a serious threat, followed by a constellation of symptoms including intrusive reexperiencing, avoidance or numbing, and hyperarousal. The 12-month prevalence has been reported to be 2.1% (Byers et al. 2010), with an estimated lifetime prevalence of 7.8% in the United States (Kessler et al. 1994). In a study using DSM-IV criteria, Kessler et al. (2005b) found that PTSD has a high rate of comorbidity with other anxiety disorders, depression, and alcohol dependence. PTSD is associated with significant chronicity, impairment, and medical comorbidity (Brunello et al. 2001; Sareen et al. 2005). There is ongoing research into predisposing factors, including gene-environment interactions, for suicide in trauma victims (Roy et al. 2009). Suicide in patients with PTSD has emerged as a major area of focus in Veterans Affairs hospitals serving veterans from Iraq and Afghanistan.

A growing number of antidepressant classes demonstrate efficacy as monotherapy for PTSD. One of the many challenges of comparing placebo-controlled trials for PTSD has been trying to understand whether the type of trauma makes a difference. For studies that single out a specific type of trauma, the type is noted in the discussion that follows.

Acute Management

SSRIs

SSRIs are considered first-line treatment for PTSD (Stein et al. 2006a; Zhang and Davidson 2007). Sertraline and paroxetine have received FDA approval for PTSD. The results of placebo-controlled trials for paroxetine have been robust. Stein et al. (2003a) pooled three placebo-controlled trials and demonstrated paroxetine's efficacy for each of the PTSD symptom clusters, for resulting disability, and for PTSD in the presence of comorbid depression. One of the pooled trials was at fixed, rather than flexible, dosing and demonstrated efficacy with paroxetine at both 20 mg/day and 40 mg/day (Marshall et al. 2001). Marshall et al. (2007) subsequently demonstrated paroxetine's efficacy in an urban, primarily minority, population. The NNT in paroxetine studies ranges from 2.5 to 12.

Despite FDA approval for sertraline in treating PTSD, the results of RCTs with this medication are mixed. In various trials, sertraline, at dosages of 50–200 mg/day, showed benefit for adults who had been victims of interpersonal trauma or childhood abuse (Stein et al. 2006b), showed efficacy for avoidance and numbing symptoms clusters (Brady et al. 2000), and was broadly efficacious in a study by Davidson et al. (2001b). However, the support was not as robust in a subsequent study by Davidson et al. (2006b), sertraline did not separate from placebo in a trial of mostly male patients with combat trauma (Friedman et al. 2007), and the drug did not demonstrate significant efficacy for PTSD symptoms in a study of patients with co-occurring alcohol dependence (Brady et al. 2005).

Similar to the data for sertraline, the results for fluoxetine in PTSD have been mixed. Several of the early placebo-controlled fluoxetine studies showed statistically significant improvement for patients (Connor et al. 1999; Martenyi et al. 2002; van der Kolk et al. 1994). However, two 2007 studies did not demonstrate significant fluoxetine efficacy (Martenyi et al. 2007; van der Kolk et al. 2007). It is interesting to note that Martenyi et al.'s (2002) positive trial was in male combat veterans, whereas Martenyi et al.'s (2007) equivocal trial was in a mostly female, noncombat population. Moreover, the mean dosage of fluoxetine in their 2002 trial was 57 mg/day, whereas the 2007 trial featured lower, fixed dosages (20 and 40 mg/day) and a very high placebo response rate.

The lone placebo-controlled study involving citalopram for PTSD failed to show efficacy (Tucker et al. 2003). No placebo-controlled studies employing escitalopram have been reported for PTSD.

SNRIs

Venlafaxine showed efficacy at a mean dosage of 225 mg/day (Davidson et al. 2006b). Pooled data were used by Stein et al. (2009) to further confirm the overall efficacy of venlafaxine ER, further parse out symptoms that respond the earliest (i.e., physiological and psychological reactivity on exposure to cues, irritability, and intrusive recollections), and identify symptoms not significantly improved (i.e., distressing dreams, avoidance, inability to recall details of traumatic event, and sleep disturbance). Further analysis of these data has also suggested that neither gender nor age (as a surrogate for menopausal status) is a predictor of venlafaxine response (Rothbaum et al. 2008).

Neither duloxetine nor desvenlafaxine has been the subject of placebo-controlled trials for PTSD.

TCAs

In a placebo-controlled trial, amitriptyline was demonstrated to be efficacious in PTSD (Davidson et al. 1990). Imipramine has also been shown to have efficacy (Frank et al. 1988; Kosten et al. 1991). The use of TCAs is out of favor, however, because of the higher rate of side effects with TCAs than with SSRIs. However, an interesting observation is that in the placebo-controlled trials for PTSD, dropout rates were not significantly different for patients taking these different classes of medications (Stein et al. 2006a), suggesting that the greater side-effect burden of TCAs may not limit clinical utility.

MAOIs

Phenelzine has demonstrated efficacy in two placebo-controlled trials (Frank et al. 1988; Kosten et al. 1991), although the medication is rarely used in patients with PTSD because of the side-effect burden and requirement that patients keep a more restrictive, low-tyramine diet.

Mirtazapine

A 29-patient, 8-week, placebo-controlled trial showed efficacy for mirtazapine (Davidson et al. 2003). Mirtazapine was initiated at 15 mg/day, although 13 of the 17 patients in the mirtazapine group were taking 45 mg/day by the end of the trial.

Nefazodone

Although the FDA has attached a black box warning regarding nefazodone's hepatotoxicity, the medication's consistent benefit for sleep disturbances, at doses of 400–600 mg, in combat veterans with PTSD (Gillin et al. 2001; Neylan et al. 2003) led to further study. A 41-patient, placebo-controlled pilot study subsequently demonstrated statistically significant improvement (Davis et al. 2004); however, the study's small sample size provides only limited confidence, and a larger study is needed.

Bupropion

Sustained-release bupropion, added to standard care, was employed in an 8-week placebo-controlled trial with 30 patients. Bupropion, at dosages up to 300 mg/day, did not separate from placebo (Becker et al. 2007), although this small study had limited power to find a difference.

Long-Term Follow-up and Relapse Prevention

Several studies have examined the efficacy of medications in PTSD for 6 months or longer using a placebo-controlled design. Venlafaxine ER, at a mean dosage of 221 mg/day, demonstrated continued efficacy against placebo when taken for 6 months (Davidson et al. 2006a). Continued efficacy and relapse prevention was also demonstrated in a 28-week placebo-controlled trial of sertraline (mean dose=137 mg/day) in patients who had undergone a 12-week placebo-controlled trial followed by a 24-week open-label continuation study (Davidson et al. 2001a). In this study, patients who received a placebo were 6.5 times more likely to experience a relapse than those given sertraline (26% vs. 5%). The use of SSRIs in relapse prevention for PTSD is supported by a meta-analysis that employed the Davidson et al. (2001a) sertraline study, as well as two longer-term fluoxetine trials (Donovan et al. 2010). Interestingly, longer-term data show that the effects of antidepressants in PTSD increase over time, with response rates increasing substantially at 6 months compared with 2 months (Londborg et al. 2001).

Comparison With Psychological Treatment and Combined Treatment

Although cognitive-behavioral forms of psychotherapy, specifically prolonged exposure, cognitive processing therapy, and stress inoculation therapy, remain a mainstay of PTSD treatment, no placebo-controlled studies have directly compared antidepressants with CBT in adult populations. More important, no studies have compared whether the combination of CBT and medication has advantages over CBT alone. Notably, the Institute of Medicine (2007), in its report on treatment for PTSD, concluded that the evidence for CBT efficacy in PTSD was much superior to evidence for antidepressant efficacy, largely because the higher dropout rates for the pharmacotherapy studies compromised the analysis.

KEY CLINICAL CONCEPTS

- For all anxiety disorders except OCD, multiple medication classes have demonstrated efficacy. In general, large meta-analyses have failed to demonstrate significant differences between the efficacious classes. Therefore, initial selection of agents should be guided by identifying the most tolerable side-effect profile for the patient. A simple rule of thumb is that SSRIs, as a class, are effective for all five of the anxiety disorders.
- For OCD, clomipramine may have a slight advantage in efficacy over SSRIs. Because of its association with more side effects, however, the slightly greater efficacy may not be enough to warrant using it as initial treatment. Nevertheless, any SSRI treatment failure should prompt a clomipramine trial.
- Although few data are available from studies of any anxiety disorder supporting better response to higher antidepressant dosages, titration to the highest tolerable dosage should always be tried in patients without an optimal response.
- For all anxiety disorders with long-term research data, but especially OCD, reasonable evidence indicates that rate of response continues to increase well past the 12-week acute clinical trial duration. Hence, patients with at least partial (25%) response may well become responders, or even remitters, by the 6-month mark.

- Relapse rate data suggest that a substantial proportion of patients with anxiety disorder will relapse when antidepressants are discontinued. Hence, decisions to discontinue should be based on whether patients are at higher or lower risk of relapse. Extant data suggest that higher symptom severity, other comorbidities, residual avoidance behavior, and ongoing medical and psychosocial stress all predict higher relapse risk.
- For OCD, behavioral treatment is superior to pharmacotherapy. Moreover, only limited data suggest that combining treatment with medication is superior to behavioral treatment alone, although adding behavioral treatment to pharmacotherapy has improved efficacy over pharmacotherapy alone.
- For panic disorder, data suggest that combined CBT and medication treatment may produce the best efficacy over the intermediate (6-month) term. In contrast, no strong data support combined treatment for the other anxiety disorders. However, for individual patients not achieving remission, combined treatment should always be tried.

References

Abramowitz JS: Effectiveness of psychological and pharmacological treatments for obsessive-compulsive disorder: a quantitative review. J Consult Clin Psychol 65:44–52, 1997

Ackerman DL, Greenland S: Multivariate meta-analysis of controlled drug studies for obsessive-compulsive disorder. J Clin Psychopharmacol 22:309–317, 2002

Ackerman DL, Greenland S, Bystritsky A: Side effects as predictors of drug response in obsessive-compulsive disorder. J Clin Psychopharmacol 19:459–465, 1999

Alamy S, Wei Zhang, Varia I, et al: Escitalopram in specific phobia: results of a placebo-controlled pilot trial. J Psychopharmacol 22:157–161, 2008

Albert U, Aguglia E, Maina G, et al: Venlafaxine versus clomipramine in the treatment of obsessive-compulsive disorder: a preliminary single-blind, 12-week, controlled study. J Clin Psychiatry 63:1004–1009, 2002

Allgulander C: Paroxetine in social anxiety disorder: a randomized placebo-controlled study. Acta Psychiatr Scand 100:193–198, 1999

Allgulander C, Dahl AA, Austin C, et al: Efficacy of sertraline in a 12-week trial for generalized anxiety disorder. Am J Psychiatry 161:1642–1649, 2004a

Allgulander C, Mangano R, Zhang J, et al: Efficacy of Venlafaxine ER in patients with social anxiety disorder: a double-blind, placebo-controlled, parallel-group comparison with paroxetine. Hum Psychopharmacol 19:387–396, 2004b

Allgulander C, Nutt D, Detke M, et al: A non-inferiority comparison of duloxetine and venlafaxine in the treatment of adult patients with generalized anxiety disorder. J Psychopharmacol 22:417–425, 2008

American Psychiatric Association: Diagnostic and Statistical Manual of Mental Disorders, 3rd Edition. Washington, DC, American Psychiatric Association, 1980

American Psychiatric Association: Diagnostic and Statistical Manual of Mental Disorders, 4th Edition. Washington, DC, American Psychiatric Association, 1994

American Psychiatric Association: Diagnostic and Statistical Manual of Mental Disorders, 4th Edition, Text Revision. Washington, DC, American Psychiatric Association, 2000

American Psychiatric Association: APA Practice Guidelines: Treatment of Patients With Obsessive-Compulsive Disorder. July 2007. Available at: www.psychiatryonline.com/pracGuide/pracGuideHome.aspx.

Baldwin D, Bobes J, Stein DJ, et al: Paroxetine in social phobia/social anxiety disorder: randomised, double-blind, placebo-controlled study. Paroxetine Study Group. Br J Psychiatry 175:120–126, 1999

Ball SG, Kuhn A, Wall D, et al: Selective serotonin reuptake inhibitor treatment for generalized anxiety disorder: a double-blind, prospective comparison between paroxetine and sertraline. J Clin Psychiatry 66:94–99, 2005

Bandelow B, Stein DJ, Dolberg OT, et al: Improvement of quality of life in panic disorder with escitalopram, citalopram, or placebo. Pharmacopsychiatry 40:152–156, 2007

Barlow DH, Gorman JM, Shear MK, et al: Cognitive-behavioral therapy, imipramine, or their combination for panic disorder: a randomized controlled trial. JAMA 283:2529–2536, 2000

Beaumont G: A large open multicentre trial of clomipramine (Anafranil) in the management of phobic disorders. J Int Med Res 5 (suppl 5):116–123, 1977

Becker ME, Hertzberg MA, Moore SD, et al: A placebo-controlled trial of bupropion SR in the treatment of chronic posttraumatic stress disorder. J Clin Psychopharmacol 27:193–197, 2007

Beesdo K, Hartford J, Russell J, et al: The short- and long-term effect of duloxetine on painful physical symptoms in patients with generalized anxiety disorder: results from three clinical trials. J Anxiety Disord 23:1064–1071, 2009

Benjamin J, Ben-Zion IZ, Kabrofsky E, et al: Double-blind placebo-controlled pilot study of paroxetine for specific phobia. Psychopharmacology (Berl) 149:194–196, 2000

Bielski RJ, Bose A, Chang CC: A double-blind comparison of escitalopram and paroxetine in the long-term treatment of generalized anxiety disorder. Ann Clin Psychiatry 17:65–69, 2005

Blanco C, Schneier FR, Schmidt A, et al: Pharmacological treatment of social anxiety disorder: a meta-analysis. Depress Anxiety 18:29–40, 2003

Blanco C, Heimberg RC, Schneier FR, et al: A placebo-controlled trial of phenelzine, cognitive behavioral group therapy, and their combination for social anxiety disorder. Arch Gen Psychiatry 67:286–295, 2010

Bögels SM, Alden L, Beidel DC, et al: Social anxiety disorder: questions and answers for the DSM-V. Depress Anxiety 27:168–189, 2010

Boshuisen ML, Slaap BR, Vester-Blokland, et al: The effect of mirtazapine in panic disorder: an open-label pilot study with a single-blind placebo run-in period. Int Clin Psychopharmacol 16:363–368, 2001

Bradwejn J, Ahokas A, Stein DJ, et al: Venlafaxine extended-release capsules in panic disorder: flexible-dose, double-blind, placebo-controlled study. Br J Psychiatry 187: 352–359, 2005

Brady K, Pearlstein T, Asnis GM, et al: Efficacy and safety of sertraline treatment of posttraumatic stress disorder: a randomized controlled trial. JAMA 283:1837–1844, 2000

Brady KT, Sonne S, Anton RF, et al: Sertraline in the treatment of co-occurring alcohol dependence and posttraumatic stress disorder. Alcohol Clin Exp Res 29:395–401, 2005

Brawman-Mintzer O, Knapp RG, Rynn M, et al: Sertraline treatment for generalized anxiety disorder: a randomized, double-blind, placebo-controlled study. J Clin Psychiatry 67:874–881, 2006

Brunello N, Davidson JR, Deahl M, et al: Posttraumatic stress disorder: diagnosis and epidemiology, comorbidity and social consequences, biology and treatment. Neuropsychobiology 43:150–162, 2001

Byers AL, Yaffe K, Covinsky KE, et al: High occurrence of mood and anxiety disorders among older adults: The National Comorbidity Survey Replication. Arch Gen Psychiatry 67:489–496, 2010

Bystritsky A, Kerwin L, Feusner JD, et al: A pilot controlled trial of bupropion XL versus escitalopram in generalized anxiety disorder. Psychopharmacol Bull 41:46–51, 2008

Clomipramine Collaborative Study Group: Clomipramine in the treatment of patients with obsessive-compulsive disorder: the Clomipramine Collaborative Study Group. Arch Gen Psychiatry 48:730–738, 1991

Connor KM, Sutherland SM, Tupler LA, et al: Fluoxetine in post-traumatic stress disorder: randomised, double-blind study. Br J Psychiatry 175: 17–22, 1999

Coric V, Feldman HH, Oren DA, et al: Multicenter, randomized, double-blind, active comparator and placebo-controlled trial of a corticotropin-releasing factor receptor-1 antagonist in generalized anxiety disorder. Depress Anxiety 27:417–425, 2010

Crino R, Slade T, Andrews G: The changing prevalence and severity of obsessive-compulsive disorder criteria from DSM-III to DSM-IV. Am J Psychiatry 162:876–882, 2005

Dahl AA, Ravindran A, Allgulander C, et al: Sertraline in generalized anxiety disorder: efficacy in treating the psychic and somatic anxiety factors. Acta Psychiatr Scand 111:429–435, 2005

Davidson J, Kudler H, Smith R, et al: Treatment of posttraumatic stress disorder with amitriptyline and placebo. Arch Gen Psychiatry 47:259–266, 1990

Davidson JR, DuPont RL, Hedges D, et al: Efficacy, safety, and tolerability of venlafaxine extended release and buspirone in outpatients with generalized anxiety disorder. J Clin Psychiatry 60:528–535, 1999

Davidson J, Pearlstein T, Londborg P, et al: Efficacy of sertraline in preventing relapse of posttraumatic stress disorder: results of a 28-week double-blind, placebo-controlled study. Am J Psychiatry 158:1974–1981, 2001a

Davidson JR, Rothbaum BO, van der Kolk BA, et al: Multicenter, double-blind comparison of sertraline and placebo in the treatment of posttraumatic stress disorder. Arch Gen Psychiatry 58:485–492, 2001b

Davidson JR, Weisler RH, Butterfield MI, et al: Mirtazapine vs. placebo in posttraumatic stress disorder: a pilot trial. Biol Psychiatry 53:188–191, 2003

Davidson J, Bose A, Korotzer A, et al: Escitalopram in the treatment of generalized anxiety disorder: double-blind, placebo controlled, flexible-dose study. Depress Anxiety 19:234–240, 2004a

Davidson JR, Foa EB, Huppert JD, et al: Fluoxetine, comprehensive cognitive behavioral therapy, and placebo in generalized social phobia. Arch Gen Psychiatry 61:1005–1013, 2004b

Davidson J, Yaryura-Tobias J, DuPont R, et al: Fluvoxamine-controlled release formulation for the treatment of generalized social anxiety disorder. J Clin Psychopharmacol 24:118–125, 2004c

Davidson J, Baldwin D, Stein DJ, et al: Treatment of posttraumatic stress disorder with venlafaxine extended release: a 6-month randomized controlled trial. Arch Gen Psychiatry 63:1158–1165, 2006a

Davidson J, Rothbaum BO, Tucker P, et al: Venlafaxine extended release in posttraumatic stress disorder: a sertraline- and placebo-controlled study. J Clin Psychopharmacol 26:259–267, 2006b

Davis LL, Jewell ME, Ambrose S, et al: A placebo-controlled study of nefazodone for the treatment of chronic posttraumatic stress disorder: a preliminary study. J Clin Psychopharmacol 24:291–297, 2004

Dell'osso B, Mundo E, Marazziti D, et al: Switching from serotonin reuptake inhibitors to duloxetine in patients with resistant obsessive-compulsive disorder: a case series. J Psychopharmacol 22:210–213, 2008

Demyttenaere K, Andersen HF, Reines EK: Impact of escitalopram treatment on Quality of Life Enjoyment and Satisfaction Questionnaire scores in major depressive disorder and generalized anxiety disorder. Int Clin Psychopharmacol 23:276–286, 2008

Denys D, van der Wee N, van Megen HJ, et al: A double blind comparison of venlafaxine and paroxetine in obsessive-compulsive disorder. J Clin Psychopharmacol 23:568–575, 2003

Denys D, van Megen HJ, van der Wee N, et al: A double-blind switch study of paroxetine and venlafaxine in obsessive-compulsive disorder. J Clin Psychiatry 65:37–43, 2004

Donovan MR, Glue P, Kolluri S, et al: Comparative efficacy of antidepressants in preventing relapse in anxiety disorders—a meta-analysis. J Affect Disord 123:9–16, 2010

Drevets WC, Furey ML: Replication of scopolamine's antidepressant efficacy in major depressive disorder: a randomized, placebo-controlled clinical trial. Biol Psychiatry 67:432–438, 2010

Eaton WW, Kessler RC, Wittchen HU, et al: Panic and panic disorder in the United States. Am J Psychiatry 151:413–420, 1994

Emmanuel NP, Brawman-Mintzer O, Morton WA, et al: Bupropion-SR in treatment of social phobia. Depress Anxiety 12:111–113, 2000

Fernandez Cordoba E, Lopez-Ibor Alino J: [Use of monochlorimipramine in psychiatric patients who are resistant to other therapy]. Actas Luso Esp Neurol Psiquiatr 26:119–147, 1967

Fineberg NA, Pampaloni I, Pallanti S, et al: Sustained response versus relapse: the pharmacotherapeutic goal for obsessive-compulsive disorder. Int Clin Psychopharmacol 22:313–322, 2007

Frank JB, Kosten TR, Giller EL Jr, et al: A randomized clinical trial of phenelzine and imipramine for posttraumatic stress disorder. Am J Psychiatry 145:1289–1291, 1988

Friedman MJ, Marmar CR, Baker DG, et al: Randomized, double-blind comparison of sertraline and placebo for posttraumatic stress disorder in a Department of Veterans Affairs setting. J Clin Psychiatry 68:711–720, 2007

Furmark T: Social phobia: overview of community surveys. Acta Psychiatr Scand 105:84–93, 2002

Furmark T, Appel L, Michelgård A, et al: Cerebral blood flow changes after treatment of social phobia with the neurokinin-1 antagonist GR205171, citalopram, or placebo. Biol Psychiatry 58:132–142, 2005

Furukawa TA, Watanabe N, Churchill R: Psychotherapy plus antidepressant for panic disorder with or without agoraphobia: systematic review. Br J Psychiatry 188: 305–312, 2006

Gambi F, De Berardis D, Campanella D, et al: Mirtazapine treatment of generalized anxiety disorder: a fixed dose, open label study. J Psychopharmacol 19:483–487, 2005

Gillin JC, Smith-Vaniz A, Schnierow B, et al: An open-label, 12-week clinical and sleep EEG study of nefazodone in chronic combat-related posttraumatic stress disorder. J Clin Psychiatry 62:789–796, 2001

Goodman WK, Bose A, Wang Q: Treatment of generalized anxiety disorder with escitalopram: pooled results from double-blind, placebo-controlled trials. J Affect Disord 87:161–167, 2005

Greist JH, Jefferson JW, Kobak KA, et al: Efficacy and tolerability of serotonin transport inhibitors in obsessive-compulsive disorder: a meta-analysis. Arch Gen Psychiatry 52:53–60, 1995

Greist JH, Bandelow B, Hollander E, et al: WCA recommendations for the long-term treatment of obsessive-compulsive disorder in adults. CNS Spectr 8 (suppl 1):7–16, 2003

Hamilton SP: Linkage and association studies of anxiety disorders. Depress Anxiety 26:976–983, 2009

Heimberg RG, Liebowitz MR, Hope DA, et al: Cognitive behavioral group therapy vs phenelzine therapy for social phobia: 12-week outcome. Arch Gen Psychiatry 55:1133–1141, 1998

Hettema JM, Prescott CA, Kendler KS: The effects of anxiety, substance use and conduct disorders on risk of major depressive disorder. Psychol Med 33:1423–1432, 2003

Hidalgo RB, Tupler LA, Davidson JR: An effect-size analysis of pharmacologic treatments for generalized anxiety disorder. J Psychopharmacol 21:864–872, 2007

Hoehn-Saric R, Ninan P, Black DW, et al: Multicenter double-blind comparison of sertraline and desipramine for concurrent obsessive-compulsive and major depressive disorders. Arch Gen Psychiatry 57:76–82, 2000

Hollander E, Kwon JH, Stein DJ, et al: Obsessive-compulsive and spectrum disorders: overview and quality of life issues. J Clin Psychiatry 57 (suppl 8):3–6, 1996

Institute of Medicine: Treatment of PTSD: An Assessment of the Evidence. Washington, DC, National Academy of Sciences/National Academies Press, 2007

Ipser JC, Kariuki CM, Stein DJ: Pharmacotherapy for social anxiety disorder: a systematic review. Exp Rev Neurother 8:235–257, 2008

Irons J: Fluvoxamine in the treatment of anxiety disorders. Neuropsychiatr Dis Treat 1:289–299, 2005

Kapczinski FFK, Silva de Lima M, dos Santos Souza JJSS, et al: Antidepressants for generalized anxiety disorder. Cochrane Database of Systematic Reviews 2003, Issue 2. Art. No.: CD003592. DOI: 10.1002/14651858.CD003592.

Katz RJ, DeVeaugh-Geiss J, Landau P, et al: Clomipramine in obsessive-compulsive disorder. Biol Psychiatry 28:401–414, 1990

Katzelnick DJ, Kobak KA, Greist JH, et al: Sertraline for social phobia: a double-blind, placebo-controlled crossover study. Am J Psychiatry 152:1368–1371, 1995

Kendler KS: Twin studies of psychiatric illness: an update. Arch Gen Psychiatry 58:1005–1014, 2001

Kendler KS, Gardner CO, Gatz M, et al: The sources of co-morbidity between major depression and generalized anxiety disorder in a Swedish national twin sample. Psychol Med 37:453–462, 2007

Kent JM: SNaRIs, NaSSAs, and NaRIs: new agents for the treatment of depression. Lancet 355:911–918, 2000

Kessler RC, McGonagle KA, Zhao S, et al: Lifetime and 12-month prevalence of DSM-III-R psychiatric disorders in the United States: results from the National Comorbidity Survey. Arch Gen Psychiatry 51:8–19, 1994

Kessler RC, Berglund P, Demler O, et al: Lifetime prevalence and age-of-onset distributions of DSM-IV disorders in the National Comorbidity Survey Replication. Arch Gen Psychiatry 62:593–602, 2005a

Kessler RC, Chiu WT, Demler O, et al: Prevalence, severity, and comorbidity of 12-month DSM-IV disorders in the National Comorbidity Survey Replication. Arch Gen Psychiatry 62:617–627, 2005b

Klein DF: Delineation of two drug-responsive anxiety syndromes. Psychopharmacologia 17:397–408, 1964

Kobak KA, Greist JH, Jefferson JW, et al: Fluoxetine in social phobia: a double-blind, placebo-controlled pilot study. J Clin Psychopharmacol 22:257–262, 2002

Koran LM, Gamel NN, Choung HW, et al: Mirtazapine for obsessive-compulsive disorder: an open trial followed by double-blind discontinuation. J Clin Psychiatry 66:515–520, 2005

Kosten TR, Frank JB, Dan E, et al: Pharmacotherapy for posttraumatic stress disorder using phenelzine or imipramine. J Nerv Ment Dis 179:366–370, 1991

Kumar S, Malone D: Panic disorder. Clin Evid (Online) pii:1010, 2008

Lader M, Stender K, Bürger V, et al: Efficacy and tolerability of escitalopram in 12- and 24-week treatment of social anxiety disorder: randomised, double-blind, placebo-controlled, fixed-dose study. Depress Anxiety 19:241–248, 2004

Leinonen E, Lepola U, Kuponen H, et al: Citalopram controls phobic symptoms in patients with panic disorder: randomized controlled trial. J Psychiatry Neurosci 25:25–32, 2000

Lenze EJ, Mulsant BH, Shear MK, et al: Efficacy and tolerability of citalopram in the treatment of late-life anxiety disorders: results from an 8-week randomized, placebo-controlled trial. Am J Psychiatry 162:146–150, 2005

Lenze EJ, Rollman BL, Shear MK, et al: Escitalopram for older adults with generalized anxiety disorder: a randomized controlled trial. JAMA 301:295–303, 2009

Lepola UM, Wade AG, Leinonen EV, et al: A controlled, prospective, 1-year trial of citalopram in the treatment of panic disorder. J Clin Psychiatry 59:528–534, 1998

Lepola U, Bergtholdt B, St Lambert J, et al: Controlled-release paroxetine in the treatment of patients with social anxiety disorder. J Clin Psychiatry 65:222–229, 2004

Liebowitz MR, Schneier F, Campeas R, et al: Phenelzine vs atenolol in social phobia: a placebo-controlled comparison. Arch Gen Psychiatry 49:290–300, 1992

Liebowitz MR, Stein MB, Tancer M, et al: A randomized, double-blind, fixed-dose comparison of paroxetine and placebo in the treatment of generalized social anxiety disorder. J Clin Psychiatry 63:66–74, 2002

Liebowitz MR, DeMartinis NA, Weihs K, et al: Efficacy of sertraline in severe generalized social anxiety disorder: results of a double-blind, placebo-controlled study. J Clin Psychiatry 64:785–792, 2003

Liebowitz MR, Gelenberg AJ, Munjack D, et al: Venlafaxine extended release vs placebo and paroxetine in social anxiety disorder. Arch Gen Psychiatry 62:190–198, 2005a

Liebowitz MR, Mangano RM, Bradwein J, et al: A randomized controlled trial of venlafaxine extended release in generalized social anxiety disorder. J Clin Psychiatry 66:238–247, 2005b

Liebowitz MR, Asnis G, Mangano R, et al: A double-blind, placebo-controlled, parallel-group, flexible-dose study of venlafaxine extended release capsules in adult outpatients with panic disorder. J Clin Psychiatry 70:550–561, 2009

Lochner C, Hemmings SM, Kinnear CJ, et al: Gender in obsessive-compulsive disorder: clinical and genetic findings. Eur Neuropsychopharmacol 14:105–113, 2004

Londborg PD, Hegel MT, Goldstein S, et al: Sertraline treatment of posttraumatic stress disorder: results of 24 weeks of open-label continuation treatment. J Clin Psychiatry 62:325–331, 2001

Lydiard RB, Morton WA, Emmanuel NP, et al: Preliminary report: placebo-controlled, double-blind study of the clinical and metabolic effects of desipramine in panic disorder. Psychopharmacol Bull 29:183–188, 1993

March JS, Entusah AR, Rynn M, et al: A randomized controlled trial of venlafaxine ER versus placebo in pediatric social anxiety disorder. Biol Psychiatry 62:1149–1154, 2007

Marshall RD, Beebe KL, Oldham M, et al: Efficacy and safety of paroxetine treatment for chronic PTSD: a fixed-dose, placebo-controlled study. Am J Psychiatry 158:1982–1988, 2001

Marshall RD, Lewis-Fernandez R, Blanco C, et al: A controlled trial of paroxetine for chronic PTSD, dissociation, and interpersonal problems in mostly minority adults. Depress Anxiety 24:77–84, 2007

Martenyi F, Brown EB, Zhang H, et al: Fluoxetine vs. placebo in prevention of relapse in post-traumatic stress disorder. Br J Psychiatry 181:315–320, 2002

Martenyi F, Brown EB, Caldwell CD: Failed efficacy of fluoxetine in the treatment of posttraumatic stress disorder: results of a fixed-dose, placebo-controlled study. J Clin Psychopharmacol 27:166–170, 2007

Mavissakalian MR: Imipramine vs. sertraline in panic disorder: 24-week treatment completers. Ann Clin Psychiatry 15:171–180, 2003

Meoni P, Salinas E, Brault Y, et al: Pattern of symptom improvement following treatment with venlafaxine XR in patients with generalized anxiety disorder. J Clin Psychiatry 62:888–893, 2001

Mitte K: A meta-analysis of the efficacy of psycho- and pharmacotherapy in panic disorder with and without agoraphobia. J Affect Disord 88:27–45, 2005

Mitte K, Noack P, Steil R, et al: A meta-analytic review of the efficacy of drug treatment in generalized anxiety disorder. J Clin Psychopharmacol 25:141–150, 2005

Modigh K, Westberg P, Eriksson E: Superiority of clomipramine over imipramine in the treatment of panic disorder: a placebo-controlled trial. J Clin Psychopharmacol 12:251–261, 1992

Montgomery SA, Kasper S, Stein DJ, et al: Citalopram 20 mg, 40 mg and 60 mg are all effective and well tolerated compared with placebo in obsessive-compulsive disorder. Int Clin Psychopharmacol 16:75–86, 2001

Montgomery SA, Tobias K, Zornberg GL, et al: Efficacy and safety of pregabalin in the treatment of generalized anxiety disorder: a 6-week, multicenter, randomized, double-blind, placebo-controlled comparison of pregabalin and venlafaxine. J Clin Psychiatry 67:771–782, 2006

Mosing MA, Gordon SD, Medland SE, et al: Genetic and environmental influences on the co-morbidity between depression, panic disorder, agoraphobia, and social phobia: a twin study. Depress Anxiety 26:1004–1011, 2009

Mountjoy CQ, Roth M, Garside RF, et al: A clinical trial of phenelzine in anxiety depressive and phobic neuroses. Br J Psychiatry 131:486–492, 1977

Muehlbacher M, Nickel MK, Nickel C, et al: Mirtazapine treatment of social phobia in women: a randomized, double-blind, placebo-controlled study. J Clin Psychopharmacol 25:580–583, 2005

Nardi AE, Lopes FL, Valença AM, et al: Double-blind comparison of 30 and 60 mg tranylcypromine daily in patients with panic disorder comorbid with social anxiety disorder. Psychiatry Res 175:260–265, 2010

Neylan TC, Lenoci M, Maglione ML, et al: The effect of nefazodone on subjective and objective sleep quality in posttraumatic stress disorder. J Clin Psychiatry 64:445–450, 2003

Nicolini H, Arnold P, Nestadt G, et al: Overview of genetics and obsessive-compulsive disorder. Psychiatry Res 170:7–14, 2009

Pallanti S, Quercioli L, Bruscoloi M, et al: Response acceleration with mirtazapine augmentation of citalopram in obsessive-compulsive disorder patients without comorbid depression: a pilot study. J Clin Psychiatry 65:1394–1399, 2004

Piccinelli M, Pini S, Bellantuono C, et al: Efficacy of drug treatment in obsessive-compulsive disorder: a meta-analytic review. Br J Psychiatry 166:424–443, 1995

Pollack MH, Worthington JJ 3rd, Otto MV, et al: Venlafaxine for panic disorder: results from a double-blind, placebo-controlled study. Psychopharmacol Bull 32:667–670, 1996

Pollack M, Mangano R, Entsuah R, et al: A randomized controlled trial of venlafaxine ER and paroxetine in the treatment of outpatients with panic disorder. Psychopharmacology (Berl) 194:233–242, 2007

Ravizza L, Maina G, Bogetto F, et al: Episodic and chronic obsessive-compulsive disorder. Depress Anxiety 6:154–158, 1997

Rickels K, Downing R, Schweizer E, et al: Antidepressants for the treatment of generalized anxiety disorder: a placebo-controlled comparison of imipramine, trazodone, and diazepam. Arch Gen Psychiatry 50:884–895, 1993

Rickels K, Mangano R, Khan A, et al: A double-blind, placebo-controlled study of a flexible dose of venlafaxine ER in adult outpatients with generalized social anxiety disorder. J Clin Psychopharmacol 24:488–496, 2004

Rickels K, Rynn M, Ivengar M, et al: Remission of generalized anxiety disorder: a review of the paroxetine clinical trials database. J Clin Psychiatry 67:41–47, 2006

Rocca P, Fonzo V, Scotta M, et al: Paroxetine efficacy in the treatment of generalized anxiety disorder. Acta Psychiatr Scand 95:444–450, 1997

Rothbaum BO, Davidson JR, Stein DL, et al: A pooled analysis of gender and trauma-type effects on responsiveness to treatment of PTSD with venlafaxine extended release or placebo. J Clin Psychiatry 69:1529–1539, 2008

Roy A, Sarchiopone M, Carli V: Gene-environment interaction and suicidal behavior. J Psychiatr Pract 15:282–288, 2009

Roy-Byrne PP, Cowley DS: Course and outcome in panic disorder: a review of recent follow-up studies. Anxiety 1:151–160, 1994

Ruscio AM, Chiu WT, Roy-Byrne P, et al: Broadening the definition of generalized anxiety disorder: effects on prevalence and associations with other disorders in the National Comorbidity Survey Replication. J Anxiety Disord 21:662–676, 2007

Sarchiapone M, Amore M, De Risio S, et al: Mirtazapine in the treatment of panic disorder: an open-label trial. Int Clin Psychopharmacol 18:35–38, 2003

Sareen J, Cox BJ, Clara I, et al: The relationship between anxiety disorders and physical disorders in the U.S. National Comorbidity Survey. Depress Anxiety 21:193–202, 2005

Sasson Y, Iancu I, Fux M, et al: A double-blind crossover comparison of clomipramine and desipramine in the treatment of panic disorder. Eur Neuropsychopharmacol 9:191–196, 1999

Schneier FR, Johnson J, Hornig CD, et al: Social phobia: comorbidity and morbidity in an epidemiologic sample. Arch Gen Psychiatry 49:282–288, 1992

Sheehan DV, Ballenger J, Jacobsen G: Treatment of endogenous anxiety with phobic, hysterical, and hypochondriacal symptoms. Arch Gen Psychiatry 37:51–59, 1980

Sheehan DV, Davidson J, Manschreck T, et al: Lack of efficacy of a new antidepressant (bupropion) in the treatment of panic disorder with phobias. J Clin Psychopharmacol 3:28–31, 1983

Simon NM, Emmanuel N, Ballenger J, et al: Bupropion sustained release for panic disorder. Psychopharmacol Bull 37(4):66–72, 2003

Simon NM, Otto MW, Worthington JJ, et al: Next-step strategies for panic disorder refractory to initial pharmacotherapy: a 3-phase randomized clinical trial. J Clin Psychiatry 70:1563–1570, 2009

Simpson HB, Schneier FR, Campeas RB, et al: Imipramine in the treatment of social phobia. J Clin Psychopharmacol 18:132–135, 1998a

Simpson HB, Schneier FR, Marshall RD, et al: Low dose selegiline (L-deprenyl) in social phobia. Depress Anxiety 7:126–129, 1998b

Simpson HB, Foa EB, Liebowitz MR, et al: A randomized, controlled trial of cognitive-behavioral therapy for augmenting pharmacotherapy in obsessive-compulsive disorder. Am J Psychiatry 165:621–630, 2008

Skoog G, Skoog I: A 40-year follow-up of patients with obsessive-compulsive disorder [see comments]. Arch Gen Psychiatry 56:121–127, 1999

Solyom C, Solyom L, LaPierre Y, et al: Phenelzine and exposure in the treatment of phobias. Biol Psychiatry 16:239–247, 1981

Solyom L, Heseltine GF, McClure DJ, et al: Behaviour therapy versus drug therapy in the treatment of phobic neurosis. Can Psychiatr Assoc J 18:25–32, 1973

Soomro GM, Altman DG, Rajagopal S, et al: Selective serotonin re-uptake inhibitors (SSRIs) versus placebo for obsessive compulsive disorder (OCD). Cochrane Database of Systematic Reviews 2008, Issue 1. Art. No.: CD001765. DOI: 10.1002/14651858.CD001765.pub3.

Stahl SM, Gergel I, Li D: Escitalopram in the treatment of panic disorder: a randomized, double-blind, placebo-controlled trial. J Clin Psychiatry 64:1322–1327, 2003

Stein DJ, Davidson J, Seedat S, et al: Paroxetine in the treatment of post-traumatic stress disorder: pooled analysis of placebo-controlled studies. Expert Opin Pharmacother 4:1829–1838, 2003a

Stein DJ, Westenberg HG, Yang H, et al: Fluvoxamine CR in the long-term treatment of social anxiety disorder: the 12- to 24-week extension phase of a multicentre, randomized, placebo-controlled trial. Int J Neuropsychopharmacol 6:317–323, 2003b

Stein DJ, Ipser JC, van Balkom AJ. Pharmacotherapy for social anxiety disorder. Cochrane Database of Systematic Reviews 2004, Issue 4. Art. No.: CD001206. DOI: 10.1002/14651858.CD001206.pub2.

Stein DJ, Ipser JC, Seedat S: Pharmacotherapy for posttraumatic stress disorder (PTSD). Cochrane Database of Systematic Reviews 2006a, Issue 1. Art. No.: CD002795. DOI: 10.1002/14651858.CD002795.pub2.

Stein DJ, van der Kolk BA, Austin C, et al: Efficacy of sertraline in posttraumatic stress disorder secondary to interpersonal trauma or childhood abuse. Ann Clin Psychiatry 18:243–249, 2006b

Stein DJ, Carey PD, Lochner C, et al: Escitalopram in obsessive-compulsive disorder: response of symptom dimensions to pharmacotherapy. CNS Spectr 13:492–498, 2008

Stein DJ, Pedersen R, Rothbaum PO, et al: Onset of activity and time to response on individual CAPS-SX17 items in patients treated for post-traumatic stress disorder with venlafaxine ER: a pooled analysis. Int J Neuropsychopharmacol 12:23–31, 2009

Stein MB, Liebowitz MR, Lydiard RB, et al: Paroxetine treatment of generalized social phobia (social anxiety disorder): a randomized controlled trial. JAMA 280:708–713, 1998

Stein MB, Fyer AJ, Davidson JR, et al: Fluvoxamine treatment of social phobia (social anxiety disorder): a double-blind, placebo-controlled study. Am J Psychiatry 156:756–760, 1999

Tucker P, Potter-Kimball R, Wyatt DB, et al: Can physiologic assessment and side effects tease out differences in PTSD trials? A double-blind comparison of citalopram, sertraline, and placebo. Psychopharmacol Bull 37:135–149, 2003

Tyrer P, Candy J, Kelly D: A study of the clinical effects of phenelzine and placebo in the treatment of phobic anxiety. Psychopharmacologia 32:237–254, 1973

Van Ameringen MA, Lane RM, Walker JR, et al: Sertraline treatment of generalized social phobia: a 20-week, double-blind, placebo-controlled study. Am J Psychiatry 158:275–281, 2001

Van Ameringen M, Mancini C, Oakman J, et al: Nefazodone in the treatment of generalized social phobia: a randomized, placebo-controlled trial. J Clin Psychiatry 68:288–295, 2007

van Apeldoorn FJ, Timmerman ME, Mersch PP, et al: A randomized trial of cognitive-behavioral therapy or selective serotonin reuptake inhibitor or both combined for panic disorder with or without agoraphobia: treatment results through 1-year follow-up. J Clin Psychiatry 71:574–586, 2010

van der Kolk BA, Dreyfuss D, Michaels M, et al: Fluoxetine in posttraumatic stress disorder. J Clin Psychiatry 55:517–522, 1994

van der Kolk BA, Spinazzola J, Blaustein ME, et al: A randomized clinical trial of eye movement desensitization and reprocessing (EMDR), fluoxetine, and pill placebo in the treatment of posttraumatic stress disorder: treatment effects and long-term maintenance. J Clin Psychiatry 68:37–46, 2007

Versiani M, Nardi AE, Mundim FD, et al: Pharmacotherapy of social phobia: a controlled study with moclobemide and phenelzine. Br J Psychiatry 161:353–360, 1992

Vulink NC, Denys D, Westenberg HG: Bupropion for patients with obsessive-compulsive disorder: an open-label, fixed-dose study. J Clin Psychiatry 66:228–230, 2005

Waxman D: The management of phobic disorders using clomipramine (Anafranil). J Int Med Res 5(suppl):24–31, 1977

Wittchen HU, Zhao S, Kessler RC, et al: DSM-III-R generalized anxiety disorder in the National Comorbidity Survey. Arch Gen Psychiatry 51:355–364, 1994

Wittchen HU, Carter RM, Pfister H, et al: Disabilities and quality of life in pure and comorbid generalized anxiety disorder and major depression in a national survey. Int Clin Psychopharmacol 15:319–328, 2000

Yeh YW, Chen CH, Kuo SC, et al: High-dose duloxetine for treatment-resistant obsessive-compulsive disorder: a case report with sustained full remission. Clin Neuropharmacol 32:174–176, 2009

Zhang W, Davidson JR: Post-traumatic stress disorder: an evaluation of existing pharmacotherapies and new strategies. Expert Opin Pharmacother 8:1861–1870, 2007

Zitrin CM, Klein DF, Woerner MG, et al: Treatment of phobias, I: comparison of imipramine hydrochloride and placebo. Arch Gen Psychiatry 40:125–138, 1983

CHAPTER 4

Schizophrenia and Schizoaffective Disorder

Rajiv Radhakrishnan, M.B.B.S., M.D.
Deepak Cyril D'Souza, M.B.B.S., M.D.

SCHIZOPHRENIA is a heterogeneous disorder of as yet obscure etiology. Adding another layer of complexity is the presence of comorbidities. Depression and anxiety are often associated with schizophrenia. The rate of comorbidity is estimated to be as high as 50% for depression, 29% for posttraumatic stress disorder, 23% for obsessive-compulsive disorder (OCD), and 15% for panic disorder (Buckley et al. 2009). About 36% of patients develop depressive symptoms within 12 months of an acute psychotic episode (Birchwood et al. 2000), and among individuals diagnosed with chronic schizophrenia, 60% had experienced at least one depressive episode over their lifetime (Martin et al. 1985).

Among individuals with schizophrenia, those with concurrent depressive symptoms have poorer long-term functional outcomes than those without depression (Conley et al. 2007). Schizophrenia patients with depression are significantly more likely to use mental health services (emergency psychiatric services, sessions with psychiatrists), adding to the economic burden of the illness (Conley et al. 2007). They are also more likely to be a safety concern (violent, arrested, victimized, or suicidal) and to have greater substance-related problems (Conley et al. 2007). Overall, they report poorer life satisfaction, quality of life, mental functioning, quality of family relationships, and medication adherence (Conley 2009). These negative outcomes underscore a need for specific treatment interventions. An improvement in mood state appears to be associated with improvement in functional outcomes.

Negative symptoms also influence functional outcome in patients with schizophrenia (Milev et al. 2005; Rosenheck et al. 2006). Unfortunately, despite half a century of psychopharmacological research, the quest for drugs that can improve negative symptoms continues.

Depression and negative symptoms are the primary reasons that antidepressants have been used in patients with schizophrenia. In this chapter, we examine the overlap between the dimensions of negative symptoms, depressive symptoms, and extrapyramidal symptoms; review the literature regarding the use of antidepressants in schizophrenia; and draw attention to specific considerations in combining antipsychotics with antidepressants. Notably, the available evidence on the use of antidepressants in patients with schizophrenia is almost exclusively (with the exception of trimipramine) from the use of antidepressants in conjunction with antipsychotics and not the use of antidepressants alone.

Overlap Between Dimensions in Schizophrenia

The overlap in the phenomenology of depression, negative symptoms, and extrapyramidal symptoms (Figure 4–1) is especially relevant to any discussion about antidepressants in schizophrenia. A significant overlap occurs between depressive symptoms and negative symptoms of schizophrenia (Lindenmayer and Kay 1989). A number of symptoms, including anhedonia, amotivation, social withdrawal, blunted affect, and poor concentration, are observed in both depression and negative symptom syndrome and, furthermore, represent core phenomena of the two syndromes. The overlap in phenomenology makes it challenging to differentiate the two syndromes.

Negative symptoms may be categorized into *primary* negative symptoms, which are thought to be part of a core deficit syndrome, and *secondary* negative symptoms, which may be symptoms that are secondary to depression, extra-

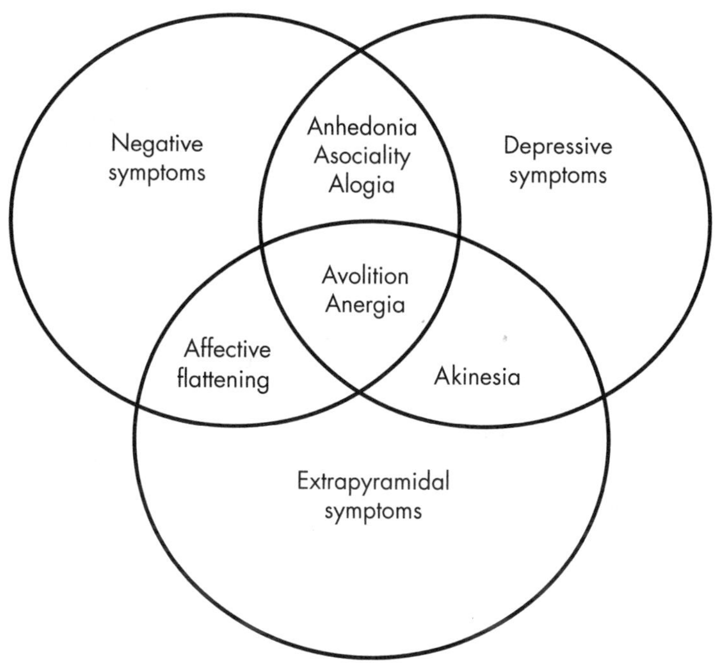

FIGURE 4–1. Overlap between symptom dimensions of schizophrenia.

pyramidal side effects of antipsychotic medication, or a psychological reaction to the experience of positive symptoms such as grief or demoralization (Carpenter et al. 1985). Core primary negative symptoms are considered to be intrinsic to the disease process and hence unresponsive to medication, whereas secondary negative symptoms can be ameliorated by treating the underlying cause (e.g., treatment of extrapyramidal symptoms with anticholinergic drugs or adjusted dosage of antipsychotic medication, treatment of depressive symptoms with antidepressants or cognitive-behavioral therapy).

One way to differentiate negative symptoms from depressive symptoms is to examine for the presence of clinical features of low mood, guilt, poor self-esteem, and appetitive symptoms such as insomnia and anorexia, all of which are more characteristic of depressive symptoms than negative symptoms (Andreasen 1998). Another clue to diagnosing depressive symptoms in a patient who has schizophrenia is the temporal correlation between the onset of depressive symptoms and a clear psychosocial stressor preceding it, even though not all episodes of depression are necessarily linked to psychosocial stressors.

Side effects of antipsychotic medication, such as extrapyramidal side effects and drowsiness, can also mimic negative symptoms, such as blunted affect, avolition, and anergia (Burrows 1998). Antipsychotic-related extrapyramidal symptoms include treatment-emergent side effects, such as akinesia, bradykinesia, rigidity, and the more chronic tardive syndromes.

Because akinesia is not a hallmark of depression or negative symptoms, the presence of akinesia indicates that the symptoms are due to drug-induced parkinsonism (Fleischhacker 1998). Another strategy that may help tease apart extrapyramidal symptoms from depression or negative symptoms is a challenge with an anticholinergic agent or reduction in the dosage of the antipsychotic. Symptoms that improve with either or both of these strategies are more likely to be due to extrapyramidal side effects than to depressive symptoms or primary negative symptoms.

Because of the significant overlap in the phenomenology of negative symptoms, depression, and drug-induced parkinsonism, even experienced clinicians have difficulty differentiating these syndromes. Also, these three syndromes are not mutually exclusive and often occur concurrently. Recognition of the overlap in these symptom dimensions may aid the clinician in deciding when treatment with an antidepressant could be of use.

Postpsychotic Depression and Depression in Schizoaffective Disorder

Following the initial description of the depressive syndrome by Bleuler in 1911, there have been many efforts to define the syndrome in schizophrenia. Mayer-Gross (1920), for example, described despair or denial of the future as a psychological reaction to psychosis.

Postpsychotic depression gained the status of a syndrome following the work of McGlashan and Carpenter (1976), but the DSM-IV-TR (American Psychiatric Association 2000) does not include it in the main classification. Instead, the DSM-IV-TR diagnostic criteria for depression in schizophrenia, called *postpsychotic depressive disorder of schizophrenia,* appear in the appendix titled "Criteria Sets and Axes Provided for Further Study." The clinical picture of postpsychotic depression is thought to be distinct from depression. Postpsychotic depression is reported to occur in approximately 25% of patients hospitalized with an acute psychotic episode, usually within 6 months of the florid psychosis. It appears less common in chronically ill patients with acute exacerbations. The clinical picture most frequently resembles that of retarded (and, less often, agitated) depression with frequent somatic complaints and complaints of emptiness, or lack of feelings. Typically, patients become socially isolated yet are found to constantly demand care and attention from all around them. Suicidal ideas and acts are common, and there is the added risk of patients discontinuing treatment during this phase.

Regardless of the distinction between depression and postpsychotic depression, the clinician needs to remember that depression can occur in all phases of schizophrenia or schizoaffective disorder. Also, the temporal association to the acute episode may be less relevant or useful in helping clinicians differentiate between the two nosological entities (Bressan et al. 2003).

Although defining a separate entity such as postpsychotic depression may alert clinicians to the possibility of depression masquerading as akinesia or negative symptoms in the phase following the acute episode, the identification and treatment of depression in any phase of schizophrenia or schizoaffective disorder remains important.

Review of Evidence for Use of Antidepressants in Schizophrenia

In the following text, we review the use of tricyclic antidepressants (TCAs), selective serotonin reuptake inhibitors (SSRIs), monoamine oxidase inhibitors (MAOIs), and other antidepressants in patients with schizophrenia. Table 4–1 summarizes findings from the studies done on the topic.

Tricyclic Antidepressants

The early studies of the addition of TCAs to typical antipsychotics were not very encouraging. TCAs were found to be ineffective during the acute phase of psychosis, when prominent positive symptoms dominate the clinical picture; to result in a modest improvement in depressive symptoms but not in negative symptoms; and to be associated with a low risk of exacerbation of psychosis (reviewed in Plasky 1991). In this section, we examine the more current literature on individual TCAs.

Trimipramine

The TCA trimipramine is interesting in that apart from being an antidepressant, it has been evaluated as monotherapy for the treatment of psychosis. It was introduced in 1962, five years after imipramine. Trimipramine is unique from other drugs in this class in that it neither inhibits the reuptake of serotonin or norepinephrine nor results in the characteristic alterations seen with

TABLE 4–1. Use of antidepressants in schizophrenia

Study	Target	Medication	Dosage (duration)	Design	*N*	Results	Side effects
TCAs							
Bender et al. 2003	Positive symptoms	Trimipramine monotherapy	300–400 mg/day (5 weeks)	DBRCT	95	No better than active control (perazine)	Well tolerated
Siris et al. 1994	Depressive symptoms	Imipramine maintenance	233±72 mg/day (1 year)	DBRCT	24	More relapse among patients receiving placebo	Well tolerated
Siris et al. 2000	Depressive symptoms	Imipramine maintenance	50 mg/day→ 200 mg/day (6 weeks)	DBRCT	70	CGI Global Improvement score superior in imipramine group but not statistically significant	Well tolerated
Berman et al. 1995	Obsessive-compulsive symptoms	Clomipramine add-on	250 mg/day (13 weeks)	DBRCT	6	Improvement on Y-BOCS and PANSS with clomipramine	Dry mouth and weight gain in 2 subjects, respectively
Prusoff et al. 1979	Depressive symptoms	Amitriptyline add-on	100–200 mg/day (4 months)	DBRCT	40	Improvement in depressive symptoms on Ham-D	Worsening of thought disorder on BPRS
Johnson 1981	Depressive symptoms	Nortriptyline add-on	75–150 mg/day (5 weeks)	DBRCT	50	No improvement in depressive symptoms	

TABLE 4–1. Use of antidepressants in schizophrenia *(continued)*

Study	Target	Medication	Dosage (duration)	Design	*N*	Results	Side effects
SSRIs							
Sepehry et al. 2007	Negative symptoms	SSRI add-on	NA	Meta-analysis	11 RCT	Within a random-effects model, a nonsignificant composite effect size estimate for (end point) negative symptoms was obtained (N=393; adjusted Hedges' g=0.178; P=0.191). However, when studies were divided according to severity of illness, a moderate and significant effect size emerged for the studies involving so-called chronic patients (N=274; adjusted Hedges' g=0.386; P=0.014).	No global support for an improvement in negative symptoms with SSRI augmentation therapy in schizophrenia

TABLE 4–1. Use of antidepressants in schizophrenia *(continued)*

STUDY	TARGET	MEDICATION	DOSAGE (DURATION)	DESIGN	*N*	RESULTS	SIDE EFFECTS
SSRIs *(continued)*							
Silver and Nassar 1992	Negative symptoms	Fluvoxamine add-on	50 mg/day→ 100 mg/day (5 weeks)	DBRCT	30	Significant improvement in negative symptoms	Well tolerated
Silver and Shmugliakov 1998	Negative symptoms	Fluvoxamine vs. maprotiline add-on	50 mg/day→ 100 mg/day (6 weeks)	DBRCT	25	Significant improvement in negative symptoms with fluvoxamine	Well tolerated
Silver et al. 2000	Negative symptoms and positive symptoms	Fluvoxamine add-on	50 mg/day→ 100 mg/day (6 weeks)	DBRCT	53	Significant improvement in negative symptoms with fluvoxamine; no change in positive symptoms	Well tolerated
Reznik and Sirota 2000	Obsessive-compulsive symptoms	Fluvoxamine add-on	100 mg/day→ 200 mg/day (8 weeks)	Open RCT	30	Improvement on Y-BOCS and PANSS with fluvoxamine	Well tolerated
Shim et al. 2003	Positive and negative symptoms	Fluoxetine add-on to haloperidol	20 mg/day→ 60 mg/day (12 weeks)	DBRCT	17	No better than placebo	Worsening of extrapyramidal symptoms in some

TABLE 4–1. Use of antidepressants in schizophrenia *(continued)*

Study	Target	Medication	Dosage (duration)	Design	*N*	Results	Side effects
SSRIs *(continued)*							
Spina et al. 1994	Negative symptoms	Fluoxetine add-on to typical antipsychotics	20 mg/day (12 weeks)	DBRCT	34	Improvement in negative symptoms and depressive symptoms	Well tolerated
Goff et al. 1995	Negative symptoms	Fluoxetine add-on to typical depot antipsychotics	20 mg/day (6 weeks)	DBRCT	20	Improvement in negative symptoms	Well tolerated
Arango et al. 2000	Negative symptoms	Fluoxetine add-on to typical depot antipsychotics	20 mg/day→ 80 mg/day (6 weeks)	DBRCT	32	No better than placebo	Well tolerated
Buchanan et al. 1996	Positive and negative symptoms	Fluoxetine add-on to clozapine	20 mg/day→ 80 mg/day (8 weeks)	DBRCT	33	No better than placebo	Well tolerated

TABLE 4–1. Use of antidepressants in schizophrenia *(continued)*

Study	Target	Medication	Dosage (duration)	Design	*N*	Results	Side effects
SSRIs *(continued)*							
Jockers-Scherübl et al. 2005	Negative symptoms	Paroxetine add-on	20 mg/day → 30 mg/day (12 weeks)	DBRCT	29	Improvement in negative symptoms	Well tolerated
Mulholland et al. 2003	Depressive symptoms	Sertraline add-on	50 mg/day→ 100 mg/day (8 weeks)	DBRCT	26	Improvement in depressive symptoms	Well tolerated
Kirli and Caliskan 1998	Postpsychotic depression	Sertraline vs. imipramine add-on	50 mg/day (5 weeks)	DBRCT	20	Improvement in depressive symptoms in both groups; more rapid onset and lower risk of relapse with sertraline	Better side-effect profile with sertraline
Lee et al. 1998	Positive and negative symptoms	Sertraline add-on to haloperidol	50 mg/day (8 weeks)	DBRCT	36	No better than placebo	Well tolerated

TABLE 4–1. Use of antidepressants in schizophrenia *(continued)*

Study	Target	Medication	Dosage (duration)	Design	*N*	Results	Side effects
SSRIs *(continued)*							
Zisook et al. 2009	Subsyndromal depression	Citalopram vs. placebo (flexible dose)	12 weeks	DBRCT (2 sites)	198	Citalopram was associated with an improvement in depressive ($P=0.002$) and negative ($P=0.049$) symptoms, mental functioning ($P=0.000$), and quality of life ($P=0.046$).	No significant differences between citalopram and placebo in suicidal ideation, positive symptoms, cognition, general medical health, physical functioning, or symptoms of movement disorders; no adverse events more frequent in participants receiving citalopram than in those receiving placebo

TABLE 4–1. Use of antidepressants in schizophrenia *(continued)*

Study	Target	Medication	Dosage (duration)	Design	*N*	Results	Side effects
SSRIs *(continued)*							
Kasckow et al. 2001	Subsyndromal depression in adults ≥40 years	Citalopram vs. placebo	Flexible dose (12 weeks)	DBRCT	198	Citalopram group had significantly higher social skills performance assessment, mental functioning (SF-12 mental component summary score), and quality of life scale scores compared with placebo group.	
Salokangas et al. 1996	Positive and negative symptoms	Citalopram vs. placebo	40 mg/day (12 weeks)	DBRCT	90	No better than placebo	Well tolerated
MAO-B inhibitors							
Bodkin et al. 2005	Negative symptoms	Selegiline vs. placebo	10 mg/day (12 weeks)	DBRCT	67	Improvement in negative symptoms	Well tolerated
Amiri et al. 2008	Positive and negative symptoms	Selegiline vs. placebo add-on to risperidone	10 mg/day (8 weeks)	DBRCT	40	Improvement in positive and negative symptoms	Well tolerated

TABLE 4–1. Use of antidepressants in schizophrenia *(continued)*

Study	Target	Medication	Dosage (duration)	Design	*N*	Results	Side effects
Newer antidepressants							
Berk et al. 2009	Negative symptoms	Mirtazapine vs. placebo add-on	30 mg/day (6 weeks)	DBRCT	40	No improvement in PANSS scores or any secondary outcome measures	Well tolerated
Berk et al. 2001	Negative symptoms	Mirtazapine vs. placebo add-on to haloperidol (5 mg/day)	30 mg/day (6 weeks)	DBRCT	30	Improvement in negative symptoms	2 patients had dry mouth, 4 experienced weight gain, 2 had sedation, and 6 suffered parkinsonism
Joffe et al. 2009	Positive and negative symptoms in partial responders	Mirtazapine vs. placebo add-on to typical antipsychotics	30 mg/day (6 weeks)	DBRCT	39	Improvement in positive and negative symptoms	Well tolerated; hypersedation in 3 patients
Abbasi et al. 2010	Negative symptoms	Mirtazapine vs. placebo add-on to risperidone (6 mg/day)	30 mg/day (8 weeks)	DBRCT	40	Improvement in positive and negative symptoms	Well tolerated

TABLE 4–1. Use of antidepressants in schizophrenia *(continued)*

Study	Target	Medication	Dosage (duration)	Design	*N*	Results	Side effects
Newer antidepressants *(continued)*							
Zoccali et al. 2004	Negative symptoms	Mirtazapine vs. placebo add-on to clozapine	30 mg/day (8 weeks)	DBRCT	24	Improvement in positive and negative symptoms	Mild and transient drowsiness in 3 patients, weight increase of 2 kg in 2 patients
Tsoi et al. 2010	Smoking cessation	Bupropion add-on	NA	Meta-analysis	9 RCTs	Increased rates of smoking abstinence	No worsening of psychosis
Englisch et al. 2010	Post-psychotic depression	Bupropion add-on	300 mg/day (10 weeks)	Case report	1	Improvement in depression and negative symptoms	EEG: diffuse slow waves, beta acceleration
Rusconi et al. 2009	Negative symptoms	Fluvoxamine + olanzapine vs. paroxetine + olanzapine			50	Improvement in negative symptoms (more so with fluvoxamine)	Well tolerated

TABLE 4–1. Use of antidepressants in schizophrenia *(continued)*

Study	Target	Medication	Dosage (duration)	Design	*N*	Results	Side effects
Newer antidepressants *(continued)*							
Poyurovsky et al. 2009	Cognitive function	(Reboxetine 4 mg/day vs. placebo)+ olanzapine (10 mg/day)	(6 weeks)	DBRCT	59	No difference in cognitive performance	Well tolerated
Bloch et al. 2010	Smoking cessation	(Bupropion vs. placebo)+ CBT+ neuroleptics	(14 weeks)	DBRCT	32	Significant difference in both groups; no significant difference between bupropion and placebo	

Note. BPRS=Brief Psychiatric Rating Scale; CBT=cognitive-behavioral therapy; CGI=Clinical Global Impression; DBRCT=double-blind randomized controlled trial; EEG=electrocardiogram; Ham-D=Hamilton Rating Scale for Depression; NA=not applicable (for meta-analyses); PANSS=Positive and Negative Syndrome Scale for Schizophrenia; RCT=randomized controlled trial; SF-12=12-Item Short Form Health Survey; SSRI=selective serotonin reuptake inhibitor; Y-BOCS=Yale-Brown Obsessive Compulsive Scale.

other TCAs such as downregulation of β_1-adrenergic receptors (Hauser et al. 1985; Kopanski et al. 1993) or desensitization of the β-adrenergic receptor–coupled adenylate cyclase system. Trimipramine acts on the dopaminergic system and binds dopamine D_1, D_2, D_3, and D_4 receptors. Although it possesses the tricyclic imidobenzyl ring structure, as do imipramine, clomipramine, and desipramine, trimipramine also possesses an aliphatic chain similar to the phenothiazine neuroleptic levomepromazine. Trimipramine also possesses a receptor-binding profile similar to that of clozapine, binding α_1-adrenergic receptors and serotonergic 5-HT_2 receptors (Gross et al. 1991). Trimipramine has been found to be efficacious in acute schizophrenia in open-label trials (Eikmeier et al. 1990, 1991), but it failed to demonstrate therapeutic equivalence to perazine at dosages of 300–400 mg/day in a randomized controlled trial (RCT) (Bender et al. 2003).

Imipramine

Chronic imipramine treatment was shown to increase amphetamine-induced dopamine release in rat nucleus accumbens (Ichikawa et al. 1998), and this hinted at a possible risk of exacerbation of positive symptoms in schizophrenia. Imipramine had no effect on phencyclidine-induced enhancement of motility in a forced swim test, a putative mouse model of depression in schizophrenia (Noda et al. 1997). However, in a double-blind RCT of antidepressant discontinuation in the maintenance phase (Siris et al. 1994), patients with postpsychotic depression who responded to imipramine plus fluphenazine decanoate/benztropine were less likely to relapse into depression and less likely to experience worsening of psychotic symptoms if the imipramine was continued. An important consideration in interpreting this disparate finding is that in the Siris et al. study, patients were carefully selected for postpsychotic depression, secondary negative symptoms were possibly excluded by the concomitant use of benztropine, and the patients had shown an initial definite improvement with imipramine. In an expansion of their study with a later cohort, Siris et al. (2000) found the benefit of adjunctive imipramine to persist, but the analysis failed to reach statistical significance.

Clomipramine

The superior efficacy of clomipramine in OCD led to its use in patients with schizophrenia and comorbid OCD or "schizo-obsessive" disorder, a separate diagnosis that is being recognized as having a distinct clinical profile (Patel et al. 2010; Rajkumar et al. 2008). In open-label trials, clomipramine (30–300 mg/day) was found to alleviate OCD, reduce the anxiety associated with compulsive rituals (Yaryura-Tobias and Neziroglu 1975), and reduce positive and negative symptoms of schizophrenia in some patients (Zohar et al.

1993), but was associated with an exacerbation of psychosis in other patients (Yaryura-Tobias and Neziroglu 1975; Zohar et al. 1993). Clomipramine was found to be efficacious in a small placebo-controlled trial (Berman et al. 1995). However, the medication's anticholinergic effects, cardiovascular side effects, and weight gain effects have pushed it further down the treatment algorithm (Poyurovsky et al. 2004).

Amitriptyline and Nortriptyline

The early studies of the use of amitriptyline in treatment of depression in schizophrenia were essentially studies that used typical antipsychotics. Prusoff et al. (1979) randomly assigned 40 patients with schizophrenia stabilized on perphenazine to receive 100–200 mg/day of amitriptyline or placebo. Patients who received amitriptyline showed a significant improvement in depression scores as measured on the Hamilton Depression Rating Scale (Ham-D) at 4 months (reduction in anxiety-depression by 55%; $P<0.05$) but at 6-month end point showed a significantly higher rating on thought disorder on the Brief Psychiatric Rating Scale (BPRS). Johnson (1981) subsequently reported a negative study of nortriptyline augmentation in patients with schizophrenia. As a result of these findings, amitriptyline and nortriptyline fell into disfavor as augmentation agents. The emergence of clozapine has led to renewed interest in the use of amitriptyline, albeit for a different indication altogether. Amitriptyline's potent anticholinergic effect has found utility in the treatment of clozapine-induced nocturia and sialorrhoea (Copp et al. 1991; Praharaj and Arora 2007); however, controlled trials for this indication are lacking.

Selective Serotonin Reuptake Inhibitors

SSRIs have been evaluated in the treatment of negative symptoms of schizophrenia. The possible role of serotonergic dysfunction in negative symptoms was suggested by the phenomenological similarities and overlap between negative symptoms and depressive symptoms such as anhedonia, motor retardation, social withdrawal, and apathy (Meltzer 1989). Some studies demonstrated abnormalities in the serotonergic system in patients with schizophrenia, such as alterations in the serotonin transporter (Naylor et al. 1996).

These findings provided the impetus for trials with SSRIs as an augmentation strategy in the treatment of negative symptoms. In a meta-analysis of 11 studies testing the use of SSRIs for negative symptoms in schizophrenia, Sepehry et al. (2007) concluded that 4–16 weeks of treatment with SSRIs had no added benefit compared with placebo. The meta-analysis evaluated adjunctive treatment with fluoxetine (5 RCTs), sertraline (2 RCTs), fluvoxamine (2 RCTs), paroxetine (1 RCT), and citalopram (1 RCT). However, when studies were categorized on the basis of severity of illness (chronic vs. nonchronic), a moderate and significant effect size emerged for the studies involving patients with chronic schizophrenia on end-point measures of negative symptoms. However, a subsequent sensitivity analysis revealed that negative symptoms improved over time, and no difference was found between SSRIs and placebo, even among patients with chronic schizophrenia. These results must be interpreted in light of the fact that the small number of studies and sample heterogeneity can confound the results of a meta-analysis (Davey Smith and Egger 1998).

The following issues are relevant to understanding the research evidence with regard to antidepressant use for negative symptoms of schizophrenia:

1. Different negative symptoms have different propensities and time courses for improvement. In a study of 16 items on the Scale for the Assessment of Negative Symptoms (SANS), Silver (2003) found a differential time course of improvement with fluvoxamine. A significant time × treatment interaction resulted for 11 of the 16 items. The first items to show significant differences between fluvoxamine and placebo (within the first 2 weeks of treatment) were decreased spontaneous movement, poverty of speech, poverty of amount of speech, grooming/hygiene, and physical anergia. Four additional items—poor eye contact, affective nonresponsivity, lack of vocal inflection, and recreational interests—showed significant improvement within 3 weeks, and paucity of gestures and facial expression showed significant improvement within 4 and 5 weeks, respectively.
2. No reliable measure exists to detect changes in specific items of the negative symptom dimension. Total scores on the SANS lack the resolution necessary to detect specific symptom change (Welham et al. 1999).
3. Although some evidence suggests that serotonergic mechanisms may contribute to the neurobiology of negative symptoms (see Silver and Shmugliakov 1998), it is not clear whether all SSRIs are equally efficacious. Individual SSRIs differ in their properties from those of the so-called class.
4. The dosage of an SSRI used for treatment of negative symptoms may be different from that used for antidepressant purposes. For example, in the case of fluvoxamine, the anti–negative symptom dosage is lower than the antidepressant dosage (Silver et al. 2000). The data on other SSRIs are lacking.
5. The type of antipsychotic (typical vs. atypical) with which the SSRI is being combined may be important. For example, the coadministration of haloperidol and fluvoxamine results in unique changes in the γ-aminobutyric acid (GABA), dopamine, and serotonin systems that are not seen with either drug used alone. Interestingly, these changes were similar to those seen with clozapine (Chertkow et al. 2006, 2007).

Individual SSRIs as Add-ons to Antipsychotic Treatment

Fluvoxamine

Studies of the use of the adjunctive fluvoxamine in schizophrenia have focused primarily on negative symptoms and obsessive-compulsive symptoms. The efficacy of add-on fluvoxamine in improving negative symptoms has been evaluated in three controlled studies (reviewed in Silver 2003).

In a study of patients with chronic schizophrenia (N=30), Silver and Nassar (1992) examined the efficacy of adjunctive fluvoxamine in a randomized double-blind design. All the patients were inpatients who had prominent negative symptoms as evidenced by SANS global item scores of 3 or more. The patients were taking typical antipsychotics at stable dosages (mean dose= 474 mg/day chlorpromazine equivalents). Patients were excluded if they had prominent depressive or positive symptoms. Extrapyramidal symptoms were minimized by adjustment of anticholinergic medication 2 weeks prior. Fluvoxamine (50 mg/day in the first week, then 100 mg/day) or placebo was added to the patients' antipsychotic regimen. After 5 weeks, patients who were receiving fluvoxamine showed significant improvement in negative symptom scores (total SANS scores) over patients who were being given placebo. Depressive, extrapyramidal, and positive symptoms did not change in either group.

In another study, Silver and Shmugliakov (1998) compared the efficacy of fluvoxamine versus maprotiline on negative symptoms in patients with chronic schizophrenia. The sample consisted of 25 inpatients with a DSM-III-R (American Psychiatric Association 1987) diagnosis of schizophrenia and prominent negative symptoms (SANS global score of at least moderate). Patients received fluvoxamine or maprotiline (50 mg/day in the first week, then 100 mg/day) for 6 weeks as add-on treatment in a double-blind randomized fashion. The patients were taking typical antipsychotics at a stable dosage (mean dosage= 502 mg/day chlorpromazine equivalents). Patients were assessed for positive symptoms, negative symptoms, depressive symptoms, and extrapyramidal symptoms. Baseline scores were low for depressive, positive, and extrapyramidal symptoms. Compared with the maprotiline group, the fluvoxamine-treated group showed significant improvement in SANS total score and on the items affective flattening and alogia. Neither group demonstrated a change in depressive symptoms, positive symptoms, or extrapyramidal symptoms.

In a third study, Silver et al. (2000) studied the effect of coadministration of fluvoxamine on both positive and negative symptoms. The sample consisted of 53 patients with a DSM-III-R diagnosis of chronic schizophrenia and scores of at least moderate severity (3 or more) on the global items of the Scale for the Assessment of Positive Symptoms (SAPS) and the SANS. The patients were randomly assigned to receive either add-on fluvoxamine (50–100 mg/day) or placebo. Patients had been taking typical antipsychotics for at least 2 months. The diagnosis of depression was an exclusion criterion. Patients in the sample had high baseline SANS and SAPS scores. Fluvoxamine treatment was associated with significant improvement in negative symptoms (SANS total score) compared with placebo. Positive, depressive, and extrapyramidal symptoms did not change with treatment.

Several open-label trials have examined the efficacy of fluvoxamine in combination with atypical antipsychotics. In a study of add-on fluvoxamine with clozapine, Silver et al. (1996) reported improvement on the affective blunting and anhedonia items of the SANS after 6 weeks of add-on treatment with fluvoxamine. The sample consisted of a small number ($n=11$) of inpatients with a DSM-III-R diagnosis of chronic schizophrenia. Patients had persistent negative symptoms despite clozapine treatment (dosage range 300–750 mg/day) and had been undergoing treatment for an average of 1.4 years. Patients received fluvoxamine 25–50 mg/day in the first week; the dosage was then titrated upward, to a maximum of 100 mg/day for 6 weeks. Depressive symptoms (depressive item of the BPRS) did not change with treatment, and the medication was well tolerated.

Lammers et al. (1999) studied 18 psychotic patients taking clozapine in an open protocol. Patients received fluvoxamine 50 mg/day in addition to clozapine, the dosage of which was titrated individually. At the 5-week assessment, significant improvement was found in cognitive speed and BPRS scores, and five patients were considered treatment responders (BPRS reduction >50%); 10 patients went on to remit from psychosis at the time of discharge. The combination was well tolerated, with no excess increase in sedation.

In a study of pharmacokinetics and tolerability, Szegedi et al. (1999) studied the effect of fluvoxamine 50 mg/day added to clozapine in 16 patients with schizophrenia and found improvement in psychopathology. Although serum clozapine levels were markedly increased, the side-effect profile remained relatively unchanged, and the combination of fluvoxamine and clozapine was well tolerated.

In a later pharmacokinetic study, Hiemke et al. (2002) added fluvoxamine to olanzapine in patients with chronic schizophrenia. Five of the seven patients showed an improvement in negative symptoms (change of 20% or more in SANS scores) after 8 weeks.

Takashi et al. (2002) added fluvoxamine to risperidone in 30 patients with schizophrenia who had failed to respond to risperidone alone. The patients demonstrated no significant change in positive or negative factors on the Positive and Negative Syndrome Scale (PANSS) at the 12-week end point.

The utility of fluvoxamine in treatment of obsessive-compulsive symptoms in patients with schizophrenia is reflected in case reports and open trials

(Dwivedi et al. 2002; Poyurovsky et al. 1996). In an open RCT of coadministration of fluvoxamine with antipsychotics in patients who had schizophrenia with prominent obsessive-compulsive symptoms, Reznik and Sirota (2000) found improvement in obsessive-compulsive symptoms and positive symptoms. The sample comprised 30 patients with a DSM-IV diagnosis of schizophrenia. Both at baseline and end point, psychotic symptoms and obsessive-compulsive symptoms were assessed using the PANSS and the Yale-Brown Obsessive Compulsive Scale (Y-BOCS), respectively. Patients who received adjunctive fluvoxamine showed a decrease in scores on both the PANSS (34.3%) and the Y-BOCS (29.4%). No patient experienced a worsening of psychosis.

Fluvoxamine has also been tested for clozapine-induced weight gain with encouraging results (Lu et al. 2004). However, the increase in serum clozapine levels with coadministration warrants concern of an increased risk of adverse effects.

Finally, fluvoxamine is unique among SSRIs in being a potent σ_1 receptor agonist. The endoplasmic reticulum σ_1 receptors are being considered important in neuroprotection and release of neurotransmitters, suggesting a potential role for fluvoxamine in preventing conversion of prodromal subjects to schizophrenia (Hashimoto 2009).

Fluoxetine

In an open trial of 17 patients with chronic schizophrenia who were taking haloperidol, fluoxetine augmentation failed to improve negative symptoms (Shim et al. 2003). Fluoxetine, being a cytochrome P450 (CYP) 2D6 inhibitor, typically increases levels of plasma haloperidol and "reduced haloperidol." However, at study end point, plasma haloperidol and "reduced haloperidol" levels were not significantly different between the two groups in this study.

The efficacy of fluoxetine as an add-on to typical antipsychotics for the treatment of negative symptoms has been evaluated in three controlled studies (Arango et al. 2000; Goff et al. 1995; Spina et al. 1994). Two of the RCTs showed a significant effect, and one showed no improvement.

In the first RCT, Spina et al. (1994) added fluoxetine 20 mg/day or placebo to typical antipsychotics in 34 inpatients with chronic schizophrenia. Patients with moderate to severe depression (Ham-D score >20) were excluded. After 12 weeks of treatment, fluoxetine was found to improve negative symptoms (SANS) and depressive symptoms (Ham-D), without worsening positive symptoms.

In another RCT, Goff et al. (1995) studied the efficacy of add-on fluoxetine 20 mg/day in 41 patients with schizophrenia who were taking stable depot antipsychotics. Patients with depression were excluded, and extrapyramidal symptoms were measured using the Simpson-Angus Scale. Patients received fluoxetine or placebo for 6 weeks after a 2-week placebo lead-in. Scores on the negative symptom subscale of the BPRS were significantly lower for the fluoxetine group at the end point, after adjustment for baseline scores. The negative symptoms were found to improve steadily over the treatment period, suggesting that treatment for a longer duration may have resulted in greater clinical improvement.

In the third RCT, Arango et al. (2000) compared the efficacy of coadministration of flexible-dose fluoxetine in patients with schizophrenia taking stable antipsychotic medication. The sample comprised 32 outpatients with DSM diagnosis of schizophrenia. Patients were required to have minimum positive symptoms (BPRS positive symptom score of at least 8) and negative symptoms (SANS minimum score of 20 or a score of 2 or more on at least one global item). After a 2-week evaluation phase, patients were randomly assigned to receive either add-on fluoxetine or placebo for 8 weeks. Fluoxetine was initiated at 20 mg/day, and clinicians were allowed to increase the dosage based on a clinical judgment of response (mean dose=36.2 mg/day, range=20–80 mg/day). The study did not find a significant difference between the fluoxetine and placebo groups, although the possibility of a Type II error, given the small sample size, cannot be ruled out.

In one of the first double-blind controlled studies of SSRI augmentation of atypical antipsychotics, Buchanan et al. (1996) studied the effect of the addition of fluoxetine to clozapine on residual positive and negative symptoms. The sample comprised 33 patients with schizophrenia who had been taking clozapine (mean dosage=457 mg/day) for at least 6 months. They had a history of partial response to at least two typical antipsychotics from different classes and currently had minimal residual symptoms (BPRS positive symptoms total score of 8, or negative symptoms SANS score of 20, or a score of 2 or more on one or more global items). Patients were randomly assigned to receive either adjunctive fluoxetine or placebo in an 8-week double-blind parallel-group design. Fluoxetine was initiated at 20 mg/day, and that dosage was maintained for the first 3 weeks, and then could be increased at the clinician's discretion to a maximum of 80 mg/day (mean maximum dosage= 48.9 mg/day). The study found no significant improvement in positive, negative, depressive, or obsessive-compulsive symptoms after 8 weeks of treatment. However, the limited efficacy of fluoxetine in this study must be interpreted in light of the low baseline levels of depressive and obsessive-compulsive symptoms in the sample.

Additionally, fluoxetine has been studied for olanzapine-induced weight gain in a double-blind RCT, but with negative results (Bustillo et al. 2003).

Paroxetine

Paroxetine showed promise for improvement of negative symptoms in a small open-label trial (Jockers-Scherübl et al. 2001). In a subsequent double-blind placebo-controlled trial, 29 patients with chronic schizophrenia and a score of

>20 on the negative subscale of the PANSS plus a score >12 on the Ham-D (to exclude depression) were randomly assigned to receive paroxetine (20 mg/day for 4 weeks, followed by 30 mg/day for 8 weeks) or placebo for 12 weeks (Jockers-Scherübl et al. 2005). Those with significant depressive symptoms (Ham-D >12) and significant extrapyramidal symptoms were excluded. At the end point, compared with the control group, the paroxetine group had a significantly lower PANSS total score. Significant improvement occurred on three items—affective blunting, impaired abstract thinking, and lack of spontaneity and flow of conversation—in the paroxetine group compared with the placebo group. The careful exclusion of patients with depression and extrapyramidal symptoms led the authors to opine that paroxetine was efficacious in improving primary negative symptoms.

Sertraline

The efficacy of sertraline for depressive symptoms in patients with chronic schizophrenia was evaluated in a double-blind RCT (Mulholland et al. 2003). Twenty-six subjects with schizophrenia who scored >15 on the Beck Depression Inventory (BDI) and 3 on the depression item of the BPRS were assigned to receive sertraline (50 mg/day for 4 weeks, followed by 100 mg/day for 4 weeks) or placebo for 8 weeks. In an intent-to-treat analysis, the sertraline group had a significant decrease in Ham-D and BDI scores and scored lower on the depression/anxiety items of the BPRS.

Sertraline has also been studied in patients with postpsychotic depression. In a randomized double-blind study of sertraline versus imipramine, 20 patients with schizophrenia and postpsychotic depression were assigned to receive 50 mg/day of sertraline or 150 mg/day of imipramine after a 10-day lead-in period. Subjects were evaluated at 5 weeks. Both drugs were associated with improvement in depressive symptoms, although sertraline had a more rapid onset, had a better side-effect profile, and was associated with a lower risk of relapse of schizophrenia (Kirli et al. 1998).

In an 8-week randomized double-blind trial (Lee et al. 1998), patients with chronic schizophrenia being treated with haloperidol were given sertraline 50 mg/day or placebo. Sertraline was not better than placebo as measured by PANSS and the Clinical Global Impressions (CGI) Scale.

Citalopram

In a two-site, double-blind, placebo-controlled study of citalopram for subsyndromal depression involving 198 middle-aged patients (older than 40 years) with schizophrenia and schizoaffective disorder, Zisook et al. (2009) found that flexible-dose treatment with citalopram resulted in a significant improvement in depressive and negative symptoms, random functioning, and quality of life.

Salokangas et al. (1996) compared citalopram 40 mg/day and placebo added to typical neuroleptics in 90 outpatients with chronic schizophrenia (diagnosed using DSM-III-R) who scored higher than 50 on the PANSS. Total PANSS scores decreased significantly after 12 weeks in both groups, with no statistically significant difference between groups.

In a single-blind trial, citalopram 20–40 mg/day was added to antipsychotics in elderly patients with schizophrenia. At the end of the 10-week study, Kasckow et al. (2001) found no improvement in positive or negative symptoms but some improvement in depressive symptoms.

Citalopram has been evaluated as an adjunct to atypical antipsychotics for the improvement of cognitive deficits of schizophrenia. In a 24-week, randomized, placebo-controlled, crossover-designed study, citalopram 40 mg/day was not found to be better than placebo on any clinical or cognitive measures (Friedman et al. 2005).

Attractive features of citalopram are its relatively safe pharmacological profile and lack of significant pharmacokinetic interactions. Citalopram is a weak inhibitor of CYP2D6 in vitro and has weak or no effects on CYPIA2, CYP2C19, and CYP3A4 (Von Moltke et al. 1999). Unlike most other SSRIs, citalopram does not cause an increase in plasma levels of antipsychotics (Syvälahti et al. 1997).

Monoamine Oxidase Inhibitors

The hypothesis that negative symptoms are a result of dopamine hypofunction makes MAOIs an attractive candidate for treatment of patients with negative symptoms of schizophrenia. MAO-B inhibitors selectively enhance dopaminergic transmission. The selective inhibition of MAO-B without inhibition of MAO-A gives MAO-B inhibitors a safer side-effect profile, because most of the side effects are mediated by inhibition of MAO-A (Finberg and Youdim 2002). The MAO-B inhibitors fared well in several open-label trials (Bodkin et al. 1996; Gupta et al. 1999; Perenyi et al. 1992) but did not yield an adequate response in two double-blind placebo-controlled trials (Goff et al. 1993; Jungerman et al. 1999). Two newer double-blind placebo-controlled studies suggest a potential use for MAO-B inhibitors in the treatment of negative symptoms.

In a 12-week, double-blind, placebo-controlled, multicenter trial of oral selegiline augmentation of antipsychotic medication, 67 subjects with prominent negative symptoms (SANS score >12) participated in a 2-week single-blind placebo run-in, followed by 1:1 random assignment to 12 weeks of treatment with oral selegiline (5 mg bid) or matched placebo (Bodkin et al. 2005). Compared with the placebo group, the selegiline group showed a significant improvement on the SANS summary total, avolition-apathy global, and anhedonia global scores; BPRS total score; and CGI severity and improvement scale scores.

Amiri et al. (2008) reported on an 8-week, randomized, double-blind, placebo-controlled study of selegiline as an add-on to risperidone. The study included 40 patients with chronic schizophrenia and a score of >15 on the negative subscale of the PANSS. Patients did not receive neuroleptics for 1 week prior to entering the study. They were randomly assigned to receive risperidone (6 mg/day) plus selegiline (5 mg bid) or risperidone (6 mg/day) alone for 8 weeks. The selegiline group had significantly lower PANSS negative subscale and PANSS total scores.

Selegiline has also been tested in patients with tardive dyskinesia (Goff et al. 1993) and sexual dysfunction (Kodesh et al. 2003), with negative results.

Other Antidepressants

Mirtazapine

Mirtazapine is the first of a new class of dual-action compounds, the noradrenergic and specific serotonergic antidepressants, whose activity is related to the enhancement of noradrenergic and serotonergic transmission through antagonism of a presynaptic α_2 receptor and antagonism of postsynaptic 5-HT_2 and 5-HT_3 receptors, respectively (de Boer et al. 1988). Mirtazapine may have inverse agonistic effects on neuronal 5-HT_{2C} (Chanrion et al. 2008), in a manner similar to that of some atypical antipsychotics (Rauser et al. 2001). Furthermore, some evidence suggests that α_2-adrenergic receptors have a role in negative symptoms of schizophrenia (Litman et al. 1996).

The utility of mirtazapine has been examined in five double-blind placebo-controlled trials, four of which yielded positive results. The potential use of mirtazapine as augmentation strategy for the treatment of negative symptoms of schizophrenia has been highlighted in a randomized, double-blind, placebo-controlled study (Berk et al. 2001). This study showed a significant decrease in negative symptoms when mirtazapine was added to haloperidol in a group of patients with schizophrenia. In a subsequent double-blind, placebo-controlled study, 40 patients with schizophrenia who were being treated with atypical antipsychotics were given either adjunctive mirtazapine 30 mg/day or placebo. Berk et al. (2009) did not find a significant difference in negative symptoms (PANSS scores) between the two groups. The overlap of receptor occupancy profiles of the atypical antipsychotics and the heterogeneity of the sample may explain these findings.

In a double-blind RCT that explored the efficacy of adjunctive mirtazapine with typical antipsychotics, Joffe et al. (2009) found a robust additive antipsychotic effect with significant improvements in PANSS positive and negative subscale scores.

In a double-blind, placebo-controlled trial of mirtazapine as add-on treatment to risperidone in inpatients in the active phase of chronic schizophrenia with prominent negative symptoms (N=40), mirtazapine 30 mg/day plus risperidone 6 mg/day was superior to risperidone 6 mg/day alone in improving PANSS total score and negative symptoms over 8 weeks (Abbasi et al. 2010). The combination was well tolerated, with no clinically significant side effects.

In an 8-week double-blind placebo-controlled trial in 24 patients with chronic schizophrenia, mirtazapine was found to augment the response to clozapine, as demonstrated by a significant improvement on the SANS avolition/apathy and anhedonia/asociality subscale scores and on the BPRS total score (Zoccali et al. 2004). The authors reported the side effects of mild and transient drowsiness in three patients and a weight increase of 2 kg in two patients.

Finally, a randomized, double-blind, placebo-controlled study has demonstrated the therapeutic effect of low-dose mirtazapine in the treatment of neuroleptic-induced akathisia (Poyurovsky et al. 2003a).

Bupropion

Bupropion is an atypical antidepressant with both dopaminergic and adrenergic actions (Stahl et al. 2004). It acts as a noncompetitive antagonist at the nicotinic acetylcholinergic receptor (Fryer and Lukas 1999). Bupropion may also have an effect on the brain reward system, which may contribute to its action on smoking cessation (Cryan et al. 2003).

Compared with the general population, people with schizophrenia have three times the odds of ever smoking and lower smoking cessation rates (de Leon and Diaz 2005). Furthermore, smokers with schizophrenia may smoke more heavily and extract more nicotine from each cigarette (Williams et al. 2005). Tobacco may also be used to alleviate some of the symptoms in schizophrenia and some of the side effects of antipsychotic medications (Sacco et al. 2004). Using nicotine to "self-medicate," together with the depressive symptoms, drug misuse, disorganized thinking, and poor task persistence in people with schizophrenia, may explain the lower motivation and the greater difficulty for smoking cessation in these individuals (Addington et al. 1997).

In a recent meta-analysis of nine RCTs comparing bupropion with placebo or alternative therapeutic control in adult smokers with schizophrenia, Tsoi et al. (2010) concluded that bupropion increased the rates of smoking abstinence in smokers with schizophrenia without causing an alteration of positive or negative symptoms. George et al. (2008) reported that the combination of bupropion and transdermal nicotine patch was more effective than transdermal nicotine patch alone.

Nefazodone, Mianserin, and Reboxetine

A therapeutic effect on neuroleptic-induced extrapyramidal symptoms and akathisia has been found using nefazodone 100 mg/day (Wynchank and Berk 2003). Mianserin has been evaluated as a possible adjunct for cognitive enhancement of typical antipsychotics, given its marked 5-HT_{2A} antagonistic activity in addition to 5-HT_{2C}, histaminergic (H_1), and α_2-adrenergic blockade (Salzman et al. 1994) and the hypothesis that atypical antipsychotics bring about an improvement in cognitive functioning because of a higher 5-HT_{2A} antagonism. In a double-blind RCT, Poyurovsky et al. (1999) found mianserin 15 mg/day to be significantly better than placebo in improving selective learning and memory. Reboxetine, a selective norepinephrine reuptake inhibitor, failed to improve negative symptoms when added to haloperidol (Schutz and Berk 2001) but has been shown to attenuate olanzapine-induced weight gain in two double-blind RCTs (Poyurovsky et al. 2003a, 2007).

Specific Considerations in Coadministration of Antidepressants and Antipsychotics

Theoretical Rationale for Use of Antidepressants in Schizophrenia

Serotonin-Dopamine Interaction

The dopamine hypothesis of schizophrenia posits that mesolimbic hyperdopaminergia and prefrontal hypodopaminergia contribute to the pathophysiology of positive and negative symptoms, respectively (Davis et al. 1991). The dopaminergic neurons receive innervation from 5-HT fibers arising from cell bodies of the dorsal raphe nuclei and the medial raphe (Van Bockstaele et al. 1994). Among the serotonin receptor subtypes, 5-HT_{1A}, 5-HT_{1B}, 5-HT_{2A}, 5-HT_3, and 5-HT_4 receptors act to facilitate neuronal dopamine function and release, whereas 5-HT_{2C} receptors mediate an inhibitory effect of 5-HT on the basal electrical activity of dopaminergic neurons and on dopamine release (Di Giovanni et al. 2010). One feature differentiating typical from atypical antipsychotics is a preferential increase of dopamine release in the medial prefrontal cortex seen with some atypical antipsychotics; this effect might be relevant for the therapeutic action of atypical antipsychotics on negative symptoms of schizophrenia (Kuroki et al. 1999), although a question that remains debatable is whether atypical antipsychotics improve so-called primary negative symptoms or seemingly improve negative symptoms because of lesser depressive and extrapyramidal symptoms. This release of cortical dopamine requires the facilitation of 5-HT_{1A} receptor stimulation, in addition to simultaneous blockade of 5-HT_{2A} and D_2 receptors (Ichikawa et al. 2001).

Effects on the GABAergic System

Converging lines of evidence, including from postmortem (Benes and Berretta 2001; Hashimoto et al. 2003; Lewis et al. 2005), genetic (reviewed in Charych et al. 2009), and brain imaging studies (Busatto et al. 1997; Schröder et al. 1997; Yoon et al. 2010), suggest that dysfunction of the GABAergic system contributes to the pathophysiology of schizophrenia. 5-HT can modulate dopaminergic neurons indirectly by modifying GABAergic and glutamatergic input to the ventral tegmental area and substantia nigra pars compacta (Di Giovanni et al. 2010). The combination of typical antipsychotics and SSRIs leads to changes in the GABAergic system not seen with either drug alone (Danovich et al. 2010). The protein expression changes that are specific to the combined treatment include glutamic acid decarboxylase 67 and protein kinase C (PKC) beta (Chertkow et al. 2006); the latter showed a similar trend following clozapine treatment. Augmentation of atypical antipsychotics with an SSRI enhances dopamine release. This effect is modulated by specific serotonergic receptors and by tyrosine hydroxylase. Modifications in the GABAergic system occur via glutamate decarboxylase 67, PKC beta, and the receptor for activated C-kinase 1 (Rack1) (reviewed in Chertkow et al. 2009).

Pharmacokinetic Interactions Between Antidepressants and Antipsychotics

Table 4–2 lists pharmacokinetics of atypical antipsychotics. Table 4–3 provides a review of interactions between antipsychotics and antidepressants. The interactions between TCAs and the newer antipsychotics have not been formally evaluated. TCAs have been reported to increase chlorpromazine plasma levels. Antipsychotics such as perphenazine, chlorpromazine, and haloperidol are known to increase the plasma concentrations of antidepressants due to inhibition of the CYP2D6 isoenzyme (Mulsant et al. 1997).

SSRIs are potent inhibitors of CYP2D6, a cytochrome P450 enzyme that is also responsible for the biotransformation of atypical antipsychotics. This

TABLE 4–2. Pharmacokinetics of atypical antipsychotics

Drug	Bioavailability (%)	Protein binding (%)	Volume of distribution (L/kg)	Half-life (hours)	Time to reach steady state (days)	Enzymes responsible for biotransformation[a]	Active metabolites
Clozapine	27–50	>90	2–7	9–17	4–8	***CYP1A2***, CYP2C19, CYP3A4, CYP2D6	*N*-desmethyl-clozapine
Risperidone	70–85	RSP=89 9-OH-RSP=77	1	3–24	4–6	***CYP2D6, CYP3A4***	9-Hydroxy-risperidone
Olanzapine	60	93	16±7	20–70	5–7	***CYP1A2***, CYP2D6	—
Quetiapine	70	83	6.1–8.8	6	2–3	***CYP3A4***	7-Hydroxy-quetiapine 7-Hydroxy-*N*-desalkyl-quetiapine
Sertindole	75	99.5		50–110	15–20	***CYP2D6, CYP3A4***	—
Ziprasidone	60	>99	1.5	8–10	2–3	CYP3A4, aldehyde oxidase	—
Aripiprazole	87	>99	4.9	48–68	14	***CYP3A4, CYP2D6***	Dehydro-aripiprazole

TABLE 4–2. Pharmacokinetics of atypical antipsychotics *(continued)*

DRUG	BIOAVAILABILITY (%)	PROTEIN BINDING (%)	VOLUME OF DISTRIBUTION (L/KG)	HALF-LIFE (HOURS)	TIME TO REACH STEADY STATE (DAYS)	ENZYMES RESPONSIBLE FOR BIOTRANSFORMATION[a]	ACTIVE METABOLITES
Amisulpride	43–48	17	5.8	12	2–3	Not clinically relevant	—
Paliperidone	28	74	487	23	4–5	***CYP2D6***	—
Asenapine	35 (sublingual) <2 (oral)	95	20–25	24	2–3	Direct glucuronidation, ***CYP1A2,*** CYP3A4, and CYP2D6	—
Iloperidone	96	98	2,527	18–33	3–4	***CYP3A4, CYP2D6***	P88

[a]Enzymes that are bold and italic are the primary enzymes responsible for biotransformation.
Source. Adapted from Mauri et al. 2007.

TABLE 4–3. Drug–drug interactions

Drug	Antipsychotic	Effect on plasma concentrations	Proposed mechanism	Comment
TCAs	Haloperidol	Increased levels of TCAs	Inhibition of CYP2D6 and P-glycoprotein by haloperidol and "reduced haloperidol"	Increased risk of arrhythmias
	Pimozide	Increased levels of TCAs	Inhibition of CYP2D6, CYP3A4, and P-glycoprotein by pimozide	Increased risk of arrhythmias
	Ziprasidone	No change		Synergistic QT prolongation
SSRIs				
Fluoxetine	Clozapine	Increase (40%–70%)	Inhibition of various CYP isoforms (CYP2D6, CYP2C19, and CYP3A4)	
	Risperidone	Increase (75%)	Inhibition of CYP2D6 and, to a lesser extent, CYP3A4	
	Olanzapine	No change or minimal increase	Inhibition of CYP2D6	
	Quetiapine	No change		

TABLE 4–3. Drug–drug interactions *(continued)*

Drug	Antipsychotic	Effect on plasma concentrations	Proposed mechanism	Comment
SSRIs *(continued)*				
Fluoxetine *(continued)*	Typical antipsychotics	Increase	Inhibition of various CYP isoforms and P-glycoprotein	Combination with mesoridazine, thioridazine, or pimozide can increase risk of arrhythmias
Paroxetine	Clozapine	Increase (20%–40%)	Inhibition of CYP2D6	
	Risperidone	Increase (40%–50%)	Inhibition of CYP2D6	
	Typical antipsychotics	Increase	Inhibition of CYP2D6 isoform and P-glycoprotein	Combination with mesoridazine, thioridazine, or pimozide can increase risk of arrhythmias
Fluvoxamine	Clozapine	Increase (up to 5–10 times)	Inhibition of CYP1A2 and, to a lesser extent, CYP2C19 and CYP3A4	
	Risperidone	Minimal increase (10%–20%)	Inhibition of CYP2D6 and CYP3A4	
	Olanzapine	Increase (up to 100%)	Inhibition of CYP1A2	
	Typical antipsychotics	Increase	Inhibition of various CYP isoforms and P-glycoprotein	Combination with mesoridazine, thioridazine, or pimozide can increase risk of arrhythmias

TABLE 4–3. Drug–drug interactions *(continued)*

Drug	Antipsychotic	Effect on plasma concentrations	Proposed mechanism	Comment
SSRIs *(continued)*				
Sertraline	Clozapine	No change		
	Risperidone	Minimal increase	Inhibition of CYP2D6	
	Olanzapine	No change		
	Pimozide	Increase	Inhibition of CYP3A4 and CYP1A2	
Citalopram/ escitalopram	Clozapine	No change		
	Risperidone	No change		
	Typical antipsychotics (phenothiazines)	Increased level of phenothiazine	Inhibition of CYP2D6	
Newer antidepressants				
Bupropion	Typical antipsychotics (phenothiazines)	Increased level of phenothiazine	Inhibition of CYP2D6	
Mirtazapine	None			
Nefazodone	Pimozide	Increase	Inhibition of CYP3A4	Increased risk of QT prolongation; potentially fatal

Note. CYP=cytochrome P450; SSRI=selective serotonin reuptake inhibitor; TCA=tricyclic antidepressant.

Source. Reviewed in Spina E, de Leon J: "Metabolic Drug Interactions With Newer Antipsychotics: A Comparative Review." *Basic and Clinical Pharmacology and Toxicology* 100:4–22, 2007; Sandson NB, Armstrong SC, Cozza KL: "An Overview of Psychotropic Drug–Drug Interactions." *Psychosomatics* 46:464–494, 2005.

inhibitory action leads to the possibility of clinically significant pharmacokinetic interactions. The various SSRIs differ in their potency to inhibit CYP enzymes. Fluoxetine and paroxetine are potent inhibitors of CYP2D6, fluvoxamine is a potent inhibitor of CYP1A2 and CYP2C19, fluoxetine and fluvoxamine are moderate inhibitors of CYP2C19 and CYP3A4, and sertraline is a moderate inhibitor of CYP2D6. Citalopram and escitalopram do not appear to significantly inhibit any CYP.

SSRIs cause an increase in plasma levels of risperidone, primarily through inhibition of CYP2D6 (and CYP3A4 to a lesser extent). Fluoxetine, paroxetine, fluvoxamine, and sertraline cause an increase in plasma risperidone levels when coadministered with risperidone. The interaction with fluoxetine is notable for the fact that norfluoxetine, the active metabolite of fluoxetine, is a potent inhibitor of CYP3A4, thus blocking both pathways of risperidone's metabolism (Spina et al. 2002). This provides a rational explanation for the clinical observation that when fluoxetine is added to risperidone, some patients develop extrapyramidal symptoms, urinary retention, and gynecomastia, all of which are accentuated side effects of risperidone. The dosage of risperidone should be reduced when fluoxetine is being coadministered. No pharmacokinetic interaction has been described with citalopram.

Clozapine is metabolized primarily by CYP1A2 and to a lesser extent by CYP2C19, CYP3A4, and CYP2D6. Fluoxetine, paroxetine, and fluvoxamine cause an increase in serum clozapine levels (Prior et al. 1999; Spina et al. 1998). The combination of clozapine and fluvoxamine warrants caution. Fluvoxamine can result in a 5- to 10-fold increase in serum clozapine levels due to its potent inhibition of CYP1A2, as well as CYP2C19 and CYP3A4. Hence, patients taking clozapine and fluvoxamine must be closely monitored with serum clozapine levels and for extrapyramidal side effects and other adverse events such as agranulocytosis. Sertraline and citalopram have not been shown to increase serum clozapine levels when used in combination. The evidence of interaction between paroxetine and clozapine is equivocal.

Olanzapine is metabolized primarily by CYP1A2 and to a lesser extent by CYP2D6. Fluoxetine and fluvoxamine are known to increase serum olanzapine levels. The interaction with fluvoxamine is particularly relevant because it causes a twofold increase in serum olanzapine levels, resulting in an increased incidence of side effects (sedation, orthostatic hypotension, tachycardia, elevation of serum transaminase, and seizures).

The newer antidepressants, with the exception of nefazodone, do not have clinically relevant pharmacokinetic interactions with atypical antipsychotics (Spina et al. 2003). Nefazodone is a potent inhibitor of CYP3A4 and has been shown to increase plasma levels of clozapine and risperidone. The pharmacokinetic interaction of mirtazapine with olanzapine, risperidone, and clozapine was found to be insignificant (Zoccali et al. 2003).

Selegiline, when administered via the transdermal system, was not found to have significant pharmacokinetic interactions with the antipsychotics risperidone and olanzapine (Azzaro et al. 2007).

Side-Effect Profiles

In evaluating the rationale for coadministration of antidepressants with antipsychotic medication in patients with schizophrenia, the clinician needs to weigh the risks against the benefits. Clinically significant drug interactions can be predicted based on the degree of overlap in receptor binding profiles of the antidepressant and antipsychotic being coadministered. Table 4–4 provides an overview of receptor binding profiles for different antipsychotic medications. Figure 4–2 illustrates the receptor binding profile for antipsychotic medications as a class and the effects thought to be mediated by individual receptors. Table 4–5 provides a list of common side effects of antipsychotic medications.

TCAs worsen the sedative and anticholinergic side effects of antipsychotics, although they may improve extrapyramidal symptoms. A case report documents an increased risk of seizure when clomipramine was coadministered with olanzapine (Deshauer et al. 2000). TCAs are also associated with an exacerbation of psychosis and with causing a delay in response to typical antipsychotics when coadministered (Kramer et al. 1989).

SSRIs increase the serum levels of antipsychotics and hence lead to an increased rate of adverse effects. The emergence of serotonin syndrome when SSRIs are coadministered with antipsychotics has been previously noted. This is a potentially fatal side effect and requires a high index of suspicion for its early recognition.

Among the newer antidepressants, mirtazapine is associated with weight gain and dyslipidemia and when combined with olanzapine may lead to an increased risk of metabolic syndrome. Bupropion is associated with an increased risk of seizures, which is particularly relevant when coadministered with clozapine, which also has an epileptogenic property.

An older theory that has been disproved but may still worry some clinicians was that the addition of antidepressants to antipsychotics worsens the course of schizophrenia during the actively psychotic phase, presumably through stimulation of the catecholamine system. Kramer et al. (1989), for example, showed that combining TCAs with typical antipsychotics for the treatment of actively psychotic patients with both schizophrenia and depression did not alleviate the depression and actually resulted in a slower resolution of psychosis. When a TCA or MAOI was the only medication given, without the presumably protective cover of an antipsychotic, some patients experienced an increase in delusions, hallucinations, and disorganization (Baldessarini and Willmuth 1968).

TABLE 4–4. Receptor binding profile of tricyclic antidepressants, selective serotonin reuptake inhibitors, newer antidepressants, and antipsychotics: uptake inhibition and receptor antagonism

	TRANSPORTERS		RECEPTOR BINDING (K_I, NMOL/L)				
DRUG	5-HT	NE	H_1	α_1	M_1	D_2	5-HT_{2A}
Tricyclic antidepressants							
Amitriptyline	20	50	1	27	11	1,460	29
Imipramine	7	60	40	32	42	620	80
Clomipramine	0.14	54	15	32	25	77.6	35
Nortriptyline	100	10	6.3	55	40	2,570	44
Desipramine*	18	0.83	110	100	110	3,500	280
SSRIs							
Fluoxetine	14	143	5,400	3,800	590	12,000	280
Norfluoxetine	25	416	11,000	3,900	810	16,000	600
Sertraline	3.4	220	24,000	380	630	10,700	9,900
Desmethylsertraline	76	420	9,000	1,200	1,430	11,000	4,800
Citalopram	1.8	6,100	350	1,600	5,600	33,000	>10,000
Desmethylcitalopram	14	740	1,700	1,500	14,000	53,000	19,000
Newer antidepressants							
Reboxetine*	58	7.2	310	>1,000	>1,000	>10,000	>1,000
Mirtazapine*	>10,000	4,600	0.14	500	670	>5,454	16
Mianserin*	>4,000	71	0.40	34	820	2,197	7

TABLE 4–4. Receptor binding profile of tricyclic antidepressants, selective serotonin reuptake inhibitors, newer antidepressants, and antipsychotics: uptake inhibition and receptor antagonism *(continued)*

	Transporters		Receptor binding (K_I, nmol/L)				
Drug	5-HT	NE	H_1	α_1	M_1	D_2	5-HT_{2A}
Antipsychotics							
Risperidone	>10,000	>10,000	5.2	2.7	>10,000	3.7	0.42
Olanzapine	3,676	>10,000	4.9	109	73	10	2.5
Quetiapine	>10,000	>10,000	7.5	8.1	858	567	31
Ziprasidone	112	44	4.6	2.6	2,440	8.5	0.3
Clozapine	1,624	3,168	2.8	6.8	14	130	11
Haloperidol	3,256	2,112	260	17	>10,000	0.35	36
Asenapine*	—	—	1	1.2	8,128	1.3	0.06
Iloperidone	—	1,479	12.3	0.31	6,000	3.3	0.2

Note. Smaller K_i values represent greater potency. Receptors: α_1=α_1 adrenoceptor; D_2=dopamine type 2; H_1=histamine type 1; 5-HT=serotonin; 5-HT_{2A}=serotonin type 2A; M_1=acetylcholine muscarinic; NE=norepinephrine; SSRI=selective serotonin reuptake inhibitor.

Source. All data have been extracted from PDSP K_i database (http://pdsp.med.unc.edu/pdsp.php), except *Richelson E: "Pharmacology of Antidepressants." *Mayo Clinic Proceedings* 76:511–527, 2001. Values for asenapine derived from Shahid M, Walker GB, Zorn SH, et al: "Asenapine: A Novel Psychopharmacologic Agent With a Unique Human Receptor Signature." *Journal of Psychopharmacology* 23:65–73, 2009.

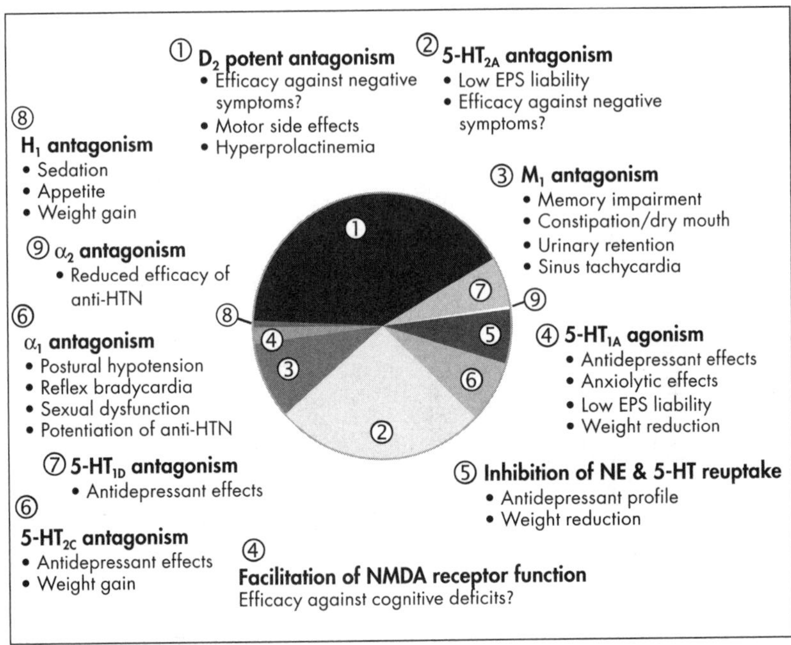

FIGURE 4–2. Receptor binding profile and clinical implications.
Note. EPS=extrapyramidal symptoms; 5-HT=serotonin; HTN=hypertension; NE=norepinephrine; NMDA=*N*-methyl-D-aspartate.

Case reports from the 1990s documented a worsening of psychotic symptoms with SSRIs. Chong et al. (1997) described the cases of two patients taking clozapine who developed obsessive-compulsive symptoms. Addition of sertraline for one patient and fluvoxamine for the other to ameliorate the obsessive-compulsive symptoms led to a worsening of psychosis. In another case report, Rocco and DeLeo (1992) described a worsening of psychosis in a patient with residual symptoms on addition of fluvoxamine to perphenazine.

The relationship between antidepressant treatment and exacerbation of psychosis is controvertible, yet it is important to remember the clinical implications of such a risk.

Conclusion

The evidence supporting the adjunctive use of antidepressants in patients with schizophrenia and comorbid depression is far from compelling. For example, the last Cochrane review on this topic concluded that overall, the literature

TABLE 4–5. Common side effects of antipsychotic medications

- Extrapyramidal symptoms
  - Parkinsonism
  - Akathisia
  - Acute dystonia
- Hyperprolactinemia
  - Gynecomastia
  - Galactorrhoea
  - Menstrual dysregulation (oligomenorrhea, amenorrhea)
  - Sexual dysfunction (decreased libido, decreased arousal, delayed orgasm)
  - Decreased bone mineral density
  - Acne and hirsutism in women
  - Infertility
- Metabolic side effects
  - Weight gain
  - Hyperglycemia
  - Dyslipidemia
- Cardiovascular side effects
  - Postural hypotension
  - QTc prolongation
  - Myocarditis (with clozapine)
- Antimuscarinic side effects
  - Dry mouth, blurred vision, urinary retention, constipation, and, in severe cases, cognitive impairment and delirium
- Blood dyscrasias (with clozapine)
  - Neutropenia
  - Agranulocytosis
- Sedation
- Seizure
- Cerebrovascular events
- Antipsychotic discontinuation symptoms
- Neuroleptic malignant syndrome

TABLE 4–6. Some conditions in which the use of antidepressants should be considered in patients with schizophrenia

Smoking cessation (bupropion)
Antipsychotic-induced obsessive-compulsive disorder (fluvoxamine, clomipramine)
Comorbid depression/anxiety disorder (SSRI)
Antipsychotic-induced sexual dysfunction (bupropion)
Clozapine-induced sialorrhea/nocturia (amitriptyline, moclobemide)

Note. SSRI=selective serotonin reuptake inhibitor.

was of poor quality. Although some evidence suggested that antidepressants may be beneficial for patients with schizophrenia and comorbid depression, the evidence was far from convincing to either support or refute the use of antidepressants (Whitehead et al. 2002).

Similarly, the 2009 Schizophrenia Patient Outcomes Research Team (PORT), in its Psychopharmacological Treatment Recommendations (Buchanan et al. 2010), decided to drop the antidepressant treatment recommendation listed in the 2004 guidelines due to the lack of rigorous studies on the effectiveness of newer antidepressants (e.g., SSRIs) for depressive symptoms in patients with schizophrenia, particularly among patients treated with second-generation antipsychotics. The guidelines, however, recommend the use of sustained-release bupropion 150 mg bid for 10–12 weeks, with or without nicotine replacement therapy, to achieve short-term abstinence accompanied by a smoking cessation education or support group. Table 4–6 lists some alternatives to antidepressant use in schizophrenia with comorbid depression. Table 4–7 lists some conditions in which the use of antidepressants should be considered in patients with schizophrenia.

The evidence supporting the use of adjunctive antidepressants for primary negative symptoms is far from compelling. For example, the last Cochrane review concluded that although the combination of antidepressants with antipsychotics may be beneficial, the amount of information was limited (Rummel-Kluge et al. 2006). The need for large, pragmatic, long-term studies was also echoed in the Cochrane review. Similarly, the PORT, in its treatment recommendations, pointed out that despite promising trials of SSRIs, mirtazapine, and MAO-B inhibitors in the treatment of negative symptoms, the level of evidence is currently insufficient to support a treatment recommendation for any of the pharmacological treatments (Buchanan et al. 2010).

TABLE 4–7. Alternatives to use of antidepressants in schizophrenia with comorbid depression

Cognitive-behavioral therapy
Antipsychotics with antidepressant properties (quetiapine, amisulpride, zotepine, asenapine)
Electroconvulsive therapy

KEY CLINICAL CONCEPTS

- Negative symptoms and comorbid depression and anxiety are important targets that would improve the functional outcome of patients with schizophrenia.
- Negative symptoms, depression, and extrapyramidal symptoms are difficult to differentiate.
- Studies of antidepressant augmentation of antipsychotic medication lack the level of evidence required to advocate their "routine" use for the treatment of negative symptoms.
- Studies of antidepressant augmentation of antipsychotic medication lack the level of evidence required to advocate their "routine" use for the treatment of depression.
- No compelling evidence indicates that the use of antidepressants is associated with exacerbation of psychosis in schizophrenia.
- The evidence is strong for the utility of bupropion as an adjunct to antipsychotics in patients with schizophrenia who smoke extensively and are keen on quitting.
- The combination of an SSRI or newer antidepressant with an atypical antipsychotic is generally safer than the combination of a TCA with a typical antipsychotic.
- The combination of fluoxetine or fluvoxamine with clozapine requires particular attention in view of the increase in plasma clozapine levels and increased risk of side effects.
- The use of SSRIs or newer antidepressants for comorbid depression and anxiety warrants careful consideration of drug-drug interactions and increased risk of side effects.

References

Abbasi SH, Behpournia H, Ghoreshi A, et al: The effect of mirtazapine add on therapy to risperidone in the treatment of schizophrenia: a double-blind randomized placebo-controlled trial. Schizophr Res 116:101–106, 2010

Addington J, el-Guebaly N, Addington D, et al: Readiness to stop smoking in schizophrenia. Can J Psychiatry 42:49–52, 1997

American Psychiatric Association: Diagnostic and Statistical Manual of Mental Disorders, 3rd Edition, Revised. Washington, DC, American Psychiatric Association, 1987

American Psychiatric Association: Diagnostic and Statistical Manual of Mental Disorders, 4th Edition, Text Revision. Washington, DC, American Psychiatric Association, 2000

Amiri A, Noorbala AA, Nejatisafa AA, et al: Efficacy of selegiline add on therapy to risperidone in the treatment of the negative symptoms of schizophrenia: a double-blind randomized placebo-controlled study. Hum Psychopharmacol 23:79–86, 2008

Andreasen NC: Mood disorders and schizophrenia. J Clin Psychiatry 16:7–8, 1998

Arango C, Kirkpatrick B, Buchanan RW: Fluoxetine as an adjunct to conventional antipsychotic treatment of schizophrenia patients with residual symptoms. J Nerv Ment Dis 188:50–53, 2000

Azzaro AJ, Ziemniak J, Kemper E, et al: Selegiline transdermal system: an examination of the potential for CYP450-dependent pharmacokinetic interactions with 3 psychotropic medications. J Clin Pharmacol 47:146–158, 2007

Baldessarini RJ, Willmuth RL: Psychotic reactions during amitriptyline therapy. Can Psychiatr Assoc J 13:571–573, 1968

Bender S, Olbrich HM, Fischer W, et al: Antipsychotic efficacy of the antidepressant trimipramine: a randomized, double-blind comparison with the phenothiazine perazine. Pharmacopsychiatry 36:61–69, 2003

Benes FM, Berretta S: GABAergic interneurons: implications for understanding schizophrenia and bipolar disorder. Neuropsychopharmacology 25:1–27, 2001

Berk M, Ichim C, Brooks S: Efficacy of mirtazapine add on therapy to haloperidol in the treatment of the negative symptoms of schizophrenia: a double-blind randomized placebo-controlled study. Int Clin Psychopharmacol 16:87–92, 2001

Berk M, Gama CS, Sundram S, et al: Mirtazapine add-on therapy in the treatment of schizophrenia with atypical antipsychotics: a double-blind, randomized, placebo-controlled clinical trial. Hum Psychopharmacol 24:233–238, 2009

Berman I, Kalinowski A, Berman S, et al: Obsessive-compulsive symptoms in chronic schizophrenia. Compr Psychiatry 36:6–10, 1995

Bleuler E: Dementia Praecox oder Gruppe der Schizophrenien. Leipzig, Deuticke, 1911

Birchwood M, Iqbal Z, Chadwick P, et al: Cognitive approach to depression and suicidal thinking in psychosis, 1: ontogeny of post-psychotic depression. Br J Psychiatry 177:516–521, 2000

Bloch B, Reshef A, Cohen T, et al: Preliminary effects of bupropion and the promoter region (HTTLPR) serotonin transporter (SLC6A4) polymorphism on smoking behavior in schizophrenia. Psychiatry Res 175:38–42, 2010

Bodkin JA, Cohen BJ, Salomon MS, et al: Treatment of negative symptoms of schizophrenia and schizoaffective disorder by selegiline augmentation of antipsychotic medication: a pilot study examining the role of dopamine. J Nerv Ment Dis 184:295–301, 1996

Bodkin JA, Siris SG, Bermanzohn PC, et al: Double-blind, placebo-controlled, multicenter trial of selegiline augmentation of antipsychotic medication to treat negative symptoms in outpatients with schizophrenia. Am J Psychiatry 162:388–390, 2005

Bressan RA, Chaves AC, Pilowsky LS, et al: Depressive episodes in stable schizophrenia: critical evaluation of the DSM-IV and ICD-10 diagnostic criteria. Psychiatry Res 117:47–56, 2003

Buchanan RW, Kirkpatrick B, Bryant N, et al: Fluoxetine augmentation of clozapine treatment in patients with schizophrenia. Am J Psychiatry 153:1625–1627, 1996

Buchanan RW, Kreyenbuhl J, Kelly DL, et al: The 2009 Schizophrenia PORT psychopharmacological treatment recommendations and summary statements. Schizophr Bull 36:71–93, 2010

Buckley PF, Miller BJ, Lehrer DS, et al: Psychiatric comorbidities and schizophrenia. Schizophr Bull 35:383–402, 2009

Burrows DG: Biology and etiology of affective disorders in schizophrenia. J Clin Psychiatry 16:4–5, 1998

Busatto GF, Pilowsky LS, Costa DC, et al: Correlation between reduced in vivo benzodiazepine receptor binding and severity of psychotic symptoms in schizophrenia. Am J Psychiatry 154:56–63, 1997

Bustillo JR, Lauriello J, Parker K, et al: Treatment of weight gain with fluoxetine in olanzapine-treated schizophrenic outpatients. Neuropsychopharmacology 28:527–529, 2003

Carpenter WT, Heinrichs DW, Alphs LD: Treatment of negative symptoms. Schizophr Bull 11:440–452, 1985

Chanrion B, Mannoury LA, Cour C, et al: Inverse agonist and neutral antagonist actions of antidepressants at recombinant and native 5-hydroxytryptamine 2C receptors: differential modulation of cell surface expression and signal transduction. Mol Pharmacol 73:748–757, 2008

Charych EI, Liu F, Moss SJ, et al: GABA(A) receptors and their associated proteins: implications in the etiology and treatment of schizophrenia and related disorders. Neuropharmacology 57:481–495, 2009

Chertkow Y, Weinreb O, Youdim MB, et al: The effect of chronic co-administration of fluvoxamine and haloperidol compared to clozapine on the GABA system in the rat frontal cortex. Int J Neuropsychopharmacol 9:287–296, 2006

Chertkow Y, Weinreb O, Youdim MB, et al: Dopamine and serotonin metabolism in response to chronic administration of fluvoxamine and haloperidol combined treatment. J Neural Transm 114:1443–1454, 2007

Chertkow Y, Weinreb O, Youdim MB, et al: Molecular mechanisms underlying synergistic effects of SSRI-antipsychotic augmentation in treatment of negative symptoms in schizophrenia. J Neural Transm 116:1529–1541, 2009

Chong SA, Tan CH, Lee HS: Worsening of psychosis with clozapine and selective serotonin reuptake inhibitor combination: two case reports. J Clin Psychopharmacol 1768–1769, 1997

Conley RR: The burden of depressive symptoms in people with schizophrenia. Psychiatr Clin North Am 32:853–861, 2009

Conley RR, Ascher-Svanum H, Zhu B, et al: The burden of depressive symptoms in the long-term treatment of patients with schizophrenia. Schizophr Res 90:186–197, 2007

Copp PJ, Lament R, Tennent TG: Amitriptyline in clozapine-induced sialorrhoea. Br J Psychiatry 159:166, 1991

Cryan JF, Bruijnzeel AW, Skjei KL, et al: Bupropion enhances brain reward function and reverses the affective and somatic aspects of nicotine withdrawal in the rat. Psychopharmacology (Berl) 168:347–358, 2003

Danovich L, Weinreb O, Youdim MB, et al: The involvement of GABAA receptor in the molecular mechanisms of combined selective serotonin reuptake inhibitor–antipsychotic treatment. Int J Neuropsychopharmacol 25:1–13, 2010

Davey Smith G, Egger M: Meta-analysis: unresolved issues and future developments. BMJ 316:221–225, 1998

Davis KL, Kahn RS, Ko G, et al: Dopamine in schizophrenia: a review and reconceptualization. Am J Psychiatry 148:1474–1486, 1991

de Boer TH, Maura G, Raitieri M, et al: Neurochemical and autonomic pharmacological profiles of the 6-aza-analogue of mianserin, Org 3770 and its enantiomers. Neuropharmacology 27:399–408, 1988

de Leon J, Diaz FJ: A meta-analysis of worldwide studies demonstrates an association between schizophrenia and tobacco smoking behaviors. Schizophr Res 76:135–157, 2005

Deshauer D, Albuquerque J, Alda M, et al: Seizures caused by possible interaction between olanzapine and clomipramine. J Clin Psychopharmacol 20:283–284, 2000

Di Giovanni G, Esposito E, Di Matteo V: Role of serotonin in central dopamine dysfunction. CNS Neurosci Ther 16:179–194, 2010

Dwivedi S, Pavuluri M, Heidenreich J, et al: Response to fluvoxamine augmentation for obsessive and compulsive symptoms in schizophrenia. J Child Adolesc Psychopharmacol 12:69–70, 2002

Eikmeier G, Muszynski K, Berger M, et al: High-dose trimipramine in acute schizophrenia: preliminary results of an open trial. Pharmacopsychiatry 23:212–214, 1990

Eikmeier G, Berger M, Lodemann E, et al: Trimipramine—an atypical neuroleptic? Int Clin Psychopharmacol 6:147–153, 1991

Englisch S, Esser A, Zink M: Bupropion for depression in schizophrenia: a case report. Pharmacopsychiatry 43:38–39, 2010

Finberg JP, Youdim MB: Pharmacological properties of the anti-Parkinson drug rasagiline: modification of endogenous brain amines, reserpine reversal, serotonergic and dopaminergic behaviours. Neuropharmacology 43:1110–1118, 2002

Fleischhacker W: Differentiation of depression, negative symptoms, and EPS in schizophrenia. J Clin Psychiatry 16:5–7, 1998

Friedman JI, Ocampo R, Elbaz Z, et al: The effect of citalopram adjunctive treatment added to atypical antipsychotic medications for cognitive performance in patients with schizophrenia. J Clin Psychopharmacol 25:237–242, 2005

Fryer JD, Lukas RJ: Noncompetitive functional inhibition at diverse, human nicotinic acetylcholine receptor subtypes by bupropion, phencyclidine, and ibogaine. J Pharmacol Exp Ther 288:88–92, 1999

George TP, Vessicchio JC, Sacco KA, et al: A placebo-controlled trial of bupropion combined with nicotine patch for smoking cessation in schizophrenia. Biol Psychiatry 63:1092–1096, 2008

Goff DC, Renshaw PF, Sarid-Segal O, et al: A placebo-controlled trial of selegiline (L-deprenyl) in the treatment of tardive dyskinesia. Biol Psychiatry 33:700–706, 1993

Goff DC, Midha KK, Sarid-Segal O, et al: A placebo-controlled trial of fluoxetine added to neuroleptic in patients with schizophrenia. Psychopharmacology (Berl) 117:417–423, 1995

Gross G, Xie X, Gastpar M: Trimipramine: pharmacological reevaluation and comparison with clozapine. Neuropharmacology 30:1159–1166, 1991

Gupta S, Droney T, Kyser A, et al: Selegiline augmentation of antipsychotics for the treatment of negative symptoms in schizophrenia. Compr Psychiatry 40:148–150, 1999

Hashimoto K: Can the sigma-1 receptor agonist fluvoxamine prevent schizophrenia? CNS Neurol Disord Drug Targets 8:470–474, 2009

Hashimoto T, Volk DW, Eggan SM, et al: Gene expression deficits in a subclass of GABA neurons in the prefrontal cortex of subjects with schizophrenia. J Neurosci 23:6315–6326, 2003

Hauser K, Olpe HR, Jones RS: Trimipramine, a tricyclic antidepressant exerting atypical actions on the central noradrenergic system. Eur J Pharmacol 111:23–30, 1985

Hiemke C, Peled A, Jabarin M, et al: Fluvoxamine augmentation of olanzapine in chronic schizophrenia: pharmacokinetic interactions and clinical effects. J Clin Psychopharmacol 22:502–506, 2002

Ichikawa J, Kuroki T, Meltzer HY: Differential effects of chronic imipramine and fluoxetine on basal and amphetamine-induced extracellular dopamine levels in rat nucleus accumbens. Eur J Pharmacol 350:159–164, 1998

Ichikawa J, Ishii H, Bonaccorso S, et al: 5-HT2A and D2 receptor blockade increases cortical DA release via 5-HT1A receptor activation: a possible mechanism of atypical antipsychotic-induced cortical dopamine release. J Neurochem 76:1521–1531, 2001

Jockers-Scherübl MC, Godemann F, Pietzcker A: Negative symptoms of schizophrenia are improved by paroxetine added to neuroleptics: a pilot study (letter). J Clin Psychiatry 62:573, 2001

Jockers-Scherübl MC, Bauer A, Godemann F, et al: Negative symptoms of schizophrenia are improved by the addition of paroxetine to neuroleptics: a double-blind placebo-controlled study. Int Clin Psychopharmacol 20:27–31, 2005

Joffe G, Terevnikov V, Joffe M, et al: Add-on mirtazapine enhances antipsychotic effect of first generation antipsychotics in schizophrenia: a double-blind, randomized, placebo-controlled trial. Schizophr Res 108:245–251, 2009

Johnson DA: Studies of depressive symptoms in schizophrenia. Br J Psychiatry 139:89–101, 1981

Jungerman T, Rabinowitz D, Klein E: Deprenyl augmentation for treating negative symptoms of schizophrenia: a double-blind, controlled study. J Clin Psychopharmacol 19:522–525, 1999

Kasckow JW, Mohamed S, Thallasinos A, et al: Citalopram augmentation of antipsychotic treatment in older schizophrenia patients. Int J Ger Psychiatry 16:1163–1167, 2001

Kirli S, Caliskan M: A comparative study of sertraline versus imipramine in postpsychotic depressive disorder of schizophrenia. Schizophr Res 33:103–111, 1998

Kodesh A, Weizman A, Aizenberg D, et al: Selegiline in the treatment of sexual dysfunction in schizophrenic patients maintained on neuroleptics: a pilot study. Clin Neuropharmacol 26:193–195, 2003

Kopanski C, Turck M, Schulz JE: Effects of long-term treatment of rats with antidepressants on adrenergic-receptor sensitivity in cerebral cortex: structure activity study. Neurochem Int 5:649–659, 1993

Kramer MS, Vogel WH, DiJohnson C, et al: Antidepressants in "depressed" schizophrenic inpatients: a controlled trial. Arch Gen Psychiatry 46:922–928, 1989

Kuroki T, Meltzer HY, Ichikawa J: Effects of antipsychotic drugs on extracellular dopamine levels in rat medial prefrontal cortex and nucleus accumbens. J Pharmacol Exp Ther 288:774–781, 1999

Lammers CH, Deuschle M, Weigmann H, et al: Coadministration of clozapine and fluvoxamine in psychotic patients: clinical experience. Pharmacopsychiatry 32:76–77, 1999

Lee MS, Kim YK, Lee SK, et al: A double-blind study of adjunctive sertraline in haloperidol-stabilized patients with chronic schizophrenia. J Clin Psychopharmacol 18:399–403, 1998

Lewis DA, Hashimoto T, Volk DW: Cortical inhibitory neurons and schizophrenia. Nat Rev Neurosci 6:312–324, 2005

Lindenmayer JP, Kay SR: Depression, affect, and negative symptoms in schizophrenia. Br J Psychiatry 155 (suppl 7):108–114, 1989

Litman RE, Su TP, Potter WZ, et al: Idazoxan and response to typical neuroleptics in treatment-resistant schizophrenia: comparison with the atypical neuroleptic, clozapine. Br J Psychiatry 168:571–579, 1996

Lu ML, Lane HY, Lin SK, et al: Adjunctive fluvoxamine inhibits clozapine-related weight gain and metabolic disturbances. J Clin Psychiatry 65:766–771, 2004

Martin RL, Cloninger CR, Guze SB, et al: Frequency and differential diagnosis of depressive syndromes in schizophrenia. J Clin Psychiatry 46:9–13, 1985

Mauri MC, Volonteri LS, Colasanti A, et al: Clinical pharmacokinetics of atypical antipsychotics: a critical review of the relationship between plasma concentrations and clinical response. Clin Pharmacokinet 46:359–388, 2007

Mayer-Gross W: Über die Stellungsnahme auf abgelaufenen akuten psychose. Zeitschrift für die Gesamte Neurologie und Psychiatrie 60:160–212, 1920

McGlashan TH, Carpenter WT: Postpsychotic depression in schizophrenia. Arch Gen Psychiatry 33:231–239, 1976

Meltzer H: Serotonergic dysfunction in depression. Br J Psychiatry Suppl December (8):25–31, 1989

Milev P, Ho BC, Arndt S, et al: Predictive values of neurocognition and negative symptoms on functional outcome in schizophrenia: a longitudinal first-episode study with 7-year follow-up. Am J Psychiatry 162:495–506, 2005

Mulholland C, Lynch G, King DJ, et al: A double-blind, placebo-controlled trial of sertraline for depressive symptoms in patients with stable, chronic schizophrenia. J Psychopharmacol 17:107–112, 2003

Mulsant BH, Foglia JP, Sweet RA, et al: The effects of perphenazine on the concentration of nortriptyline and its hydroxymetabolites in older patients. J Clin Psychopharmacol 17:318–321, 1997

Naylor L, Dean B, Opeskin K, et al: Changes in the serotonin transporter in the hippocampus of subjects with schizophrenia identified using [3H]paroxetine. J Neural Transm 103:749–757, 1996

Noda Y, Mamiya T, Furukawa H, et al: Effects of antidepressants on phencyclidine-induced enhancement of immobility in a forced swimming test in mice. Eur J Pharmacol 324:135–140, 1997

Patel DD, Laws KR, Padhi A, et al: The neuropsychology of the schizo-obsessive subtype of schizophrenia: a new analysis. Psychol Med 40:921–933, 2010

Perenyi A, Goswami U, Frecksa E, et al: L-Deprenyl in treating negative symptoms of schizophrenia. Psychiatry Res 42:189–191, 1992

Plasky P: Antidepressant usage in schizophrenia. Schizophr Bull 17:649–657, 1991

Poyurovsky M, Hermesh H, Weizman A: Fluvoxamine treatment in clozapine-induced obsessive-compulsive symptoms in schizophrenic patients. Clin Neuropharmacol 19:305–313, 1996

Poyurovsky M, Shardorodsky M, Fuchs C, et al: Treatment of neuroleptic-induced akathisia with the 5-HT2 antagonist mianserin: double-blind, placebo-controlled study. Br J Psychiatry 174:238–242, 1999

Poyurovsky M, Epshtein S, Fuchs C, et al: Efficacy of low-dose mirtazapine in neuroleptic-induced akathisia: a double-blind randomized placebo-controlled pilot study. J Clin Psychopharmacol 23:305–308, 2003a

Poyurovsky M, Isaacs I, Fuchs C, et al: Attenuation of olanzapine-induced weight gain with reboxetine in patients with schizophrenia: a double-blind, placebo-controlled study. Am J Psychiatry 160:297–302, 2003b

Poyurovsky M, Koren D, Gonopolsky I, et al: Effect of the 5-HT2 antagonist mianserin on cognitive dysfunction in chronic schizophrenia patients: an add-on, double-blind placebo-controlled study. Eur Neuropsychopharmacol 13:123–128, 2003c

Poyurovsky M, Weizman A, Weizman R: Obsessive-compulsive disorder in schizophrenia: clinical characteristics and treatment. CNS Drugs 18:989–1010, 2004

Poyurovsky M, Fuchs C, Pashinian A, et al: Attenuating effect of reboxetine on appetite and weight gain in olanzapine-treated schizophrenia patients: a double-blind placebo-controlled study. Psychopharmacology (Berl) 192:441–448, 2007

Poyurovsky M, Faragian S, Fuchs C, et al: Effect of the selective norepinephrine reuptake inhibitor reboxetine on cognitive dysfunction in schizophrenia patients: an add-on, double-blind placebo-controlled study. Isr J Psychiatry Relat Sci 46:213–220, 2009

Praharaj SK, Arora M: Amitriptyline for clozapine-induced nocturnal enuresis and sialorrhoea. Br J Clin Pharmacol 63:128–129, 2007

Prior TI, Chue PS, Tibbo P, et al: Drug metabolism and atypical antipsychotics. Eur Neuropsychopharmacol 9:301–309, 1999

Prusoff BA, Williams DH, Weissman MM, et al: Treatment of secondary depression in schizophrenia. A double-blind, placebo-controlled trial of amitriptyline added to perphenazine. Arch Gen Psychiatry 36:569–575, 1979

Rajkumar RP, Reddy YC, Kandavel T: Clinical profile of "schizo-obsessive" disorder: a comparative study. Compr Psychiatry 49:262–268, 2008

Rauser L, Savage JE, Meltzer HY, et al: Inverse agonist actions of typical and atypical antipsychotic drugs at the human 5-hydroxytryptamine(2C) receptor. J Pharmacol Exp Ther 299:83–89, 2001

Reznik I, Sirota P: Obsessive and compulsive symptoms in schizophrenia: a randomized controlled trial with fluvoxamine and neuroleptics. J Clin Psychopharmacol 20:410–416, 2000

Richelson E: Pharmacology of antidepressants. Mayo Clin Proc 76:511–527, 2001

Rocco PL, DeLeo D: Fluvoxamine-induced acute exacerbation in residual schizophrenia. Pharmacopsychiatry 25:245, 1992

Rosenheck R, Leslie D, Keefe R: Barriers to employment for people with schizophrenia. Am J Psychiatry 163:411–417, 2006

Rummel-Kluge C, Kissling W, Leucht S: Antidepressants for the negative symptoms of schizophrenia. Cochrane Database of Systematic Reviews 2006, Issue 3. Art. No.: CD005581. DOI: 10.1002/14651858.CD005581.pub2.

Rusconi AC, Carlone C, Muscillo M, et al: [SSRI antidepressants and negative schizophrenic symptoms: differences between paroxetine and fluvoxamine in patients treated with olanzapine.] (in Italian). Riv Psichiatr 44:313–319, 2009

Sacco KA, Bannon KL, George TP: Nicotinic receptor mechanisms and cognition in normal states and neuropsychiatric disorders. J Psychopharmacol 18:457–474, 2004

Salokangas RK, Saarijarvi S, Taiminen T, et al: Citalopram as an adjuvant in chronic schizophrenia: a double-blind placebo-controlled study. Acta Psychiatr Scand 94:175–180, 1996

Salzman SK, Kelly G, Chavin J, et al: Characterization of mianserin neuroprotection in experimental spinal trauma: dose/route response and late treatment. J Pharmacol Exp Ther 269:322–328, 1994

Sandson NB, Armstrong SC, Cozza KL: An overview of psychotropic drug-drug interactions. Psychosomatics 46:464–494, 2005

Schröder J, Bubeck B, Demisch S, et al: Benzodiazepine receptor distribution and diazepam binding in schizophrenia: an exploratory study. Psychiatry Res 68:125–131, 1997

Schutz G, Berk M: Reboxetine add on therapy to haloperidol in the treatment of schizophrenia: a preliminary double-blind randomized placebo-controlled study. Int Clin Psychopharmacol 16:275–278, 2001

Sepehry AA, Potvin S, Elie R, et al: Selective serotonin reuptake inhibitor (SSRI) add-on therapy for the negative symptoms of schizophrenia: a meta-analysis. J Clin Psychiatry 68:604–610, 2007

Shahid M, Walker GB, Zorn SH, et al: Asenapine: a novel psychopharmacologic agent with a unique human receptor signature. J Psychopharmacol 23:65–73, 2009

Shim JC, Kelly DL, Kim YH, et al: Fluoxetine augmentation of haloperidol in chronic schizophrenia. J Clin Psychopharmacol 23:520–522, 2003

Silver H: Selective serotonin reuptake inhibitor augmentation in the treatment of negative symptoms of schizophrenia. Int Clin Psychopharmacol 18:305–313, 2003

Silver H, Nassar A: Fluvoxamine improves negative symptoms in treated chronic schizophrenia: an add-on double-blind, placebo-controlled study. Biol Psychiatry 31:698–704, 1992

Silver H, Shmugliakov N: Augmentation with fluvoxamine but not maprotiline improves negative symptoms in treated schizophrenia: evidence for a specific serotonergic effect from a double-blind study. J Clin Psychopharmacol 18:208–211, 1998

Silver H, Kushnir M, Kaplan A: Fluvoxamine augmentation in clozapine resistant schizophrenia: an open pilot study. Biol Psychiatry 40:671–674, 1996

Silver H, Barash I, Aharon N, et al: Fluvoxamine augmentation of antipsychotics improves negative symptoms in psychotic chronic schizophrenic patients: a placebo-controlled study. Int Clin Psychopharmacol 15:257–261, 2000

Siris SG, Bermanzohn PC, Mason SE, et al: Maintenance imipramine therapy for secondary depression in schizophrenia: a controlled trial. Arch Gen Psychiatry 51:109–115, 1994

Siris S, Pollack S, Bermanzohn P, et al: Adjunctive imipramine for a broader group of post-psychotic depressions in schizophrenia. Schizophr Res 44:187–192, 2000

Spina E, de Leon J: Metabolic drug interactions with newer antipsychotics: a comparative review. Basic Clin Pharmacol Toxicol 100:4–22, 2007

Spina E, De Domenico P, Ruello C, et al: Adjunctive fluoxetine in the treatment of negative symptoms in chronic schizophrenic patients. Int Clin Psychopharmacol 9:281–285, 1994

Spina E, Avenoso A, Facciolà G, et al: Effect of fluoxetine on the plasma concentrations of clozapine and its major metabolites in patients with schizophrenia. Int Clin Psychopharmacol 13:141–145, 1998

Spina E, Avenoso A, Scordo MG, et al: Inhibition of risperidone metabolism by fluoxetine in patients with schizophrenia: a clinically relevant pharmacokinetic drug interaction. J Clin Psychopharmacol 22:419–423, 2002

Spina E, Scordo M, D'Arrigo C: Metabolic drug interactions with new psychotropic agents. Fundam Clin Pharmacol 17:517–538, 2003

Stahl SM, Pradko JF, Haight BR, et al: A review of the neuropharmacology of bupropion, a dual norepinephrine and dopamine reuptake inhibitor. Prim Care Companion J Clin Psychiatry 6:159–166, 2004

Syvälahti EK, Taiminen T, Saarijärvi S, et al: Citalopram causes no significant alterations in plasma neuroleptic levels in schizophrenic patients. J Int Med Res 25:24–32, 1997

Szegedi A, Anghelescu I, Wiesner J, et al: Addition of low-dose fluvoxamine to low-dose clozapine monotherapy in schizophrenia: drug monitoring and tolerability data from a prospective clinical trial. Pharmacopsychiatry 32:148–153, 1999

Takashi H, Sugita T, Higuchi H, et al: Fluvoxamine augmentation in risperidone-resistant schizophrenia: an open trial. Hum Psychopharmacol 17:95–98, 2002

Tsoi DT, Porwal M, Webster AC: Efficacy and safety of bupropion for smoking cessation and reduction in schizophrenia: systematic review and meta-analysis. Br J Psychiatry 196:346–353, 2010

Van Bockstaele EJ, Cestari DM, Pickel VM: Synaptic structure and connectivity of serotonin terminals in the ventral tegmental area: potential sites for modulation of mesolimbic dopamine neurons. Brain Res 647:307–322, 1994

Von Moltke LL, Greenblatt DJ, Grassi JM, et al: Citalopram and desmethylcitalopram in vitro: human cytochromes mediating transformation, and cytochrome inhibitory effects. Biol Psychiatry 46:839–849, 1999

Welham J, Stedman T, Clair A: Choosing negative symptom instruments: issues of representation and redundancy. Psychiatry Res 87:47–56, 1999

Whitehead C, Moss S, Cardno A, et al: Antidepressants for people with both schizophrenia and depression. Cochrane Database of Systematic Reviews 2002, Issue 2. Art. No.: CD002305. DOI: 10.1002/14651858.CD002305.

Williams JM, Ziedonis DM, Abanyie F, et al: Increased nicotine and cotinine levels in smokers with schizophrenia and schizoaffective disorder is not a metabolic effect. Schizophr Res 79:323–335, 2005

Wynchank D, Berk M: Efficacy of nefazodone in the treatment of neuroleptic induced extrapyramidal side effects: a double-blind randomised parallel group placebo-controlled trial. Hum Psychopharmacol 18:271–275, 2003

Yaryura-Tobias JA, Neziroglu F: The action of chlorimipramine in obsessive-compulsive neurosis: a pilot study. Curr Ther Res Clin Exp 17:111–116, 1975

Yoon JH, Maddock RJ, Rokem A, et al: GABA concentration is reduced in visual cortex in schizophrenia and correlates with orientation-specific surround suppression. J Neurosci 30:3777–3781, 2010

Zisook S, Kasckow JW, Golshan S, et al: Citalopram augmentation for subsyndromal symptoms of depression in middle-aged and older outpatients with schizophrenia and schizoaffective disorder: a randomized controlled trial. J Clin Psychiatry 70:562–571, 2009

Zoccali R, Muscatello MR, La Torre D, et al: Lack of pharmacokinetic interaction between mirtazapine and the newer antipsychotics clozapine, risperidone and olanzapine in patients with chronic schizophrenia. Pharmacol Res 48:411–414, 2003

Zoccali R, Muscatello MR, Cedro C, et al: The effect of mirtazapine augmentation of clozapine in the treatment of negative symptoms of schizophrenia: a double-blind, placebo-controlled study. Int Clin Psychopharmacol 19:71–76, 2004

Zohar J, Kaplan Z, Benjamin J: Clomipramine treatment of obsessive compulsive symptomatology in schizophrenic patients. J Clin Psychiatry 54:385–388, 1993

CHAPTER 5

Personality Disorders

Kenneth R. Silk, M.D.
Michael D. Jibson, M.D., Ph.D.

THE ROLE of antidepressant medications in patients with personality disorders has been studied since the mid-1970s. Although used for a wide array of symptoms these patients experience, antidepressants were initially used primarily for chronic dysphoria. They now are used for anxiety, impulsivity, anger, irritability, and mood lability. Substantial evidence exists regarding the use of antidepressants for the social phobia attendant to avoidant personality disorder or for the rigidity of obsessive-compulsive personality disorder, but data are confounded by diagnostic disagreement and uncertainty in the former and a lack of any real data in the latter. Although it is often dysphoria that brings patients with personality disorders to clinical attention, the antidepressants as a class appear to be less effective for these dysphoric or depressive symptoms in patients with personality disorders than for these symptoms in patients who do not have an Axis II comorbidity.

In this chapter, we briefly review the use of antidepressants for the range of mood disturbances that occur both across and within specific personality disorders. We also review the range of other symptoms among personality disorder patients that have responded to antidepressant medications in patients without personality disorder. We discuss the use of antidepressant medications in the personality disorders in general and for specific personality disorders. We review the use of this medication class in particular diagnostic groups—patients with borderline personality disorder (BPD), schizotypal personality disorder (STPD), and avoidant personality disorder (AvPD)—for which some empirical data might provide useful clinical information. We touch briefly on obsessive-compulsive personality disorder (OCPD), although evidence for pharmacological treatment is very weak. Additionally, we briefly cover the purported use of antidepressants in other personality disorders; we say "purported" because limited empirical data are available for the use of antidepressants for personality disorders other than BPD, STPD, and AvPD.

This overview might be simpler if antidepressants were used solely for mood dysregulation and/or depression in patients with personality disorders. However, they have been used for a wide array of symptoms, including impulsivity, aggression, emotional lability, irritability and anger, social anxiety and phobia, and overall functioning in these patients. Although all of these symptoms do not occur in all of the specific personality disorder syndromes, they all occur in BPD, and the most and best empirical data addressing these problems are found in studies of BPD.

Understanding Mood Disturbance in Personality Disorders

Although the antidepressant medications, particularly the selective serotonin reuptake inhibitors (SSRIs), have been found to be useful pharmacological agents for a wide array of symptoms, including depression, mood or emotional lability, irritability, anger, impulsivity, anxiety, and panic, the role of these medications, as their name implies, is for the treatment of depression. Thus, a good place to begin is to examine how to look at and/or understand depression in personality disorders. Most of what is known about personality disorders comes primarily from research into BPD, which is extended by inference to personality disorders in general. Although such inference makes some sense, because most of the empirical research in personality disorders is with patients who have BPD, and some from patients with STPD and antisocial personality disorder (ASPD) (Blashfield and Intoccia 2000), a number of reasons exist why BPD may not be the best proxy or prototype for the study of personality disorders (Mulder 2009; Tyrer 2009). Nonetheless, much of what we discuss in this chapter comes from work done with BPD, which is then extracted to other personality disorders. Although the multicenter Collaborative Longitudinal Personality Disorders Study has begun to accumulate data for AvPD and OCPD in addition to STPD and BPD (Skodol et al. 2005), not enough data are currently available to add substantially to the pharmacological database.

The experience of most of the affect of depression in BPD has usually been seen as qualitatively different from depression as experienced in a major depressive episode, although patients with BPD may endorse severity levels of depressive affect that equal or exceed those endorsed by patients with major depression. Often, the chronic dysphoria, emptiness, and loneliness about which borderline patients complain is mistaken for being active or residual symptoms of a major depressive episode (Silk 2010; Westen et al. 1992). This dysphoria is frequently triggered by external events that are related to actual or anticipated (whether real or imagined) separation or abandonment (Gunderson 1984, 1996). Patients with BPD rate their depression higher on self-rated scales than observers rate them on corresponding observer-rated scales (Levy et al. 2007; Stanley and Wilson 2006). Patients with BPD often experience the affect of anger accompanying the depression, as well as the feeling that they are bad, in contrast to the sadness and guilt often felt by patients experiencing an uncomplicated major depressive episode without significant personality disorder comorbidity (Gunderson 1984; Wilson et al. 2007). Furthermore, the depressive symptoms in a patient with BPD do not respond as readily or completely to antidepressants as do depressive symptoms in a patient with a major depressive episode without a comorbid personality disorder. Table 5–1 provides a summary of evidence that differentiates depression in BPD from a major depressive episode.

General Considerations

Some Historical Considerations

Few studies have examined the overlap between various personality disorders and major affective disorder, and most of the existing studies have merely recorded the comorbidity of the two disorders, either at intake into a study or at points of reassessment during the course of the study. Essentially, no data exist regarding antidepressant medication intervention for most of the specific personality disorders. Most available studies suggest that patients with major depression have a worse prognosis or a longer time to improvement when they have a comorbid personality disorder, although conflicting data exist with re-

TABLE 5–1. Uniqueness of reported depressive symptoms in patients with borderline personality disorder (BPD)

1. The dysphoric mood in BPD appears to be triggered by environmental issues, especially upon fear of separation, fear of abandonment, or actual separation.
2. The dysphoric mood often involves chronic feelings of boredom, emptiness, loneliness, and desperation (Gunderson 1984, 1996).
3. Patients with BPD without major depression can score on rating scales of depression as high as or even higher than patients with BPD with major depression (Levy et al. 2007).
4. Patients with BPD often score themselves higher on self-rating scales of depression than scores on their corresponding observer-rated scales suggest (Stanley and Wilson 2006).
5. The depression is more often experienced as a mad-bad depression than as a sad-guilty depression (Gunderson 1984; Wilson et al. 2007).
6. When the depression in BPD is qualitatively different from a major depressive episode, it does not respond as uniformly or as effectively to standard antidepressant treatment (Duggan et al. 2008; Nose et al. 2006).
7. All of the above-listed findings suggest that careful questioning will lead to appreciating that the quality of depression in BPD is different from the quality of depression as experienced in major depression without a comorbid personality disorder (Silk 2010; Westen et al. 1992).

spect to whether or not it is the comorbid presence of personality disorder and major depressive episode that delays, impedes, or prevents such pharmacological response (Mulder 2002; Newton-Howes et al. 2006).

Two theoretical speculations by clinicians are that patients with ASPD experience depression unconsciously, for which their acting-out behavior serves as a form of denial, and that patients with narcissistic personality disorder "allow" themselves to experience depression in response to even the slightest narcissistic injury. In the Collaborative Longitudinal Personality Disorders Study, Skodol et al. (1999) found co-occurrences of major depressive disorder and the following personality disorders: AvPD, 35% (n=324); BPD, 31% (n=240); OCPD, 24% (n=261); ASPD, 20% (n=49); narcissistic personality disorder, 15% (n=26); paranoid personality disorder, 14% (n=81); STPD, 13% (n=96); dependent personality disorder, 9% (n=49); schizoid personality disorder, 4% (n=18); and histrionic personality disorder, 1% (n=13). Eighty-five percent of those subjects had episodes of depression during a 6-year follow-up, with BPD subjects just as likely as subjects with other personality disorders to have new onsets (41% [*n*=15] vs. 45% [*n*=57]) but much more likely to have recurrences (92% [*n*=61] vs. 82% [*n*=126]) (Gunderson et al. 2008). Zanarini et al. (2004) found that comorbidity with major depression occurred at intake in 86% of subjects with BPD, decreasing 6 years later to 61%, in comparison to an "other personality disorders" group, which showed 76% of such comorbidity at baseline, decreasing 6 years later to 37%.

It would make sense that the major studies of pharmacological treatment of depression in patients with personality disorders would involve patients with BPD because there has been a long-standing argument since the publication of DSM-III (American Psychiatric Association 1980) as to whether BPD would be better classified as a mood disorder. Although the focus of this argument was mainly on the overlap between BPD and major depression (Akiskal 1981; Gunderson and Phillips 1991), more recently the discussion of the relationship of mood disorders and BPD has focused on the bipolar-BPD connection, particularly because much attention has been paid to the emotional dysregulation or instability found in patients with BPD and its similarity to or difference from bipolar disorder (Gunderson et al. 2006; Koenigsberg et al. 2002; Linehan 1993; Paris et al. 2007; Perugi et al. 2003; Putnam and Silk 2005; Sripada and Silk 2007; Wilson et al. 2007).

Mechanism of Action

Antidepressant medications operate primarily through modulation of the central serotonin and norepinephrine systems. Through a variety of mechanisms, such as presynaptic reuptake or blockade of enzymatic degradation, antidepressants directly or indirectly increase the level of these neurotransmitters available to postsynaptic receptors. These actions appear to have direct beneficial effects for depressed and anxious patients, but less attention has been given to how the mechanisms might impact personality disorders.

The neurobiology of BPD and STPD has been the subject of numerous studies, some of which may shed light on the role of antidepressant medications in their treatment. In this section, we focus on evidence for the involvement of specific neurotransmitter systems that might be affected by antidepressant treatment.

Borderline Personality Disorder

Although the dysphoria and affective instability of BPD suggest a common underlying neuropathology with mood disorders, the additional issues of impulsivity, interpersonal difficulties, and self-directed aggression suggest a unique basis for the disorder. Several lines of evidence point to dysregulation of serotonergic systems in BPD.

Early studies noted a correlation between low serum markers of serotonin and acts of aggression, impulsivity, disinhibition, suicidality, and feelings of emptiness in patients with BPD (Brown et al. 1982; Verkes et al. 1997, 1998). Central serotonin dysregulation was suggested by a blunted prolactin response to fenfluramine, an inhibitor of serotonin release and reuptake (Coccaro et al. 1989). Low serotonin metabolites in cerebrospinal fluid were observed directly in patients with BPD who had made serious suicide attempts (Gardner et al. 1990).

The prominent role of genetic factors was demonstrated by twin studies that yielded estimates of genetic heritability of BPD from 0.42 to 0.76 (Coolidge et al. 2001; Distel et al. 2008). Several genes have shown significant associations with BPD, including those coding for the serotonin transporter responsible for reuptake (5-HTT); serotonin 5-HT_{1A} and 5-HT_{2A} receptors; monoamine oxidase A; and tryptophan hydroxylase, the rate-limiting enzyme in serotonin synthesis (Ni et al. 2009; Wilson et al. 2009; Zaboli et al. 2006; Zetzsche et al. 2008).

Functional imaging studies have shown reduced serotonin responses in areas of the prefrontal cortex associated with impulse control in BPD patients specifically (Soloff et al. 2000) and in individuals with high levels of impulsive aggression generally (New et al. 2002). Most important from the perspective of treatment, the SSRI fluoxetine was found to normalize prefrontal activity in BPD patients with high levels of impulsive aggression (New et al. 2004).

On the basis of these studies, it has been hypothesized that the affective hyperresponsiveness and disinhibition seen in BPD arise from hypersensitivity of the limbic system and a failure of serotonergic functions in the prefrontal cortex (New et al. 2008; Siever 2008). This model suggests that antidepressants with primary serotonergic activity may be most effective in the treatment of at least some aspects of the disorder.

Schizotypal Personality Disorder

Studies of the biological basis of STPD have focused on aberrations of the dopamine system similar to those found in schizophrenia (Siever et al. 1993). Genetic studies show a strong overlap between the disorders, as do neuropsychological factors such as abnormalities in information processing, attention, and executive functions (Fanous and Kendler 2004). Structural brain abnormalities, including enlarged ventricles and increased ventricle-brain ratios, have likewise been reported in patients with STPD. Thus, modulation of dopamine pathways has been the focus of pharmacological treatment of the disorder.

With the exception of bupropion, which increases dopamine transmission via reuptake blockade, antidepressant medications show minimal dopaminergic activity and would be expected to have little beneficial effect on the core symptoms of STPD. Symptoms of depression and anxiety, however, are more common in both schizophrenia and STPD than in the general population. Some evidence suggests that an increased susceptibility to anxiety and mood disturbance contributes to the cognitive and functional deficits associated with schizophrenia spectrum disorders (Dickey et al. 2005; Mohanty et al. 2008). Thus, antidepressants may be of benefit both for comorbid anxiety and depression, and for the cognitive impairments associated with STPD.

Indications and Efficacy

The only controlled studies for the use of antidepressant medications in patients with personality disorders have occurred in patients with BPD and AvPD. The medications used have included the antidepressant categories of tricyclic antidepressants (TCAs), SSRIs, monoamine oxidase inhibitors (MAOIs), and mianserin, a tetracyclic antidepressant studied in the United Kingdom but not available in the United States. No controlled studies of bupropion have been done in patients with personality disorders. Although certain atypical antipsychotic medications have been shown to have some impact against the depression and/or emotion dysregulation found in BPD, the results of those studies are inconsistent, so we do not discuss them. Furthermore, we have restricted the medications discussed here to those medications or medication classes that are usually thought of and generally classified as antidepressants. The use of these atypical antipsychotic medications in patients with personality disorders has been reviewed in the first volume in this Evidence-Based Guide series (Silk and Jibson 2010).

We also have restricted the discussion (and the listing of relevant studies in the tables) to controlled studies. By doing this, we have limited ourselves essentially to studies of BPD. Although a number of studies have used antidepressant medications in patients with social phobia, and although there may be some reasons to think of AvPD and social phobia as being related and as overlapping in some patients, we commit only a brief paragraph to summarizing randomized controlled trials (RCTs) with respect to social phobia because the treatment of that disorder is covered elsewhere in this volume (see Chapter 3, "Anxiety Disorders").

In considering the use of antidepressants as a group, we find that within each class of antidepressants, no prototypical antidepressant has been used in RCTs. Also, no specific class of antidepressants has been used as the prototypic class. Thus, generalizability is limited. Furthermore, although some studies are methodologically sound, they suffer from having small numbers of subjects (Saunders and Silk 2009).

Other sources of inconsistency that limit generalizability are that different instruments are used to measure the same outcome in different studies and that more than one outcome measure may be used for the same outcome parameter in the same study. Also, at times, results from the different measures do not agree. The clinician is then left with trying to figure out the subtle (or at times not so subtle) distinction between two instruments that essentially study the same outcome or improvement in a specific outcome parameter. This inconsistency leads to a variation in outcomes across studies that is difficult to explain and leaves the field not much better informed than before the study was initiated (Duggan et al. 2008; Saunders and Silk 2009).

In RCTs, antidepressants have been employed primarily for the following indications: depression, emotional lability, anger, irritability, impulsivity, impulsive aggression, and anxiety, but outcome measures have also been applied to study suicidal behavior and ideation, dysphoria, global outcome, hostility, mood shifts, and abstinence or decreased use of alcohol or cocaine (Bellino et al. 2008; Duggan et al. 2008; Herpertz et al. 2007). In patients with social phobia, antidepressants have been shown to impact primarily social functioning and social anxiety, although outcome measures have been applied to measure general anxiety, avoidance, and depression (Herpertz et al. 2007) (Table 5–2).

Clinical Use

The use of antidepressants in patients with personality disorders is no different from their use in psychiatric patients in general. One can use the same starting dosage as one would use in any psychiatric patient and titrate dosages upward, again as one would with any psychiatric patient. Although there is some thought that the SSRI dosages needed to treat patients with personality disorders may be higher than those used to treat major depression (perhaps because of the prominent anxiety symptoms present in many of these patients), no systematic dosing studies have been done. Some people think that patients with personality disorders may be more prone to the activating or anxiogenic effects of the antidepressants, particularly the SSRIs, but again, no systematic studies have been performed. Early reports suggested that increased affective dysregulation occurred in patients with BPD in response to the TCAs (Soloff et al. 1987), but no systematic studies of TCAs have been done since that possibility was first observed. However, because TCAs are quite lethal, one must employ caution combined with careful monitoring when using this class of drugs among patients who can be both chronically suicidal and suddenly impulsive.

As mentioned earlier in the section "Indications and Efficacy," antidepressants, particularly the SSRIs, have been known to impact a broad array of symptoms, especially in patients with BPD. The major issue with respect to using these medications in patients with personality disorder is that therapeutic response, even when present, may be quite modest. Before increasing

TABLE 5–2. Symptoms that have been studied with respect to their pharmacological responsivity in personality disorders

Depression (±phenelzine, ±fluoxetine, ±amitriptyline [more effective when comorbid major depressive episode is present])
Dysphoria
Emotional lability (+fluvoxamine, ±fluoxetine)
Mood shifts (+fluvoxamine, ±fluoxetine)
Suicidal behavior
Suicidal ideation
Anger (+phenelzine, ±fluoxetine [perhaps more effective in aggressive patients])
Irritability (±fluoxetine)
Impulsivity
Impulsive aggression (+phenelzine, +fluoxetine [more effective when significant aggression/hostility is present])
Hostility (+phenelzine, ±fluoxetine [more effective when significant aggression/hostility is present])
Anxiety (+phenelzine, ±fluoxetine [more effective when actual anxiety disorder diagnosis is present])
Social phobia (+SSRIs)
Social functioning (+SSRIs in AvPD)
Social anxiety (+SSRIs in AvPD)
Avoidance (+SSRIs in AvPD)
Global outcome (+tranylcypromine, ±phenelzine)
Abstinence or decreased use of alcohol (+nortriptyline)
Abstinence or decreased use of cocaine

Note. + indicates moderate evidence for effectiveness, and ± indicates weak or contradictory evidence for effectiveness.
AvPD=avoidant personality disorder; SSRI=selective serotonin reuptake inhibitor.
Source. Bellino et al. 2008; Duggan et al. 2008; Herpertz et al. 2007.

the dosage or augmenting with a second medication, the treating physician needs to stop and consider 1) whether the medication resulted in some form of a decent therapeutic response given the patient's diagnosis and the (limited) knowledge of the therapeutic response to the medications in patients with personality disorder, and 2) whether the patient's remaining (or continuing) symptoms can be effectively treated pharmacologically or are more chronic, persistent symptoms representing the personality pathology (Westen et al. 1992; Zanarini et al. 2010). We do not intend to suggest that some of these remaining symptoms might not respond to medications; rather, we want to emphasize that the prescriber needs to appreciate that even the best response to pharmacological agents in the best of circumstances may be quite modest. Clinicians may have a tendency to use polypharmacy in patients with personality disorders, but no evidence exists supporting such prescribing practices in these patients.

As stated, the antidepressants as a group have been used in patients with personality disorders for a wide variety of symptomatic outcomes. Combining recent reviews by Bellino et al. (2008), Duggan et al. (2008), and Herpertz et al. (2007), we summarize in Table 5–2 the symptoms that have been targeted and the antidepressant medications that have been used and been found to be somewhat effective (though often not impressively so and often not in all studies). The antidepressant medications and the symptoms to which they have been applied are summarized in Table 5–3. (Table 5–2 is organized by symptom, whereas Table 5–3 is organized by medication.) Unfortunately, for most of these symptoms or behaviors, there are at least as many negative studies of pharmacological interventions as there are positive studies. Also, this listing does not mean that only these particular antidepressants are effective, but they are the only ones that have been found to be effective in RCTs. Clinicians should keep in mind that although antidepressant drugs in some instances can be used for a wide array of symptoms found among patients with personality disorder, the positive outcomes found in some studies have not been duplicated in other studies.

Guidelines for Selection and Use

Because no specific guidelines exist indicating which antidepressant medication a clinician might use preferentially for any given personality disorder, a clinician might wish to restrict use to those medications that have been shown to have at least some partial effectiveness in an RCT. To date, the medications that have shown some effectiveness are the SSRIs fluoxetine and fluvoxamine, the MAOIs phenelzine and tranylcypromine, and the TCA amitriptyline in BPD, and to all the SSRIs and venlafaxine in AvPD/social phobia. We again note caution in using a TCA in patients who have chronic suicidal and impulsive behavior and further note that in the United States, the MAOIs (i.e., phenelzine, tranylcypromine) currently appear to be out of favor.

The clinician might then choose among these medications with respect to side-effect profile. Although the side-effect profile of SSRIs appears more benign than the profile for either the MAOIs (weight gain and low blood pressure are common side effects, with adverse effects occurring in the face of tyramine-containing compounds that consist of high blood pressure and possible hypertensive crises) or the TCAs (cardiac arrhythmias; anticholinergic

TABLE 5–3. Antidepressants that have been found to ameliorate symptoms in patients with personality disorder

MEDICATION(S)	SYMPTOM(S)
Fluoxetine	Depression, anger, irritability, aggressiveness, anxiety, overall functioning
Fluvoxamine	Affective instability
Phenelzine	Depression, anger, hostility, anxiety, obsessiveness, psychoticism, schizotypal symptoms, overall functioning
Tranylcypromine	Overall functioning
Amitriptyline	Depression
Nortriptyline	Reduction in alcohol use
SSRIs[a]/venlafaxine	Social phobia, social anxiety, social functioning

Note. Although substantial multistudy support exists for improvement in social functioning, social phobia, and social anxiety, many studies do not show improvement in these other listed symptoms when treated with antidepressants. There is much contradictory evidence across studies.
SSRI=selective serotonin reuptake inhibitor.
[a]SSRIs include citalopram, escitalopram, fluoxetine, fluvoxamine, and paroxetine; clinical population studied was primarily patients with social phobia rather than avoidant personality disorder.
Source. Bellino et al. 2008; Duggan et al. 2008; Herpertz et al. 2007.

effects including headache, fatigue, urinary retention, and dry mouth; weight gain), the SSRIs do have side effects that can be quite distressing or disruptive to patients (gastrointestinal disturbances; substantial weight gain or weight loss; increased fatigue or anxiety; sleep difficulties; possibly increased suicidal ideation; sexual side effects that include difficulty or impossibility of reaching orgasm, impotence, delayed or retrograde ejaculation, or decreased libido; withdrawal symptoms upon discontinuation). Overall, however, the SSRIs are certainly more benign in overdose than are the MAOIs or the TCAs. The following is perhaps more important when considering the modest impact that SSRIs have in effectively treating the array of symptoms found in personality disorders: the cost-benefit ratio that appears to favor active pharmacological intervention with these agents in patients with major depression without confounding personality disorder can be thought of as changing substantially in patients when personality disorder is present. A clinician might be more cautious about prescribing in patients with comorbid major depression and personality disorder because the medication's overall effectiveness is decreased and sensitivity to side effects is increased.

Notably, studies of antidepressant medication in personality disorders, leaving aside the AvPD/social phobia diagnostic category, were much more prevalent in the 1980s and 1990s than they have been recently. Of the eight RCTs most frequently cited in reviews of pharmacotherapy of personality disorders, particularly BPD, six of the studies were completed by 1997. Only two RCTs of antidepressants have been conducted since then (Table 5–4).

The only study that has examined the long-term use of an antidepressant among patients with personality disorders is that by Soloff et al. (1993), who found decreased effectiveness of phenelzine for depression and irritability over time. Without more research to provide guidance, one must rely on clinical wisdom, which would suggest that if a medication does not appear to be impacting the identified target symptoms or, by extension, other symptoms by 12–16 weeks, then the medication should be stopped. Consideration should be given to using another antidepressant or switching to a different category of medications, either a mood stabilizer or an atypical antipsychotic.

The choice of a specific antidepressant medication may depend on a number of factors: 1) the actual cost of the medication to the patient, 2) the side-effect profile of the medication, 3) the potential or actual interactions of the medication with other medications that the patient is currently taking, and 4) the coexisting medical problems or medical status of the patient. Although all the SSRIs might be thought of as being "the same" in terms of their efficacy in patients with personality disorders, no data are available to support that conclusion, and drug-drug interactions also differ among the SSRIs. Only fluoxetine and fluvoxamine have been subjected to RCTs in the BPD population; whereas data suggest that fluvoxamine improves mood lability, only scant evidence suggests that fluoxetine has a similar impact, and most of the RCTs involving fluoxetine did not measure improved mood lability as an outcome. Also, despite some evidence for fluoxetine improving anger and anxiety in these patients (and perhaps having some impact on depressed mood), Rinne et al. (2002) did not explore those specific outcome measures in the only fluvoxamine RCT that has been published.

Side Effects and Their Management

The side effects of antidepressant medications in patients with personality disorders are no different from the side effects these medications might induce among patients with any diagnosis (and probably among nonpatients as well). In both sexes, SSRIs can cause sexual side effects, as mentioned in the previous section, "Guidelines for Selection and Use." Although the topic remains controversial, some evidence suggests that SSRIs result in increased suicidality, particularly when the drug is initiated or when it is stopped suddenly. The MAOIs can cause significant weight gain and/or hypertension when taken

TABLE 5–4. Randomized controlled trials that included antidepressants in the treatment of borderline personality disorder

RCT	Subject number and description	Methods	Medication and dosage	Outcome
Montgomery and Montgomery 1983	N=58 Suicidal behavior	6-month RCT	Mianserin Placebo	Drug=placebo
Cowdry and Gardner 1988	N=25 BPD; no comorbid depression	Randomized crossover trial, with each trial lasting 6 weeks	Tranylcypromine Trifluoperazine Alprazolam Carbamazepine Placebo	Patients taking tranylcypromine: global improvement noted by both patients and staff
Soloff et al. 1989	N=90 No comorbid bipolar disorder	5-week RCT	Haloperidol Amitriptyline 100–175 mg/day Placebo	Haloperidol>placebo and >amitriptyline for depressive/anxiety symptoms, hostility, paranoia, psychotic, and other behaviors; no advantage for haloperidol over amitriptyline or phenelzine on follow-up

TABLE 5–4. Randomized controlled trials that included antidepressants in the treatment of borderline personality disorder *(continued)*

RCT	Subject number and description	Methods	Medication and dosage	Outcome
Soloff et al. 1993	*N*=108 acute *N*=54 continuation	5-week RCT acute 16-week continuation	Phenelzine 15–90 mg/day Haloperidol	Phenelzine>haloperidol Phenelzine>placebo for depression, anxiety, anger, and hostility acutely; much less effect on irritability and depression during continuation phase
Salzman et al. 1995	*N*=22	13-week RCT	Fluoxetine 20–60 mg/day Placebo	Fluoxetine>placebo for anxiety, anger, and depression
Coccaro and Kavoussi 1997	*N*=40 Mixed PD with impulsive and/or aggressive issues Approximately one-third with BPD	12-week RCT	Fluoxetine 20–60 mg/day Placebo	Fluoxetine>placebo for verbal and impulsive aggression, and irritability; no effect on global functioning

TABLE 5–4. Randomized controlled trials that included antidepressants in the treatment of borderline personality disorder *(continued)*

RCT	Subject number and description	Methods	Medication and dosage	Outcome
Rinne et al. 2002	*N*=38; many with mood and anxiety disorders; none with bipolar disorder	6-week RCT	Fluvoxamine 150–250 mg/day Placebo	Fluvoxamine>placebo for rapid mood shifts; no effect on aggression or impulsivity
Simpson et al. 2004	*N*=25 No bipolar disorder	10- to 11-week RCT	Fluoxetine 40 mg/day+DBT Placebo+DBT Fluoxetine 40 mg/day	No additional benefit of fluoxetine over placebo on depression, anxiety, dissociation, aggression, and global functioning

Note. BPD=borderline personality disorder; DBT=dialectical behavior therapy; PD=personality disorder; RCT=randomized controlled trial.
Source. Adapted from Herpertz et al. 2007 with modifications from Mercer et al. 2009 and Ingenhoven et al. 2010.

in combination with foods that contain tyramine or with prescription or over-the-counter medications that can interact with the MAOIs. When patients are exposed to those adverse conditions, severe and life-threatening hypertension can occur. The primary troubling side effects of the TCAs include anticholinergic effects (see previous section, "Guidelines for Selection and Use"), as well as prolongation of the QT interval on electrocardiogram (ECG), and decreased transit time of the cardiac impulse through the atrioventricular node that can, in overdose, lead to fatal arrhythmias and orthostasis.

Cluster A Personality Disorders

Cluster A includes schizoid, schizotypal, and paranoid personality disorders. There are no empirical data on the use of antidepressants to address the core pathology of any of these disorders. Although some of the empirical studies of antidepressants in BPD included subjects who were comorbid for STPD, no data were reported to indicate whether those with comorbid STPD had response rates to antidepressants that were different from those of subjects without comorbid STPD. Some studies were done with subjects with "mixed" personality disorders, but those studies did not differentiate the study population sufficiently to determine the effectiveness of antidepressants with Cluster A personality disorders.

Antidepressants may be useful, however, for the treatment of comorbid depression and anxiety in patients with Cluster A personality disorders. Up to 50% of STPD patients have comorbid depression (Dickey et al. 2005), which contributes significantly to the functional impairment they experience (Mohanty et al. 2008). Although no studies have addressed the effectiveness of antidepressants for these symptoms in STPD, antidepressants are commonly used in patients with schizophrenia (Kasckow and Zisook 2008), and at least weak evidence suggests that they are beneficial in patients with schizophrenia (Whitehead et al. 2003).

Cluster B Personality Disorders (Excluding Borderline Personality Disorder)

Cluster B includes borderline, antisocial, histrionic, and narcissistic personality disorders. BPD is discussed more fully in the section "Borderline Personality Disorder" below. No empirical studies have been reported of the effectiveness of antidepressant medication in patients with either narcissistic or histrionic personality disorder. In the two empirical studies of the use of TCAs in patients with ASPD, the TCA was used to study its impact on addictive behavior. In one of these studies (Powell et al. 1995), 65 subjects with ASPD and alcohol dependence were treated with nortriptyline (which was compared with bromocriptine or placebo). The nortriptyline patients fared better in terms of decreased alcohol abuse. In the second study (Leal et al. 1994), 19 subjects who were being treated with methadone for cocaine abuse were randomly assigned to receive desipramine, amantadine, or placebo plus standard care in each instance. In the antisocial subset, there was no difference between medicated or placebo-exposed subjects with respect to drug-free urine samples.

Cluster C Personality Disorders

Cluster C includes dependent, obsessive-compulsive, and avoidant personality disorders. There are no empirical RCTs of the use of antidepressants in dependent personality disorders and only one study, whose methodology is unclear, of their use in OCPD. Most open studies reveal that comorbid OCPD does not appear to be associated with a better response to serotonergic antidepressants used in patients with OCD and could even represent a negative predictor. However, a 3-month, double-blind RCT of 24 outpatients assigned to either fluvoxamine (50–100 mg/day) or placebo found significant improvement in DSM-III-R (American Psychiatric Association 1987) OCPD symptoms in the fluvoxamine group compared with the placebo group (Ansseau et al. 1993).

Some studies have examined antidepressant use in patients with AvPD, but most of those studies involve social phobia. Some studies have "separated out" those patients who are both socially phobic as well as avoidant, but no empirical studies have looked only at AvPD. Four studies (Katchnig 1995; Noyes et al. 1997; Schneier et al. 1998; van Ameringen et al. 2001) reported the percentage of subjects who were also comorbid for AvPD in their social phobic sample (49% of 578, 48% of 583, 38% of 77, and 61% of 204, respectively). The earliest three studies involved moclobemide, an MOAI not approved for use in the United States, and the van Ameringen et al. (2001) study involved sertraline. In all four studies, there was essentially no difference in the percentage of subjects who improved between the non-AvPD and the AvPD comorbid groups. The range of improvement was from 18% to 53% in the medication-treated groups and from 13% to 34% in the placebo groups.

Borderline Personality Disorder

Choice of Antidepressant

RCTs with BPD have been conducted with SSRIs, TCAs, and MAOIs (see Tables 5–3 and 5–4). The results of these studies are not consistent. The data appear to suggest that among the antidepressants, phenelzine has the broadest effectiveness, as demonstrated by RCTs that support improvement for depression, anxiety, anger, hostility, and overall functioning; unfortunately, these data come from a single RCT (Soloff et al. 1993). Although fluoxetine, amitriptyline, and phenelzine have been shown to improve depression, the results of these studies are not overpowering. Even though some RCTs reveal that fluoxetine may improve anger, irritability, aggressiveness, and anxiety, Stoffers et al. (2010) concluded in a recent Cochrane review that for the symptom of depression, patients treated with fluoxetine did worse. This Cochrane review suggests that although phenelzine may improve overall functioning and fluvoxamine may improve affective instability, no further claims can be made for effectiveness of antidepressant medication in BPD. The data for effectiveness overall are often quite weak, and the sample sizes have been quite small. In light of such "weak" data, perhaps a good rule of thumb is to choose the medication based on the side-effect profile.

Indications and Efficacy

Although we have listed the various symptoms for which measures of outcome have been studied (see Table 5–2), the improvement in symptoms by drug (see Table 5–3), and the studies that led to these conclusions (see Table 5–4), we caution the reader against placing too much emphasis on the findings from these studies. The two most recent Cochrane reviews on BPD remain very cautious (Binks et al. 2006; Stoffers et al. 2010), especially with respect to effectiveness of antidepressants in BPD. A number of other reviews found contradictory evidence as to whether this broad class of drugs, despite the American Psychiatric Association (2001) guidelines that emphasized the use of SSRIs, can be labeled as being effective in this patient population. Those reviews and meta-analyses are listed in Table 5–5; although they all involved essentially the same eight studies or a subset of those studies (Table 5–6), the conclusions contradict one another. The National Institute for Health and Clinical Excellence (2011) study included the studies by Soloff et al. (1989, 1993), Cowdry and Garner (1988), Salzman et al. (1995), and Rinne et al. (2002). In general, however, these studies suggest that the evidence for antidepressant effectiveness in this population remains quite weak.

TABLE 5–5. Reviews and meta-analyses of randomized controlled trials that included antidepressants in the treatment of borderline personality disorder

Study and type	Comment	Conclusion for clinicians
Nose et al. 2006 (meta-analysis)	"Pharmacotherapy can exert a modest positive effect on specific core traits of BPD. Treatment with antidepressants, in particular fluoxetine, was effective against affective instability and impulsivity, although the finding on impulsivity was obtained by means of a post-hoc sensitivity analysis.... Treatment effects were particularly evident when subgroup analyses included patients with BPD only" (p. 352).	Effective for affective instability Possibly effective for impulsivity
Herpertz et al. 2007 (review, guideline)	"No class of psychopharmacological agents appears to improve BPD psychopathology in general" (p. 214). Some evidence indicates that they may influence emotion dysregulation that can include depression and anxiety, but perhaps only when these are comorbid Axis I conditions. No evidence of effectiveness for loneliness, emptiness, or boredom.	Weak evidence for antidepressant effectiveness in the absence of comorbid Axis I depressive or anxiety disorders
Duggan et al. 2008 (systematic review)	Weak evidence exists for some effectiveness for anger and depression, although other drug classes appear more effective.	Perhaps some weak evidence for anger and/or depression

TABLE 5–5. Reviews and meta-analyses of randomized controlled trials that included antidepressants in the treatment of borderline personality disorder *(continued)*

STUDY AND TYPE	COMMENT	CONCLUSION FOR CLINICIANS
National Institute for Health and Clinical Excellence 2011 (guideline)	"Drug treatment should not be used specifically for borderline personality disorder or for the individual symptoms or behaviour associated with the disorder (for example, repeated self-harm, marked emotional instability, risk-taking behaviour and transient psychotic symptoms)" (p. 10).	Little evidence for effectiveness for any symptoms
Mercer et al. 2009 (meta-analysis)	Antidepressants have a medium effect size for anger and a small effect size for depression.[a]	Perhaps some role for SSRIs or MAOIs, particularly in subjects with high levels of aggression
Binks et al. 2006 (Cochrane review)	Antidepressants do not seem to have an effect over placebo with regard to global functioning. Although scores on anger and depression may be improved, replication is needed. No evidence indicates reduction in suicidality, impulsivity, or hostility, except that hostility may respond to MAOIs. "If offered medication, people with BPD should know that this is not based on good evidence from clinical trials. This does not mean it may not do considerable good and there is no indication of significant harm" (p. 19).	Evidence is weak for anger and depression No evidence for improved global functioning Perhaps some effectiveness for MAOIs with hostility

TABLE 5–5. Reviews and meta-analyses of randomized controlled trials that included antidepressants in the treatment of borderline personality disorder *(continued)*

Study and type	Comment	Conclusion for clinicians
Lieb et al. 2010 (Cochrane review)	"There is little evidence for the effectiveness of antidepressant treatment.... There was only one significant effect for...amitriptyline in the reduction of depressive pathology. No significant effect was found for mianserin, the SSRIs fluoxetine and fluvoxamine or...phenelzine" (p. 7).	Little evidence for treatment with antidepressants Perhaps some evidence that amitriptyline may help with depression
Ingenhoven et al. 2010 (meta-analysis)	No effect was found for impulsivity or depression. Small effect was found for anxiety and anger.	Little substantial evidence for effectiveness but perhaps some for anxiety or anger

Note. BPD=borderline personality disorder; MAOI=monoamine oxidase inhibitor; SSRI=selective serotonin reuptake inhibitor.
[a]Only anger and depression were examined.

TABLE 5–6. Randomized controlled trials included in meta-analyses and/or systematic reviews

	Meta-analysis or review							
RCT	Nose et al. 2006	Herpertz et al. 2007	Duggan et al. 2008	Mercer et al. 2009	Binks et al. 2006	Lieb et al. 2010	Ingenhoven et al. 2010	NICE 2011
Montgomery and Montgomery 1983		+	+		+	+	+	
Cowdry and Gardner 1988		+		+			+	
Soloff et al. 1989	+	+	+	+	+	+	+	+
Soloff et al. 1993	+	+	+	+	+	+	+	+
Salzman et al. 1995	+	+	+	+	+	+	+	+
Coccaro and Kavoussi 1997	+	+	+	+			+	
Rinne et al. 2002	+	+	+	+		+	+	+
Simpson et al. 2004	+	+	+	+		+	+	

Note. NICE=National Institute for Health and Clinical Excellence; RCT=randomized controlled trial.

The following list summarizes the evidence for the use of antidepressants in patients with specific symptoms of BPD.

- *Depression*—The strongest evidence appears to be for phenelzine, with some weaker evidence for amitriptyline. The evidence for fluoxetine is contradictory, with one meta-analysis suggesting that it makes the symptom worse. Fluoxetine may be more effective when an established comorbid major depression is present.
- *Anxiety*—Some evidence supports the use of phenelzine or fluoxetine, but the evidence is not strong. These agents appear more effective when a comorbid anxiety disorder is present.
- *Anger*—There is probably more evidence for the use of antidepressants (phenelzine and fluoxetine) for anger than for any other symptom. Antidepressants appear to be most effective when aggression is clearly present.
- *Irritability, hostility, and aggressiveness*—Some evidence supports fluoxetine for irritability and aggressiveness and phenelzine for hostility, but the evidence is not strong and is at times contradictory.
- *Affective instability*—Fluvoxamine has been shown to be effective for affective instability, and fluoxetine has some support, although other classes of medications appear to have superior effectiveness.
- *Overall functioning*—The strongest evidence indicates that the MAOIs (i.e., phenelzine or tranylcypromine) result in greater improvement in global functioning. There is some, but weaker and contradictory at best, evidence for fluoxetine (see Table 5–2).

Clinical Use

The clinical use of antidepressant medications in patients with BPD is no different from that in an Axis I population. Care must be taken with respect to overdose with the TCAs and MAOIs, especially if the clinician is concerned about "acting-out" behavior. Compliance with dietary restrictions and clear warnings about the concomitant use of some other medications and supplements are important with MAOIs. Dosing is similar to that with patients without personality disorders, although some people think that SSRIs might be more effective at the higher end of the dosage range, at levels that might be used in patients with anxiety disorders.

Not only do patients with BPD present with a wide array of symptoms of varying severity, but the symptoms may come and go and the severity may change dramatically from session to session. Before deciding on a pharmacological strategy for a particular patient, the clinician might be wise to wait until he or she has a reasonably confident picture of what symptom or symptom complex appears to be the most persistent or the least varying from session to session. Once identified (not always an easy task), then this symptom or symptom complex can become the target for the pharmacological intervention. Rating scales may be useful to determine the overall trend of symptom change because the scales may help "see through" crises when all symptoms appear to be exacerbated. Full medication effectiveness may take 12–16 weeks, and for patients with BPD who appear to have incomplete response, switching rather than augmenting medication might be more useful. However, the clinician needs to be able to distinguish residual or remaining depressive symptoms from rage or anxiety that stems from the emptiness and loneliness of BPD.

No recent guidelines have been published for choosing among antidepressant medications for patients with BPD, and the American Psychiatric Association's (2001) "Practice Guideline for the Treatment of Patients with Borderline Personality Disorder" may be out of date (Abraham and Calabrese 2008). However, if one chooses to go the antidepressant route, the information in the subsection "Indications and Efficacy" above and in Table 5–2 might be informative. The guidelines of the National Institute for Health and Clinical Excellence (2011) do not recommend medication: "Drug treatment should not be used specifically for borderline personality disorder or for the individual symptoms or behaviour associated with the disorder (for example, repeated self-harm, marked emotional instability, risk-taking behaviour and transient psychotic symptoms)" (p. 10). Although other classes of medications can be used in treating BPD symptoms, the focus in this chapter is on the evidence for antidepressants.

In Table 5–2, we list the specific antidepressants subjected to RCTs and their impact on the symptoms of patients with personality disorders. No listing after a symptom means no evidence was found supporting the use of an antidepressant. Although at least one RCT has examined the impact of antidepressants on each symptom listed, lack of evidence may be because the symptom has only rarely been subjected to an outcome study in an RCT. Again, in general, the best advice is to choose the medication based primarily on the side-effect profile. Additional considerations are these: How much sedation is desirable? How much orthostasis might the medication induce? How much will the antidepressant cost (taking into account both the health plan and the patient)? Will it interact with other medications the patient is currently taking? Will the patient follow dietary restrictions? How impulsive is the patient?

Although more evidence may be available regarding the effectiveness of other classes of medications (mood stabilizers and atypical antipsychotics) for some of these symptoms, these categories of medications may be more problematic to take, and it may be harder to comply with such a regimen, because they tend to have more troubling short-term and long-term side effects. When

Soloff (1998) published his algorithms for the treatment of patients with personality disorders, the highest priority was given to proven effectiveness, and the secondary priority was given to safer medications. If clinicians think about the antidepressants according to this hierarchy, there may be some good clinical reasons to at least try SSRI antidepressants before trying other antidepressants or other categories of medications in patients with BPD.

Before Starting Medications

The advantages and disadvantages as well as the side effects of the medication should be discussed thoroughly with the patient, and the patient should be given adequate opportunity and encouragement to ask questions. The patient may wish to read about the particular medication on the Internet, although the reliability of the information found on the Internet is always questionable. Nonetheless, this collaborative approach is important to establish, especially for patients with BPD who may have also experienced significant abuse and/or invalidation (Linehan 1993; Ogata et al. 1990) in their past. Before prescribing, the clinician should also talk with the patient about the possibility of increased suicidality and/or anxiety for some people with BPD, particularly when they start taking SSRIs or abruptly stop taking them.

General laboratory screening is useful but not mandatory before initiating any medications so as to have some baseline measures as well as to rule out any baseline abnormalities. Complete blood count with differential and electrolytes, blood urea nitrogen, creatinine, liver function, and glucose are suggested. A baseline ECG is useful when a clinician is thinking of prescribing TCAs.

Side Effects, Drug-Drug Interactions, and Other Adverse Events

The side effects of antidepressants in patients with BPD are no different from the side effects of antidepressants in general. No specific unusual or untoward events should be anticipated because of the BPD diagnosis. Nonetheless, mention needs to be made that patients with BPD are thought to be both very sensitive to the side effects of psychotropic medication (although there are no empirical studies that support this observation) and impulsive. The management of these side effects is no different in this patient population than in any other patient population.

Because patients with BPD are often treated with polypharmacy, drug-drug interactions are important to consider. The clinician should talk with the patient about the increased risk of suicidality and anxiety with the SSRIs, and about hypotension and weight gain with the MAOIs, in addition to the hypertension that can occur when certain foods, over-the-counter medications, prescribed medications, or supplements are taken concurrently with MAOIs. The toxicity of the TCAs and the MAOIs should be addressed as well.

Fortunately, the SSRIs are reasonably safe in overdose, but the TCAs and MAOIs can be quite lethal (the TCAs are probably more lethal). The clinician should never ignore an accidental or attempted overdose, even with a relatively benign medication. Because the patient had an unsuccessful overdose attempt or did not choose a lethal enough agent or dosage for one attempt does not mean that the next attempt will have the same outcome. Furthermore, because patients with BPD are often taking multiple psychopharmacological agents, some of which may be more dangerous in overdose than the SSRIs, the clinician needs to make sure that the patient did not also overdose with other medications and that the patient understands the lethality of the other medications being taken or available to the patient.

Even when the patient is medically safe after an overdose, the clinician must not ignore or merely briefly touch on the act and the behavior leading up to the act. It is very important to discuss the proper use of medications and to emphasize that the patient needs to be serious and conscientious in their use. Patients must be honest with the clinician when they have been noncompliant with prescriptions; they should not stop taking medications without letting the clinician know; and they should inform the clinician immediately should they take more than the prescribed dosage.

KEY CLINICAL CONCEPTS

- There are no specific indications for the use of any psychotropic medication in any specific personality disorder or in the group of disorders as a whole.
- No solid indications exist for the use of any specific antidepressant medication for any personality disorder (except perhaps for AvPD and socially phobic/avoidant behavior). Therefore, the use of antidepressant medication in any personality disorder is using the medication off label.
- Although there are RCTs examining the use of antidepressant medications in BPD and AvPD and a single RCT for OCPD, no RCTs have been reported for the other personality disorders.
- In patients with BPD, antidepressant medications have been found in some studies to be effective for a wide array of symptoms and behaviors. These include global functioning, aggression, hostility, irritability, anxiety, and in some studies mood

lability and depression. Unfortunately, the evidence is not strong and is often contradictory.

- Good evidence suggests that in AvPD, SSRIs can improve social phobia and anxiety.
- Conventional wisdom suggests that when antidepressant medications (particularly the SSRIs) are used in patients with BPD, the dosages should be at the higher end of the dosage range.
- The side effects of antidepressant medication in patients with personality disorders are no different from the side effects of these medications in any patient population.
- General laboratory screening (blood, urine) is useful but not mandatory prior to initiating these medications. It is always good for the clinician to have some sense of the patient's general medical condition before prescribing medication.
- No studies have reported the long-term use of antidepressant medications in patients with personality disorders.

References

Abraham PF, Calabrese JR: Evidenced-based pharmacologic treatment of borderline personality disorder: a shift from SSRIs to anticonvulsants and atypical antipsychotics? J Affect Disord 111:21–30, 2008

Akiskal HS: Subaffective disorders: dysthymic, cyclothymic and bipolar II disorders in the "borderline" realm. Psychiatr Clin North Am 4:25–46, 1981

American Psychiatric Association: Diagnostic and Statistical Manual of Mental Disorders, 3rd Edition. Washington, DC, American Psychiatric Association, 1980

American Psychiatric Association: Diagnostic and Statistical Manual of Mental Disorders, 3rd Edition, Revised. Washington, DC, American Psychiatric Association, 1987

American Psychiatric Association: Practice guideline for the treatment of patients with borderline personality disorder. Am J Psychiatry 158(suppl):1–52, 2001

Ansseau M, Troisfontaines B, Papart P, et al: Compulsive personality and serotonergic drugs. Eur Neuropsychopharmacol 3:288–289, 1993

Bellino S, Paradiso E, Bogetto F: Efficacy and tolerability of pharmacotherapies for borderline personality disorder. CNS Drugs 22:671–692, 2008

Binks CA, Fenton M, McCarthy L, et al: Pharmacological interventions for people with borderline personality disorder. Cochrane Database Syst Rev 1:CD005653, 2006

Blashfield RK, Intoccia V: Growth of the literature on the topic of personality disorders. Am J Psychiatry 157:472–473, 2000

Brown GL, Ebert MH, Goyer PF, et al: Aggression, suicide, and serotonin: relationships to CSF amine metabolites. Am J Psychiatry 139:741–746, 1982

Coccaro EF, Kavoussi RJ: Fluoxetine and impulsive aggressive behavior in personality-disordered subjects. Arch Gen Psychiatry 54:1081–1088, 1997

Coccaro EF, Siever LJ, Klar HM, et al: Serotonergic studies in patients with affective and personality disorders: correlates with suicidal and impulsive aggressive behavior. Arch Gen Psychiatry 46:587–599, 1989

Coolidge FL, Thede LL, Jang KL: Heritability of personality disorders in childhood: a preliminary investigation. J Pers Disord 15:33–40, 2001

Cowdry RW, Gardner DL: Pharmacotherapy of borderline personality disorder: alprazolam, carbamazepine, trifluoperazine, and tranylcypromine. Arch Gen Psychiatry 45:111–119, 1988

Dickey CC, McCarley RW, Niznikiewicz MA, et al: Clinical, cognitive, and social characteristics of a sample of neuroleptic-naive persons with schizotypal personality disorder. Schizophr Res 78:297–308, 2005

Distel MA, Trull TJ, Derom CA, et al: Heritability of borderline personality disorder features is similar across three countries. Psychol Med 38:1219–1229, 2008

Duggan C, Huband N, Smailagic N, et al: The use of pharmacological treatments for people with personality disorder: a systematic review of randomized controlled trials. Personal Ment Health 2:119–170, 2008

Fanous AH, Kendler KS: The genetic relationship of personality to major depression and schizophrenia. Neurotox Res 6:43–50, 2004

Gardner DL, Lucas PB, Cowdry RW: CSF metabolites in borderline personality disorder compared with normal controls. Biol Psychiatry 28:247–254, 1990

Gunderson JG: Borderline Personality Disorder. Washington, DC, American Psychiatric Press, 1984

Gunderson JG: The borderline patient's intolerance of aloneness: insecure attachments and therapist availability. Am J Psychiatry 153:752–758, 1996

Gunderson JG, Phillips KA: A current view of the interface between borderline personality disorder and depression. Am J Psychiatry 148:967–975, 1991

Gunderson JG, Weinberg I, Davevsa MT, et al: Descriptive and longitudinal observations on the relationship of borderline personality disorder and bipolar disorder. Am J Psychiatry 163:1173–1178, 2006

Gunderson JG, Stout RL, Sanislow CA, et al: New episodes and new onsets of major depression in borderline and other personality disorders. J Affect Disord 111:40–45, 2008

Herpertz SC, Zanarini M, Schulz CS, et al: World Federation of Societies of Biological Psychiatry (WFSBP) guidelines for biological treatment of personality disorders. World J Biol Psychiatry 8:212–244, 2007

Ingenhoven T, Lafay P, Rinne T, et al: Effectiveness of pharmacotherapy for severe personality disorders: meta-analyses of randomized controlled trials. J Clin Psychiatry 71:14–25, 2010

Kasckow JW, Zisook S: Co-occurring depressive symptoms in the older patient with schizophrenia. Drugs Aging 25:631–647, 2008

Katchnig H, Amering M, Stolk JM, et al: Long-term follow-up after a drug trial for panic disorder. Br J Psychiatry 167:487–494, 1995

Koenigsberg HW, Harvey PD, Mitropoulou V, et al: Characterizing affective instability in borderline personality disorder. Am J Psychiatry 159:784–788, 2002

Leal J, Zedonis D, Kosten T: Antisocial personality disorder as a prognostic factor for pharmacotherapy of cocaine dependence. Drug Alcohol Depend 35:31–35, 1994

Levy KN, Edell WS, McGlashan TH: Depressive experiences in inpatients with borderline personality disorder. Psychiatr Q 78:129–143, 2007

Lieb K, Völlm B, Rücker G, et al: Pharmacotherapy for borderline personality disorder: Cochrane systematic review of randomised trials. Br J Psychiatry 196:4–12, 2010

Linehan MM: Cognitive-Behavioral Treatment of Borderline Personality Disorder. New York, Guilford, 1993

Mercer M, Douglass AB, Links PS: Meta-analyses of mood stabilizers, antidepressants and antipsychotics in the treatment of borderline personality disorder: effectiveness for depression and anger symptoms. J Pers Disord 23:156–174, 2009

Mohanty A, Heller W, Koven NS, et al: Specificity of emotion-related effects on attentional processing in schizotypy. Schizophr Res 103:129–137, 2008

Montgomery SA, Montgomery D: The prevention of recurrent suicidal acts. Br J Clin Psychopharmacol 15 (suppl 2):183–188, 1983

Mulder RT: Personality pathology and treatment outcome in major depression: a review. Am J Psychiatry 159:359–371, 2002

Mulder R: Is borderline personality disorder really a personality disorder? Personality Ment Health 3:85, 2009

National Institute for Health and Clinical Excellence: Borderline personality disorder: treatment and management. March 22, 2011. Available at: www.nice.org.uk/CG78. Accessed May 10, 2011.

New AS, Hazlett EA, Buchsbaum MS, et al: Blunted prefrontal cortical 18fluorodeoxyglucose positron emission tomography response to meta-chlorophenylpiperazine in impulsive aggression. Arch Gen Psychiatry 59:621–629, 2002

New AS, Buchsbaum MS, Hazlett EA, et al: Fluoxetine increases relative metabolic rate in prefrontal cortex in impulsive aggression. Psychopharmacology 176:451–458, 2004

New AS, Goodman M, Triebwasser J, et al: Recent advances in the biological study of personality disorders. Psychiatr Clin North Am 31:441–461, vii, 2008

Newton-Howes G, Tyrer P, Johnson T: Personality disorder and the outcome of depression: meta-analysis of published studies. Br J Psychiatry 188:13–20, 2006

Ni X, Chan D, Chan K, et al: Serotonin genes and gene-gene interactions in borderline personality disorder in a matched case-control study. Progr Neuropsychopharmacol Biol Psychiatry 33:128–133, 2009

Nose M, Cipriani A, Biancosino B, et al: Efficacy of pharmacotherapy against core traits of borderline personality disorder: meta-analysis of randomized controlled trials. Int J Clin Psychopharmacol 21:345–353, 2006

Noyes R Jr, Moroz G, Davidson J, et al: Moclobemide in social phobia: a controlled dose-response trial. J Clin Psychopharmacol 17:247–254, 1997

Ogata S, Silk KR, Goodrich S, et al: Childhood sexual and physical abuse in adult patients with borderline personality disorder. Am J Psychiatry 147:1008–1013, 1990

Paris J, Gunderson J, Weinberg I: The interface between borderline personality disorder and bipolar spectrum disorders. Compr Psychiatry 48:145–154, 2007

Perugi G, Toni C, Travierso MC, et al: The role of cyclothymia in atypical depression: toward a data-based reconceptualization of the borderline–bipolar II connection. J Affect Disord 73:87–98, 2003

Powell DJ, Campbell LJ, Landn JF, et al: A double-blind, placebo-controlled study of nortriptyline and bromocriptine in male alcoholics subtyped by comorbid psychiatric disorders. Alcohol Clin Exp Res 19:462–468, 1995

Putnam K, Silk KR: Emotion dysregulation and the development of borderline personality disorder. Dev Psychopathol 17:899–925, 2005

Rinne T, van den Brink W, Wouters L, et al: SSRI treatment of borderline personality disorder: a randomized, placebo-controlled clinical trial for female patients with borderline personality disorder. Am J Psychiatry 159:2048–2054, 2002

Salzman C, Wolfson AN, Schatzberg A, et al: Effect of fluoxetine on anger in symptomatic volunteers with borderline personality disorder. J Clin Psychopharmacol 15:23–29, 1995

Saunders EFH, Silk K: Personality trait dimensions and the pharmacologic treatment of borderline personality disorder. J Clin Psychopharmacol 29:461–467, 2009

Schneier FR, Gortz D, Campeas R, et al: Placebo-controlled trial of meclobemide in social phobia. Br J Psychiatry 172:70–77, 1998

Siever LJ: Neurobiology of aggression and violence. Am J Psychiatry 165:429–442, 2008

Siever LJ, Kalus OF, Keefe RSE: The boundaries of schizophrenia. Psychiatr Clin North Am 16:217–244, 1993

Silk KR: The quality of depression in borderline personality disorder and the diagnostic process. J Pers Disord 24:25–37, 2010

Silk KR, Jibson MD: Personality disorders, in The Evidence-Based Guide to Antipsychotic Medications. Edited by Rothschild AJ. Washington, DC, American Psychiatric Publishing, 2010, pp 101–124

Simpson EB, Yen S, Costello E, et al: Combined dialectical behavior therapy and fluoxetine in the treatment of borderline personality disorder. J Clin Psychiatry 65:379–385, 2004

Skodol AE, Stout RL, McGlashan T, et al: Co-occurrence of mood and personality disorders: a report from the Collaborative Longitudinal Personality Disorders Study (CLPS). Depress Anxiety 10:175–182, 1999

Skodol AE, Gunderson JG, Shea MT, et al: The Collaborative Longitudinal Personality Disorders Study (CLPS): overview and implications. J Pers Disord 19:487–504, 2005

Soloff PH: Algorithms for pharmacological treatment of personality dimensions: symptom-specific treatments for cognitive-perceptual, affective, and impulsive-behavioral dysregulation. Bull Menninger Clin 62:195–214, 1998

Soloff PH, George A, Nathan RS, et al: Behavioral dyscontrol in borderline patients treated with amitriptyline. Psychopharmacol Bull 23:177–181, 1987

Soloff PH, George A, Nathan S, et al: Amitriptyline versus haloperidol in borderlines: final outcomes and predictors of response. J Clin Psychopharmacol 9:238–246, 1989

Soloff PH, Cornelius J, George A, et al: Efficacy of phenelzine and haloperidol in borderline personality disorder. Arch Gen Psychiatry 50:377–385, 1993

Soloff PH, Meltzer CC, Greer PJ, et al: A fenfluramine-activated FDG-PET study of borderline personality disorder. Biol Psychiatry 47:540–547, 2000

Sripada CS, Silk KR: The role of functional neuroimaging in exploring the overlap between borderline personality disorder and bipolar disorder. Curr Psychiatry Rep 9:40–45, 2007

Stanley B, Wilson ST: Heightened subjective experience of depression in borderline personality disorder. J Pers Disord 20:307–318, 2006

Stoffers J, Völlm BA, Rücker G, et al: Pharmacological interventions for borderline personality disorder. Cochrane Database of Systematic Reviews 2010, Issue 6. Art. No.: CD005653. DOI: 10.1002/14651858.CD005653.pub2.

Tyrer P: Why borderline personality disorder is neither borderline nor a personality disorder. Personal Ment Health 3:86–95, 2009 van Ameringen AM, Lane RM, Waloker JR, et al: Sertraline treatment of generalized social phobia: a 20-week, double-blind, placebo-controlled study. Am J Psychiatry 158:275–281, 2001

Verkes RJ, Fekkes D, Zwinderman AH, et al: Platelet serotonin and [3H]paroxetine binding correlate with recurrence of suicidal behavior. Psychopharmacology 132:89–94, 1997

Verkes RJ, Van der Mast RC, Kerkhof AJ, et al: Platelet serotonin, monoamine oxidase activity, and [3H]paroxetine binding related to impulsive suicide attempts and borderline personality disorder. Biol Psychiatry 43:740–746, 1998

Westen D, Moses MJ, Silk KR, et al: Quality of depressive experience in borderline personality disorder and major depression: when depression is not just depression. J Pers Disord 6:382–393, 1992

Whitehead C, Moss S, Cardno A, et al: Antidepressants for the treatment of depression in people with schizophrenia: a systematic review. Psychol Med 33:589–599, 2003

Wilson ST, Stanley B, Oquendo MA, et al: Comparing impulsiveness, hostility, and depression in borderline personality disorder and bipolar II disorder. J Clin Psychiatry 68:1533–1539, 2007

Wilson ST, Stanley B, Brent DA, et al: The tryptophan hydroxylase-1 A218C polymorphism is associated with diagnosis, but not suicidal behavior, in borderline personality disorder. Am J Med Genet B Neuropsychiatr Genet 150B:202–208, 2009

Zaboli G, Gizatullin R, Nilsonne A, et al: Tryptophan hydroxylase-1 gene variants associate with a group of suicidal borderline women. Neuropsychopharmacology 31:1982–1990, 2006

Zanarini MC, Frankenburg FR, Hennen J, et al: Axis I co-morbidity in patients with borderline personality disorder: 6-year follow-up and prediction of time to remission. Am J Psychiatry 161:2108–2114, 2004

Zanarini MC, Frankenburg FR, Reich DB, et al: The subsyndromal phenomenology of borderline personality disorder: a 10-year follow-up study. Am J Psychiatry 164:929–935, 2010

Zetzsche T, Preuss UW, Bondy B, et al: 5-HT1A receptor gene C-1019 G polymorphism and amygdala volume in borderline personality disorder. Genes Brain Behav 7:306–313, 2008

CHAPTER 6

Substance-Related Disorders

Avram H. Mack, M.D., F.A.P.A.

THE SUBSTANCE-RELATED disorders (SRDs) are perhaps the most prevalent of the psychiatric disorders. They result in a tremendous amount of morbidity and mortality and are associated with other societal costs (e.g., crime, absenteeism). With their high prevalence and societal cost, SRDs present as a major medical and psychiatric challenge for which successful pharmacological treatments have, with some exceptions, been elusive.

The SRDs are a large, heterogeneous group of disorders that have varied neurobiological states, pharmacology, and natural history. Substantial efforts have addressed the possible value of using antidepressants to reduce substance use or to alleviate substance-related or substance-induced symptoms. When considering the application of antidepressant medications to treat any SRD, clinicians need to keep in mind these basic points: with a few exceptions, the use of antidepressants in persons misusing substances tends to present dangers in misattribution of effect, is not typically approved according to U.S. Food and Drug Administration (FDA) labeling, and is based on little to no data. Therefore, this chapter is structured in a way that lays out the many clinical SRD situations in which an antidepressant might be used, but it also may be based on lesser evidence than for other conditions. This chapter is divided into two sections: the indications for antidepressants in SRDs and any information available about the use of antidepressant medications in SRDs. A few topics of great interest include bupropion for nicotine dependence, selective serotonin reuptake inhibitors (SSRIs) for comorbid alcohol dependence and depression, and other agents for cocaine depression. This sporadic grouping of therapies not only underlines the heterogeneity of the natural history and biology of the various substances of abuse, but also belies the vast number of attempts to find methods to treat these destructive conditions.

Indications for Antidepressant Medications

When considering indications for medication use for SRDs, one needs to rely on DSM-IV-TR (American Psychiatric Association 2000) diagnoses. Many different medication therapies are available, but one must have a target syndrome before use. It can be helpful to divide such indications into three types: 1) treatment of a substance use disorder (dependence, abuse, intoxication, or withdrawal); 2) treatment of substance-induced psychiatric disorders, such as alcohol-induced mood disorder; and 3) treatment of diagnoses or nonspecific conditions associated with substance use disorders. These specific indications are discussed after the following general review of SRDs.

In DSM-IV-TR, the term *substances* refers to drugs of abuse, medications, or toxins, and it need not be limited to those that are "psychoactive." The DSM-IV-TR classification provides diagnostic groups for multiple substances: alcohol; amphetamines; caffeine; cannabis; cocaine; hallucinogens; inhalants; nicotine; opioids; phencyclidine; sedatives, hypnotics, and anxiolytics; multiple substances (polysubstance); and other or unknown substances. The "other" group covers substances that are typically abused, but it also may be used for medications that are infrequently misused, such as quetiapine. A key point is that awareness of the substance being used by a patient is of great importance for a clinician to properly determine the basis for the patient's status or to predict the likely short- or long-term course.

The SRDs are classified in DSM-IV-TR as either *substance use disorders* or *substance-induced disorders,* and this distinction is vital. After determining the substance being misused, the clinician who is considering treatment of a person with an SRD turns attention to diagnosis and neurobiological status.

The classification and nomenclature of the SRDs are not trivial, and clinicians should be aware of distinctions in DSM-IV-TR, which provides generic definitions of conditions associated with the various substances. The substance use disorders include two conditions—substance dependence and substance abuse—in which there is a clinically significant syndrome due to the specific form of maladaptive use. Substance-induced disorders include intoxication or withdrawal syndromes that are characteristic for the substance in question, as well as several other substance-induced conditions, such as mood, anxiety, psychosis, sexual dysfunctions, and others. Not all substances cause all of the SRDs, as can be seen in a careful review of Tables 6–1 and 6–2. For example, no DSM-IV-TR diagnostic category exists for polysubstance abuse or for caffeine abuse. Although DSM-IV-TR does not include a withdrawal syndrome for cannabis, evidence has accumulated that there is a recognizable cannabis withdrawal syndrome (Budney and Hughes 2006), and the syndrome might be included in the forthcoming DSM-5. Table 6–2 indicates that psychotic disorders may be induced by sedatives, hypnotics, or anxiolytics during either intoxication or withdrawal, but that psychotic disorders are not recognized as being induced by caffeine. Readers of this book might be especially interested in reviewing the substances that are recognized by DSM-IV-TR as causative of either mood or anxiety disorders or sleep dysfunction. (See Mack et al. 2010 for other sources for reviews.)

Substance Use Disorders

Perhaps the foremost question that continues to be addressed in the literature and in clinical settings is whether any medications can modify, treat, or cure the substance use disorders (i.e., abuse and dependence). Some medications are useful for each of the substances of abuse, such as naltrexone for opioid dependence or disulfiram for alcohol dependence or abuse. The focus in this subsection is on evidence that supports the use of the various antidepressants for substance abuse or dependence.

Substance dependence is a state of cognitive, behavioral, and physiological features that together signify continued use despite significant substance-related problems. It is a pattern of repeated self-administration that can result in tolerance, withdrawal, and compulsive drug-taking behavior. According to DSM-IV-TR, over a 12-month period, the patient must exhibit three behaviors out of a seven-item polythetic criteria set. Neither tolerance nor withdrawal is necessarily required or sufficient for a diagnosis of substance dependence. Usually, a past history of tolerance or withdrawal is associated with a more severe clinical course. When substance dependence is present, the individual is assumed to have experienced alteration of central nervous system pathways, in particular the reinforcement of the cortico-mesolimbic/mesocortical dopamine

TABLE 6–1. Diagnoses associated with class of substances

	Intoxication	Withdrawal	Intoxication delirium	Withdrawal delirium	Dementia	Amnestic disorder	Psychotic disorders	Mood disorders	Anxiety disorders	Sexual dysfunctions	Sleep disorders
Alcohol	X	X	I	W	P	P	I/W	I/W	I/W	I	I/W
Amphetamines	X	X	I				I	I/W	I	I	I/W
Caffeine	X								I		I
Cannabis	X		I				I		I		
Cocaine	X	X	I				I	I/W	I/W	I	I/W
Hallucinogens	X		I				I*	I	I		
Inhalants	X		I		P		I	I	I		
Nicotine		X									
Opioids	X	X	I				I	I		I	I/W
Phencyclidine	X		I				I	I	I		
Sedatives, hypnotics, or anxiolytics	X	X	I	W	P	P	I/W	I/W	W	I	I/W
Polysubstance											
Other	X	X	I	W	P	P	I/W	I/W	I/W	I	I/W

*Also Hallucinogen Persisting Perception Disorder (Flashbacks).

Note. X, I, W, I/W, or P indicates that the category is recognized in DSM-IV. In addition, *I* indicates that the specifier With Onset During Intoxication may be noted for the category (except for Intoxication Delirium); *W* indicates that the specifier With Onset During Withdrawal may be noted for the category (except for Withdrawal Delirum); and *I/W* indicates that either With Onset During Intoxication or With Onset During Withdrawal may be noted for the category. *P* indicates that the disorder is Persisting.

Source. Reprinted from American Psychiatric Association: *Diagnostic and Statistical Manual of Mental Disorders,* 4th Edition, Text Revision. Washington, DC, American Psychiatric Association, 2000.

TABLE 6–2. Substance use disorders associated with class of substances

	DEPENDENCE	ABUSE
Alcohol	X	X
Amphetamines	X	X
Caffeine		
Cannabis	X	X
Cocaine	X	X
Hallucinogens	X	X
Inhalants	X	X
Nicotine	X	
Opioids	X	X
Phencyclidine	X	X
Sedatives, hypnotics, or anxiolytics	X	X
Polysubstance	X	
Other	X	X

Note. X indicates that the category is recognized in DSM-IV-TR.
Source. Reprinted from American Psychiatric Association: *Diagnostic and Statistical Manual of Mental Disorders,* 4th Edition, Text Revision. Washington, DC, American Psychiatric Association, 2000. Copyright 2000. Used with permission.

projections; increased activation of this tract is considered the final common pathway of the various types of dependence. It is unclear whether this alteration occurs in persons diagnosed with substance abuse, which is use despite significant problems caused by the use in those who do not meet criteria for substance dependence. One criterion is the failure to fulfill major role obligations. To fulfill a criterion for DSM-IV-TR substance abuse, the substance-related problem must have occurred repeatedly or persistently during the same 12-month period. The criteria for abuse do not include tolerance, withdrawal, or compulsive use.

The development of pharmacological approaches to the substance use disorders has not derived a pharmacological mechanism that is usable for all substances. Despite the understanding of the neurobiology of the dependent state, medication therapies have mostly created action at receptors away from the central mesocortical/mesolimbic tracts. Instead, the various therapies have tended to act neurochemically at other sites, such as portions of the nicotine receptor in the case of varenicline in the treatment of nicotine dependence. And these medications effect the end of dependence or abuse in different ways—from creating a behavioral aversion to use (disulfiram) to reducing cravings (naltrexone). Some medication therapies are an established central part of the treatment of alcohol, opioid, and nicotine use disorders. These medications are given in other conditions despite moderate to low evidence bases. This characterization applies to antidepressant medications as well. In the following subsections, I review three types of substance dependence for which evidence suggests that an antidepressant is helpful in treatment. Notwithstanding the many trials, ideas, and investigations to find treatments for the substance use disorders, the literature contains insufficient information to discuss use of antidepressants to treat other types of substance use disorders.

Nicotine Dependence

The pharmacological treatment of nicotine dependence might include nicotine replacement therapies or varenicline or the antidepressant bupropion in the sustained-release (SR) form. Bupropion SR, which has FDA approval for smoking cessation, is a first-line pharmacological treatment for nicotine dependence. The goals of treatment with bupropion in nicotine dependence include cessation, reduction of craving and withdrawal symptoms, and prevention of cessation-induced weight gain. In addition, evidence suggests that other antidepressants, including monoamine oxidase inhibitors (MAOIs) (George et al. 2003) and nortriptyline (Fiore et al. 2000), are helpful in nicotine dependence. The mechanism by which these antidepressants alter nicotine use is not precisely known, but one might speculate about the depressive syndrome that often follows smoking cessation and whether or not these interact with that development.

Cocaine Dependence

Much study has been done on the use of antidepressants in cocaine dependence. Overall, the efficacy of the pharmacological treatments in use is poorly supported. The first-line medications include dopaminergic agents; antidepressants are a second-line choice, based on the theory that they would counteract the alterations in catecholamine receptors that occur due to chronic stimulant exposure. SSRIs, including fluoxetine, have not been shown to be effective. At this time, support for this indication exists only for desipramine, a tricyclic antidepressant (TCA) (Oliveto et al. 1999).

Methamphetamine Dependence

In actuality, methamphetamines fall under the category of amphetamines (which are very similar pharmacologically to cocaine). However, only methamphetamine has a small evidence base to support the use of bupropion as a treatment of dependence (Newton et al. 2006).

Substance-Induced Disorders

Substance-induced disorders are those disorders that cover the psychiatric manifestations that are caused by the substances themselves. A substance-induced disorder is akin to a psychiatric condition that is due to a general medical condition; in this case, the condition is the presence of the substance in the body. Besides substance intoxication and withdrawal, which are defined according to the substance being used, several other descriptively defined conditions (e.g., substance-induced delirium, substance-induced mood disorder) are included elsewhere in DSM-IV-TR. Because substances do not necessarily cause some of these categories of illness, the clinician must refer to Tables 6–1 and 6–2 to ensure that he or she is making a bona fide diagnosis. The clinician should keep in mind that antidepressant medications might be indicated among these conditions for states other than depressed mood (e.g., for anxiolysis) and should consider whether using antidepressants for these indications is approved by the FDA.

Intoxication

Overconsumption of a substance may lead to immediate symptoms, signs, and disability that are characteristic of the substance. Clinicians may see intoxication states in emergency rooms, in cases of iatrogenic overdose, or elsewhere. Some substances pose risks of violence or suicide during intoxication (e.g., phencyclidine), whereas others result in sedate calm (e.g., cannabis). Most types of intoxication require supportive care; situations that lapse into overdose require more intensive attention. Antidepressant medications are rarely included in the armamentarium for intoxication. Amphetamines (witness children on methylphenidate) and cocaine may cause dysphoria, but such substance-induced mood disorders are not candidates for intervention with antidepressant medications.

Withdrawal

Upon any relative drop in exposure to most substances of abuse, the human body may follow with a characteristic set of symptoms and signs. In some cases the condition is mainly uncomfortable (e.g., opioid withdrawal), but in other cases there are dangers of morbidity or mortality. Most of the withdrawal syndromes are treated with nonspecific supportive measures (except that specific replacement treatment regimens are used for sedative/hypnotic, nicotine, alcohol, or opioid withdrawal). The example of withdrawal from benzodiazepines is a special case, because detoxification from benzodiazepines may last several weeks and mood symptoms may occur during this protracted period (as well as a resumption of underlying anxiety, as discussed in subsection "Anxiety Disorders" later in this chapter). The use of antidepressants during this protracted period has been shown to improve outcome (Rickels et al. 1999). Similarly, some clinical experience suggests that antidepressants are helpful to counter the depressive feelings that arise in nicotine withdrawal. Antidepressants with a soporific effect, such as trazodone, may play an adjunctive role in withdrawal from alcohol, sedatives, or opioids; trazodone's lack of activity in the γ-aminobutyric acid (GABA) or opioid systems makes it ideal. Withdrawal from cocaine frequently results in depressed mood; although interventions to protect safety and other methods of supportive care are necessarily part of the treatment plan, there is little support for use of antidepressants for cocaine withdrawal.

Other Substance-Induced Conditions

Other substance-induced conditions are psychiatric syndromes that arise during ongoing substance use; the psychiatric manifestations are assumed to be due to the direct physiological effects of the substance. This group of conditions does not include situations in which the individual has begun to experience depression or anxiety regarding the biopsychosocial losses that have resulted from the substance. In situations where the substance is a prescribed medication, these manifestations might be termed side or adverse effects. Substance-induced anxiety, mood, or sleep disorders would naturally seem to be indications for antidepressants. The clinician must remember, however, that a basic clinical approach in such cases would be to press toward abstinence and to provide reassurance that improvement would come through cessation of use (although other pharmacological or psychosocial treatments might be required nonetheless). If detoxification is likely to be slow, the clinician might consider choosing an appropriate antidepressant for substance-induced sleep, anxiety, or depressive conditions, although this situation is rare except in the case of protracted benzodiazepine withdrawal.

Psychiatric Comorbidity

Patients with a dual diagnosis have a substance use disorder and another major psychiatric diagnosis. Clinicians need to pay close attention to distinguishing between comorbid states and substance-induced states, which are conceptually different.

The connections between a substance use disorder and a comorbid psychiatric state may be manifold. Major psychiatric disorders may precede the development of substance abuse, develop concurrently, or manifest secondarily. Psychiatric disorders may precipitate the onset or modify the course of a substance abuse disorder. Psychiatric disorders and substance abuse may present as independent conditions. Thus, it is difficult at any one cross-section of time to differentiate symptoms of withdrawal, intoxication, and secondary cognitive, affective, perceptual, or personality changes from underlying psychiatric disorders. Important tools in differential diagnosis include careful history taking, laboratory analysis, and determining the course or sequence of symptoms. Information obtained from third parties, including family history, is critical.

By determining the presence of a comorbid state, the clinician may enact a treatment plan that addresses both conditions. Although the process of diagnosis needs to be done serially, if and when comorbid conditions have been ascertained, treatment may well be required on a parallel basis. Antidepressants may play a part in such care, either in treating the comorbid psychiatric condition or as adjunctive treatments. Ultimately, better treatment matching may be needed. Several comorbid situations are discussed in the following subsections.

Mood Disorders

Regardless of the patient's expectation or experiences of euphoria during chronic use, chronic major depression occurs late in the course of addiction. Mood disorders may be the result of altered neurochemistry, hormonal or metabolic changes, chronic demoralization, grief from personal losses, or result from stresses of the addictive lifestyle.

Mood disorder comorbid with alcohol misuse

Differentiating between alcohol-induced depressive disorder and a comorbid primary depressive disorder is vital. Untreated major depression in a primary alcoholic patient or secondary alcoholism in a primary depressive patient worsens prognosis. Although the majority of alcoholics will not have an independent diagnosis of major depressive disorder, other less severe depressive disorders may persist in a large proportion of alcoholics after cessation of drinking. Drinking may be more of a problem during a hypomanic or manic phase of a bipolar disorder than during a depressed phase. In the majority of cases, depressive symptomatology subsides after 3–4 weeks of abstinence and usually needs no pharmacological intervention. Use of antidepressants is indicated after diagnosis during a drug-free period, and abstinence is required for efficacy (see Mack et al. 2010 for a review of diagnosis).

A moderately large literature exists on the treatment of depressive conditions comorbid with alcohol misuse. However, the findings have been inconsistent, with only some groups demonstrating improvement. One study in this clinical situation showed that only the depression improved when treatment included an antidepressant (Pettinati 2004). Later studies reviewed the outcomes of combined treatment with naltrexone and an SSRI. One placebo-controlled, double-blind study showed that each medication improved its intended indication (Farren et al. 2009).

Depression comorbid with opioid misuse

Considerable evidence indicates that rates of depression are higher in active opioid users than in the general population. Prevalence of major depression ranges from 17% to 30% among heroin addicts and is considerably higher among methadone clients. Affective disorders in general have ranged as high as 60%. Many depressive episodes are mild, may be related to treatment seeking, and are related to stress. Depression has been found to be a poor prognostic sign in a 2.5-year follow-up, except in cases of coexistent antisocial personality, in which depression improves prognosis. In terms of antidepressant use for depression among patients undergoing long-term methadone maintenance therapy, most studies show little improvement in either condition (Nunes and Levin 2004).

Mood disorder comorbid with cocaine misuse

Affective disorders have been reported concurrently in 30% of cocaine-dependent individuals, with a significant proportion of these patients having bipolar or cyclothymic disorder. Bipolar manic patients may use cocaine to heighten feelings of grandiosity. The profound dysphoric mood related to cocaine binges will resolve in the majority of cocaine addicts. A minority of patients may have underlying unipolar or bipolar disorder, which needs to be treated separately. This abstinence dysphoria may be secondary to depletion of brain catecholamines (e.g., dopamine) or to alteration in neural receptors, with resultant postsynaptic supersensitivity. Some research suggests that comorbid cocaine abuse acts as a robust predictor of poor outcome among depressed alcoholics (Rounsaville 2004).

Anxiety Disorders

Anxiety disorders are common among people who misuse a variety of substances. In many such cases, the substance use may be self-medication. In treatment of addicted patients with anxiety disorders, benzodiazepines should be avoided if possible. Although many patients with preexisting anxiety disorders experience alcohol use as self-medication, alcohol use actually exacerbates an underlying anxiety disorder and can alter the course of one. The best approach to persons with comorbid anxiety disorders would be to treat the comorbid condition, ideally without any substances that may be abused. Antidepressants sometimes play a role in such situations, particularly in the anxiety disorders for which SSRIs or TCAs have either been indicated with FDA approval or been used with great degrees of experience. Anxiety disorders need to be clearly differentiated from substance-induced disorders, including from alcohol or sedative withdrawal and from hallucinogen intoxication.

Attention-Deficit/Hyperactivity Disorder

Attention-deficit/hyperactivity disorder (ADHD) is an important comorbid condition because 1) second-line treatments for ADHD include bupropion and TCAs, especially desipramine; 2) ADHD frequently is comorbid with substance use and with depressed mood; and 3) ADHD carries risk for future substance use. Although the literature has been clear that treatment of ADHD with stimulants should not be avoided due to fears over initiating substance misuse, there are many cases of individuals with ADHD who are administered these second-line medications due to concern about future or past real substance misuse.

Pathological Gambling

Pathological gambling is not an addictive disorder per se, but it is recognized as an impulse control disorder and is frequently considered an addiction; it is certainly closely associated with addictions. Antidepressants have been well studied in patients with pathological gambling, and clomipramine has been reported to have been effective at 125 mg/day. Larger studies have been performed with fluvoxamine; less robust findings were made with paroxetine and sertraline (see Mack et al. 2010, p. 139).

Medications Used to Treat Substance-Related Disorders

In this section, I review knowledge and support for specific antidepressant medications and issues in their use. The following are not included in this discussion: alprazolam (although its antidepressant effects were noted in the past), the neuroleptics that have received approval as antidepressants, and the mood stabilizers that sometimes are used as well.

Medication Selection

Besides evidence related to efficacy, several considerations are important in choosing the correct agent for patients with a substance use disorder. In a multimodal treatment plan for a substance use disorder, uses for pharmacological agents include detoxification via short-term tapered drug substitution (e.g., methadone, benzodiazepines), treatment of comorbid psychiatric and medical disorders, relapse prevention through aversive treatment (e.g., disulfiram in alcoholics), and attenuation of craving or euphoria (e.g., acamprosate, naltrexone). Generally, medications are used as adjuncts to psychosocial treatment and education. Physicians should have a clear understanding of differential diagnosis and natural history of substance abuse disorders, the limitations of medications, drug-drug interactions (Table 6–3), and side effects. Issues of dosing are also important: hepatic damage from alcohol, for example, may produce altered medication levels either during active alcohol use (hepatic induction) or after chronic abuse (hepatic insufficiency). Because some antidepressants, as well as other medications, can affect methadone metabolism, coadministration can lead to overdose or underdose and serum level variation of TCAs: methadone may increase plasma desipramine or amitriptyline. Drugs that can increase methadone include fluoxetine, fluvoxamine, and sertraline (see Table 6–3). In addition, reactions to drug treatments may differ according to sex. For example, evidence shows that women may respond differently than men to SSRIs. One study showed that in a group of nondepressed alcohol users treated with sertraline, women did not respond but men did on several drinking measures (Pettinati et al. 2004).

Antidepressant Medications

Heterocyclic Compounds

The literature includes studies of several off-label applications of the various TCAs in treating SRDs. Of course, this group of antidepressants has several inherent risks for side or adverse effects. Desipramine has been used to treat patients with comorbid ADHD and cocaine dependence. The literature includes discussion of the use of nortriptyline as an agent in smoking cessation. Nortriptyline has been studied in comparison to bupropion (Hall et al. 2002). The specific mechanism of action may include blockade of norepinephrine and serotonin 5-HT reuptake. Imipramine may be helpful as an adjunct in benzodiazepine withdrawal, especially for patients with underlying comorbid conditions, withdrawal-induced depression, or comorbid generalized anxiety disorder (Rickels et al. 2000). In addition, desipramine has been shown to be helpful in maintaining abstinence in individuals dependent on amphetamines but not in those dependent on phencyclidine (Tennant et al. 1986).

Monoamine Oxidase Inhibitors

MAOIs also are used off label for several purposes. For example, short-term smoking cessation was seen in a trial of moclobemide (Berlin et al. 1995) and later for selegiline in combination with the nicotine patch, although the patch plus selegiline demonstrated only an insignificant superiority over the patch

TABLE 6–3. Significant drug-drug/substance interactions

Substance	Drug	Interaction
Alcohol	SSRI/venlafaxine	Anecdotal reports of being "more" drunk, easier blackouts; possible basis is increased 5-HT transport, decreased intoxication effects
Opioids	Fluoxetine, MAOIs	Death, fulminant reaction
Methadone	Any QTc-prolonging medication or condition (e.g., many antipsychotic medications or hypokalemia)	Extension of QTc toward torsades de pointes
Methadone	Benzodiazepines	
Methadone, buprenorphine	Any medication that affects CYP3A4 enzyme activity	

Note. CYP=cytochrome P450; 5-HT=serotonin; MAOI=monoamine oxidase inhibitor; SSRI=selective serotonin reuptake inhibitor.
Source. Adapted from Mack et al. 2010.

alone (George et al. 2003). MAOIs should be avoided in cocaine withdrawal or intoxication because they inhibit the degradation of cocaine and can produce a hypertensive crisis. Extreme caution should be used in administering MAOIs to alcoholic patients for depression, especially because wine contains tyramine. Also, intoxication may further impair judgment and increase the risk of using tyramine-containing products. Additionally, clinicians should note that the prohibition of opioids and MAOIs stemmed from mortalities due to coadministration of meperidine and phenelzine.

Selective Serotonin Reuptake Inhibitors

Although ample support from animal studies indicates that SSRIs reduce ethanol consumption in animals, the evidence on the effect of SSRIs in humans has been disappointing. When given alone, SSRIs have shown limited effect in nondepressed alcohol-dependent humans and resulted in worse outcomes in patients with Type B alcoholism. In some populations, sertraline may be of some benefit as an adjunct to naltrexone in treating alcohol dependence (O'Malley et al. 2008). Studies have suggested that naltrexone plus fluoxetine is better for alcohol dependence than naltrexone alone, and this may be due to the distinction between their mechanisms of action (Le et al. 1999), in that an antidepressant would reduce the capacity of stress to reinstate drinking and naltrexone would reduce the capacity of alcohol to do so. A study of depressed alcohol-dependent patients did not find an advantage for sertraline plus naltrexone over sertraline alone (Oslin 2005). In a double-blind placebo-controlled study, Pettinati et al. (2010) evaluated the efficacy of combining sertraline and naltrexone in treating patients with depression and alcohol dependence. Although this was the strongest study yet, the authors found little effect on either dependence or depression, indicating that in patients diagnosed with comorbid conditions, sertraline (50–150 mg/day), or at least sertraline alone, may not be of assistance. Studies comparing sertraline with fluoxetine appear to be needed. There is little data to support the use of fluoxetine as treatment for cocaine dependence.

Serotonin-Norepinephrine Reuptake Inhibitors

The serotonin-norepinephrine reuptake inhibitor venlafaxine may be a safe, well-tolerated, rapidly acting, and effective treatment for patients with a dual diagnosis of depression and cocaine dependence. Venlafaxine's potential to cause diastolic hypertension at higher dosages indicates the importance of blood pressure monitoring. No evidence has been published on using desvenlafaxine or duloxetine in patients with SRDs, although duloxetine may be helpful in patients with pain accompanying these disorders.

Other

Nefazodone, an antidepressant with dual action on norepinephrine and serotonin reuptake, as well as antagonist effects at the 5-HT_{2A} receptor, reduces anxiety and can help with insomnia. It has no reported abuse potential. Nefazodone is no longer marketed, however, due to concerns about hepatic injury, but it may have been efficacious in improving outcomes in cannabis cessation.

Bupropion, a blocker of norepinephrine uptake and of dopamine reuptake, is an effective antidepressant, and its use among SRDs has been wide. It has been studied as an agent to induce cannabis cessation in dependent users, but compared with placebo, it led to increased irritability and depressed mood during a period of abstinence (Haney et al. 2001). Bupropion has been successful in reducing cocaine use (Levin et al. 2002) and methamphetamine use (Elkashef et al. 2008). The most important role for bupropion for SRDs is in its first-line indication for smoking cessation. With the sustained-release preparation, the target dosage is 300 mg/day. Typically, dosing is begun 7 days before an identified quit date at 150 mg/day, and the dosage is increased to

150 mg bid 3–4 days later. Side effects include headache, nausea, vomiting, dry mouth, insomnia, and agitation. The main contraindication is a history of seizures. Bupropion can be combined with various nicotine replacement therapies. Treatment-emergent hypertension occurred in patients using both the patch and bupropion (Jorenby et al. 1999).

Trazodone may be helpful in benzodiazepine withdrawal (Rickels et al. 1999). Trazodone has many benefits as a soporific in patients who cannot be given abusable substances, such as benzodiazepines.

Mirtazapine

The benefits of mirtazapine as a withdrawal agent are not clear based on findings from two randomized controlled trials. One report showed that amphetamine withdrawal symptoms improved more with mirtazapine than with placebo; a second report showed no differences in withdrawal symptoms between mirtazapine and placebo (Shoptaw et al. 2009).

KEY CLINICAL CONCEPTS

- Treatment of substance abuse or dependence with antidepressant medications has a small but growing evidence base.
- Clinicians should be aware that most use of antidepressants for SRDs would be off label.
- Approaching any patient who may have been using substances requires a firm understanding of what substance is being used and in what time frame, as well as the neurobiological mechanisms of the substance.
- Assessment of suicidality should occur in all substance-using patients.
- Before prescribing for an individual who is misusing substances, the clinician should contemplate both substance-induced mood disorders as well as other features and make as many comorbid diagnoses as warranted.
- Antidepressant therapy for a comorbid condition can be given concurrently with substance misuse provided that there is firm diagnostic clarity.
- Any treatment plan for an individual with an SRD should optimize both medication and psychosocial therapies concurrently.

References

American Psychiatric Association: Diagnostic and Statistical Manual of Mental Disorders, 4th Edition, Text Revision. Washington, DC, American Psychiatric Association, 2000

Berlin I, Saïd S, Spreux-Varoquaux O, et al: A reversible monoamine oxidase A inhibitor (moclobemide) facilitates smoking cessation and abstinence in heavy, dependent smokers. Clin Pharmacol Ther 58:444–452, 1995

Budney AJ, Hughes JR: The cannabis withdrawal syndrome. Curr Opin Psychiatry 19:233–238, 2006

Elkashef AM, Rawson RA, Anderson AL, et al: Bupropion for the treatment of methamphetamine dependence. Neuropsychopharmacology 33:1162–1170, 2008

Farren CK, Scimeca M, Wu R, et al: A double-blind, placebo-controlled study of sertraline with naltrexone for alcohol dependence. Drug Alcohol Depend 99:317–321, 2009

Fiore MC, Bailey WC, Cohen SJ, et al: Treating Tobacco Use and Dependence. Clinical Practice Guideline No 18. Rockville, MD, U.S. Department of Health and Human Services, Public Health Service, 2000

George TP, Vessicchio JC, Termine A, et al: A preliminary placebo-controlled trial of selegiline hydrochloride for smoking cessation. Biol Psychiatry 53:136–143, 2003

Hall SM, Humfleet GL, Reus VI, et al: Psychological intervention and antidepressant treatment in smoking cessation. Arch Gen Psychiatry 59:930–936, 2002

Haney M, Ward AS, Comer SD, et al: Bupropion SR worsens mood during marijuana withdrawal in humans. Psychopharmacology (Berl) 155:171–179, 2001

Jorenby DE, Leischow SJ, Nides MA, et al: A controlled trial of sustained-release bupropion, a nicotine patch, or both for smoking cessation. N Engl J Med 340:685–691, 1999

Le AD, Poulos CX, Harding S, et al: Effects of naltrexone and fluoxetine on alcohol self-administration and reinstatement of alcohol-seeking induced by priming injections of alcohol and exposure to stress. Neuropsychopharmacology 21:435–444, 1999

Levin F, Evans S, McDowell D, et al: Bupropion treatment for cocaine abuse and adult attention-deficit/hyperactivity disorder. J Addict Disord 21:1–16, 2002

Mack A, Harrington A, Frances R: Clinical Manual for the Treatment of Alcoholism and Addictions. Washington, DC, American Psychiatric Press, 2010

Newton TF, Roache JD, De La Garza II R, et al: Bupropion reduces methamphetamine-induced subjective effects and cue-induced craving. Neuropsychopharmacol 31:1537–1544, 2006

Nunes EV, Levin FR: Treatment of depression in patients with alcohol or other drug dependence: a meta-analysis. JAMA 291:1887–1896, 2004

Oliveto AH, Feingold A, Schottenfeld R, et al: Desipramine in opioid-dependent cocaine users maintained on buprenorphine vs methadone. Arch Gen Psychiatry 56:812–820, 1999

O'Malley SS, Robin RW, Levenson AL, et al: Naltrexone alone and with sertraline for the treatment of alcohol dependence in Alaska natives and non-Natives residing in rural settings: a randomized controlled trial. Alcohol Clin Exp Res 32:1271–1283, 2008

Oslin DW: Treatment of late-life depression complicated by alcohol dependence. Am J Geriatr Psychiatry 13:491–500, 2005

Pettinati HM: Antidepressant treatment of co-occurring depression and alcohol dependence. Biol Psychiatry 56:785–792, 2004

Pettinati HM, Dundon W, Lipkin C: Gender differences in response to sertraline pharmacotherapy in type A alcohol dependence. Am J Addict 13:236–247, 2004

Pettinati HM, Oslin DW, Kampman K, et al: A double-blind, placebo-controlled trial combining sertraline and naltrexone for treating co-occurring depression and alcohol dependence. Am J Psychiatry 167:668–675, 2010

Rickels K, Schweizer E, Garcia España F, et al: Trazodone and valproate in patients discontinuing long-term benzodiazepine therapy: effects on withdrawal symptoms and taper outcome. Psychopharmacology (Berl) 141:1–5, 1999

Rickels K, DeMartinis N, Garcia España F, et al: Imipramine and buspirone in treatment of patients with generalized anxiety disorder who are discontinuing long-term benzodiazepine therapy. Am J Psychiatry 157:1973–1979, 2000

Rounsaville BJ: Treatment of cocaine dependence and depression. Biol Psychiatry 56:803–809, 2004

Shoptaw SJ, Kao U, Heinzerling K, et al: Treatment for amphetamine withdrawal. Cochrane Database of Systematic Reviews 2009, Issue 2. Art. No.: CD003021. DOI: 10.1002/14651858.CD003021.pub2.

Tennant FS Jr, Tarver A, Pumphrey E, et al: Double-blind comparison of desipramine and placebo for treatment of phencyclidine or amphetamine dependence. NIDA Res Monogr 67:310–317, 1986

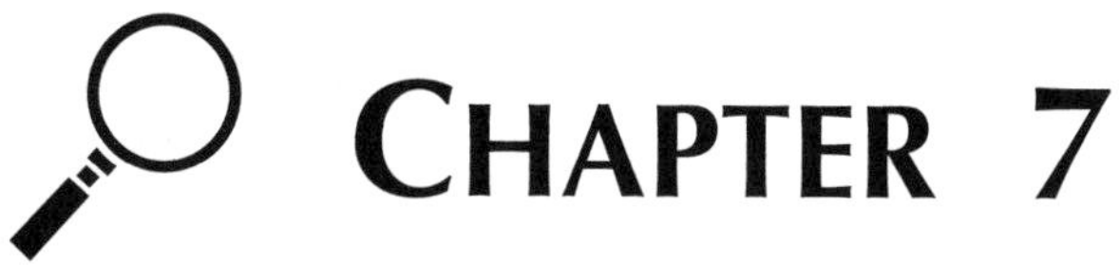

CHAPTER 7

Use of Antidepressants in Children and Adolescents

Mary S. Ahn, M.D.
Lauren Yakutis, B.A.
Jean A. Frazier, M.D.

ANTIDEPRESSANTS are classified into several categories: 1) selective serotonin reuptake inhibitors (SSRIs), 2) tricyclic antidepressants (TCAs), 3) serotonin-norepinephrine reuptake inhibitors (SNRIs), 4) monoamine oxidase inhibitors (MAOIs), and 5) other antidepressants. The other antidepressants category consists of a heterogeneous group of medications that do not fit in the first four categories; these include buspirone, trazodone, reboxetine, mirtazapine, nefazodone, and bupropion. SSRIs are the primary antidepressant type prescribed for children and adolescents because of their favorable side-effect profile and lower risk of toxicity if accidentally or intentionally ingested in high amounts. Many controlled studies have evaluated both the safety and efficacy of TCAs in children; however, with the emergence of SSRIs, the TCAs are less commonly prescribed given their cardiovascular side-effect profile. SNRIs and other antidepressants are also less often prescribed because limited controlled studies have been reported to date and these medications have less favorable side-effect profiles in general when compared to SSRIs. MAOIs are not used in children and adolescents given the high risk for nonadherence to the low-tyramine dietary restrictions. Furthermore, no efficacy data have been reported to support the use of MAOIs in youth. Therefore, a discussion about MAOIs is not included in this chapter.

In this chapter, we review the developmental considerations that are necessary when prescribing antidepressant medications for children and a discussion of the background and challenges of conducting psychotropic medication trials in children and adolescents. In addition, indications for various antidepressants are reviewed. The published controlled studies of antidepressants in youth are outlined, with special attention given to safety in light of the warning from the U.S. Food and Drug Administration (FDA) regarding the potential association between antidepressants and suicidal ideation and behaviors.

Developmental Considerations

Data regarding the safety and efficacy of antidepressants in adults are fairly extensive and can provide some framework for use of these medications in children and adolescents. However, youth are not simply small adults, and studies need to be done regarding medication use in children to fully inform prescriptive practice. Youth undergo considerable developmental changes that can have an impact on pharmacokinetics and pharmacodynamics. For example, compared with adults, children have faster metabolism and elimination of medications secondary to larger liver volumes (in proportion to total body volume) and more efficient kidney glomerular filtration rate. Therefore, children may require higher weight-adjusted dosages of some medications. On the other hand, children are often more sensitive to the side effects of medications. For example, children are more likely to have symptoms of activation or manic switching secondary to antidepressants (Safer and Zito 2006).

In light of the developmental issues around pediatric psychopharmacology and the relative lack of studies to establish safety and support for the use of medications in children, the federal government provided some initiatives to support furthering evidence-based knowledge. The United States Congress in 1997 passed the Food and Drug Administration Modernization Act, which gives incentives to pharmaceutical companies for the conduct of clinical trials in children by extending their market exclusivity for 6 additional months. The FDA now requires that pharmaceutical companies study their products in youth if they are likely to be prescribed for them. Additionally, the National Institutes of Health (NIH) has committed funding to allow large multiple-site studies to be conducted in children.

Despite the policies and incentives aimed at increasing clinical trials in children, other developmental issues make clinical trials difficult to conduct in youth. Compared with adults, children have higher levels of comorbid psychiatric diagnoses. Children often present with multiple psychiatric symptoms that cluster around several different diagnoses at the time of clinical presentation, and the "diagnostic outcome" of these syndromes may not become clear until late adolescence or adulthood. Furthermore, there are limitations to the current nosological system of classification, which clusters around symptom complexes rather than etiology. Compared with adult disorders, childhood psychiatric disorders are more heterogeneous, a fact that can confound the evaluation of safety and efficacy of medications.

When evaluating and treating children and adolescents, the clinician needs to carefully review each individual's biopsychosocial context. Youth are often more vulnerable to family, educational, and peer and social stressors. Therefore, medication interventions are only one part of a multimodal treatment plan aimed at addressing a child's needs. Ideally, medication treatment trials should take into account the various nonmedication interventions that may occur concurrently with medication administration. In the evidence-based review of the various antidepressants in this chapter, the studies that control for or include psychotherapeutic interventions are given special attention.

Another important consideration is that the placebo response in clinical trials for youth is robust. In antidepressant studies, the placebo response rate varies widely across different studies and diagnoses (36%–71% in depression, 21%–65% in obsessive-compulsive disorder [OCD], 56%–78% in anxiety) (Martin and Volkmar 2007, pp. 760–768). Therefore, it has been a challenge for controlled antidepressant trials in children to demonstrate clear separation of active drug from placebo in terms of efficacy.

Indications

Of all the antidepressants, only fluoxetine is approved by the FDA to treat depression in preadolescent children as young as 8 years. Escitalopram has recently received approval for the treatment of depression in children ages 12–17 years.

For OCD, four SSRIs and one TCA are FDA approved. Fluoxetine and paroxetine are indicated for children ages 7–17 years. Similarly, sertraline is approved by the FDA for use in OCD for patients ages 6–17, and fluvoxamine has an indication for OCD for children ages 8–17. Clomipramine, a tertiary amine TCA, is approved for use in OCD starting at age 10.

For attention-deficit/hyperactivity disorder (ADHD), atomoxetine is approved by the FDA for children 6 years and older.

Although several controlled trials support the use of antidepressants in treating a spectrum of anxiety disorders, none has FDA approval for this purpose to date. A complete list of the FDA-approved pediatric indications for antidepressants is provided in Table 7–1.

Depression

Over the past several decades, rates of depression in children and adolescents have increased and the age at onset has decreased steadily. Although cases of depression in youth were described as far back as the 17th century, not until 1975 was depression finally recognized and diagnosed in youth. Currently, depression is estimated to occur in approximately 1% of preschool-age children (ages 3–5 years), 2% of school-age children (ages 6–12 years), and 8% of adolescents (ages 13–18 years) (Son and Kirchner 2000).

Depression in young children can manifest with unique symptoms compared with depression in adolescents and adults. Irritability, reactive mood, and externalizing disruptive behaviors are more typically seen in the younger cohort. In sharp contrast, the clinical manifestation of adolescent depression is very similar to that of adult depression, with accompanying functional impairment, anxiety, and substance use disorders (Weller and Weller 1986). Although depression presents similarly in adults and adolescents, pharmacological management for adolescents cannot simply be inferred from adult clinical trials, because youth exhibit different pharmacodynamic and pharmacokinetic activity.

In the following subsections, we describe the controlled studies of depression in children and adolescents by antidepressant agent. A summary of the studies is provided in Table 7–2.

Fluoxetine

Fluoxetine has been the most extensively studied SSRI to date for children with major depressive disorder (MDD), and this agent is FDA approved for pediatric MDD. Simeon et al. (1990) conducted the first double-blind placebo-controlled study of fluoxetine for DSM-III diagnosed MDD (American Psychiatric Association 1980). Forty adolescents (inpatient and outpatient; ages 13–18 years) were given fluoxetine (20–60 mg/day) or placebo. Fluoxetine was

TABLE 7–1. U.S. Food and Drug Administration–approved pediatric indications for antidepressants

Medication	Indication	Age (years)	Usual starting dosage	Dosage range	Side effects in the pediatric population[a]
Fluoxetine	Depression	8–18	10 mg/day	10–20 mg/day	Headache, vomiting, insomnia, tremor (Simeon et al. 1990); manic symptoms, severe rash (Emslie et al. 1997); headache, trend for increased attention problems and dizziness in fluoxetine vs. placebo (Emslie et al. 2002); headache, sedation, upper abdominal pain, insomnia (March et al. 2004); insomnia, fatigue, and nausea (Riddle et al. 1992)
	OCD	7–17	10 mg/day	20–60 mg/day	Palpitations, weight loss, drowsiness, tremors, nightmares, muscle aches (Liebowitz et al. 2002); headache, tremor, insomnia, hypomanic episode (Alaghband-Rad and Hakimshooshtary 2009)
Escitalopram	Depression	12–17	10 mg/day	10–20 mg/day	No significant side effects when compared to placebo (Emslie et al. 2009; Wagner et al. 2006)

TABLE 7–1. U.S. Food and Drug Administration–approved pediatric indications for antidepressants *(continued)*

Medication	Indication	Age (years)	Usual starting dosage	Dosage range	Side effects in the pediatric population[a]
Paroxetine	OCD	7–17	10 mg/day	10–60 mg/day	Somnolence (Keller et al. 2001); headache, nausea, vomiting, agitation, anxiety, somnolence, decreased appetite (Berard et al. 2006); increased cough, dyspepsia, vomiting, dizziness (Emslie et al. 2006); hyperkinesia, decreased appetite, diarrhea, asthenia, vomiting, agitation, neurosis, pain, dysmenorrhea (Geller et al. 2004)
Sertraline	OCD	6–12 13–17	25 mg/day 50 mg/day	25–200 mg/day 50–200 mg/day	Diarrhea, vomiting, anorexia, agitation (Wagner et al. 2003a); fatigue, concentration, insomnia, drowsiness, restlessness, headache, yawning, increased appetite, nausea (Melvin et al. 2006); insomnia, nausea, agitation, tremor (March et al. 1998); decreased appetite, diarrhea, enuresis, motor overactivity, nausea, stomachache (Pediatric OCD Treatment Study Team 2004)

TABLE 7–1. U.S. Food and Drug Administration–approved pediatric indications for antidepressants *(continued)*

Medication	Indication	Age (years)	Usual starting dosage	Dosage range	Side effects in the pediatric population[a]
Fluvoxamine	OCD	8–11	25 mg at bedtime	50–200 mg divided bid	Insomnia, asthenia (defined by investigators as "fatigue, loss of energy, tired, tiredness, or weak") (Riddle et al. 2001)
		12–17	25 mg at bedtime	50–300 mg divided bid	
Clomipramine	OCD	10–17	25 mg/day	Max 3 mg/kg/day up to 100 mg/day in first 2 weeks, 200 mg/day maintenance	Tremor, dry mouth, dizziness constipation (Flament et al. 1985); fatigue, anticholinergic side effects (March et al. 1990)
Atomoxetine	ADHD	6–17	<70 kg: 0.5 mg/kg/day	1.2–1.4 mg/kg/day	A trend in somnolence and anorexia (Michelson et al. 2001); decreased appetite, vomiting, nausea, asthenia, dyspepsia (Michelson et al. 2002); decreased appetite, headache, vomiting, APU, irritability, nasopharyngitis, nausea, cough, influenza, sinusitis (Geller et al. 2007)
			>70 kg: 40 mg daily	80–100 mg/day	

Note. ADHD=attention-deficit hyperactivity disorder; APU=abdominal pain upper; bid=twice a day; OCD=obsessive-compulsive disorder.
[a]Side effects listed are those that were significantly greater than placebo unless otherwise noted.

TABLE 7–2. Controlled studies of antidepressants in children and adolescents with major depression

Study	Medication	*N*	Age (years)	Dosage (mg/day)	Duration	Outcome
Simeon et al. 1990	Fluoxetine	40	13–18	20–60	7 weeks	Fluoxetine=PBO
Emslie et al. 1997	Fluoxetine	96	7–17	20	8 weeks	Fluoxetine=PBO
Emslie et al. 2002	Fluoxetine	219	8–17	20	9 weeks	Fluoxetine>PBO
Emslie et al. 2004	Fluoxetine	40	8–17	20–60	9 weeks acute treatment; responders randomly assigned to 10 weeks titration and 32 weeks relapse prevention (fluoxetine or PBO)	Fluoxetine>PBO (time to relapse)
March et al. 2004	Fluoxetine	439	12–17	10–40	12 weeks 36 weeks	Fluoxetine+CBT>fluoxetine >PBO
Emslie et al. 2008	Fluoxetine	168	7–18	10–40	12 weeks; responders randomly assigned to 26 weeks fluoxetine or PBO	Fluoxetine>PBO (time to relapse)
Wagner et al. 2006	Escitalopram	264	6–17	10–20	8 weeks	Escitalopram>PBO (adolescents only)
Emslie et al. 2009	Escitalopram	316	12–17	10–20	8 weeks	Escitalopram>PBO

TABLE 7–2. Controlled studies of antidepressants in children and adolescents with major depression *(continued)*

Study	Medication	*N*	Age (years)	Dosage (mg/day)	Duration	Outcome
Keller et al. 2001	Paroxetine vs. imipramine vs. PBO	275	13–17	20–40 (paroxetine) 200–300 (imipramine)	8 weeks	Paroxetine > imipramine Paroxetine > PBO
Berard et al. 2006	Paroxetine	286	13–18	20–40	12 weeks	Paroxetine = PBO
Emslie et al. 2006	Paroxetine	149	7–17	10–50	8 weeks	Paroxetine = PBO
Wagner et al. 2003a	Sertraline	376	6–17	50–200	10 weeks	Sertraline > PBO
Cheung et al. 2008	Sertraline	22	13–19	50–200	36 weeks; responders randomly assigned to 55 weeks fluoxetine or PBO	Sertraline > PBO (recurrence-free)
Wagner et al. 2004b	Citalopram	174	7–17	20–40	8 weeks	Citalopram > PBO
von Knorring et al. 2006	Citalopram	244	13–18	10–40	12 weeks	Citalopram = PBO

Note. CBT = cognitive-behavioral therapy; PBO = placebo.

dosed initially at 20 mg and was increased by 20 mg weekly up to 60 mg by week 2. No significant difference was found between interventions, with both active drug and placebo groups having response rates of 66%. Of note, both groups were receiving psychosocial interventions independent of the study. Despite the higher-than-usual dosing of fluoxetine in this study, no significant side effects were reported, and no patients discontinued secondary to any side effects. The most common side effects were headache, vomiting, insomnia, and tremor.

Subsequent large-scale controlled studies have been published, including 1) a multicenter series of studies of fluoxetine consisting of three phases (9-week acute treatment phase, 10-week dose titration phase, and 32-week relapse prevention phase) funded by Eli Lilly and Company, and 2) Treatment for Adolescents with Depression Study (TADS), a multicenter trial of fluoxetine and cognitive-behavioral therapy (CBT) funded by the National Institute of Mental Health (NIMH). The aim of TADS was to study the acute and long-term effectiveness of treatments.

The first study was a double-blind placebo-controlled trial of fluoxetine (Emslie et al. 1997). The study was an 8-week trial using either fluoxetine 20 mg/day or placebo in 96 nonpsychotic outpatient children, ages 7–17 years, who had MDD as defined by the DSM-IV (American Psychiatric Association 1994). The mean Children's Depression Rating Scale—Revised (CDRS-R) score was 58 at baseline. Fluoxetine (56% response rate) was found to be superior to placebo (33% response rate) in reducing the symptoms of depression. Response was defined as being rated "much" or "very much" improved on the Clinical Global Impression Improvement Scale (CGI-I; Guy 1976) at study exit. Despite the positive findings, there was a low rate of complete remission with fluoxetine (31%) compared with placebo (23%)—as defined by a CDRS-R score of ≤28—a finding that is similar to those in adult studies (Poznanski et al. 1984). Fluoxetine was both efficacious and well tolerated. Discontinuation secondary to side effects occurred in only four patients taking fluoxetine (and one receiving placebo). Three of the four patients taking fluoxetine discontinued secondary to manic symptoms and one due to a severe rash.

Emslie et al. (2002) extended their earlier study of fluoxetine with a 9-week, double-blind, placebo-controlled multisite study. Subjects were outpatients, ages 8–17 years, who met criteria for DSM-IV nonpsychotic MDD. The mean CDRS-R score upon enrollment was 56. Patients in the fluoxetine group received 10 mg/day for 1 week and then 20 mg/day for 8 weeks of treatment. Fluoxetine was found to be superior to placebo; 52% and 37% of patients taking fluoxetine and placebo, respectively, received ratings of "much" or "very much" improved on the CGI-I. Furthermore, fluoxetine was found to be superior to placebo when using the CDRS-R score, averaging response rates of ≥20%–

60% from baseline. Fluoxetine was very well tolerated, with no significant side effects. There was a trend for fluoxetine to be associated with attention problems ($P=0.088$) and dizziness ($P=0.092$). The only side effect that patients named unsolicited was headache, which occurred more often in the fluoxetine group ($P=0.017$).

The nonresponders to Dr. Emslie's aforementioned study were randomly given fluoxetine 40–60 mg day versus a fixed dosage of 20 mg/day (Heiligenstein et al. 2006). Treatment response was defined as a CDRS-R score decrease to ≤30. Patients ($N=29$) included children and adolescents ages 9–17 years in outpatient settings. After 9 weeks of fluoxetine 20 mg/day, nonresponders were rerandomly assigned in a double-blind fashion either to continue 20 mg/day or to take 40 mg/day (with an option to increase to 60 mg/day if no response occurred after another 4 weeks of treatment). Response rate in the group that received increased dosages of 40–60 mg/day was 71% as defined by a CDRS-R score of ≤30. The response rate in the group that continued taking 20 mg/day was only 30%. Although the difference in these response rates did not reach statistical significance ($P=0.128$), likely because of the small number of subjects, the results do suggest that dosage increases of fluoxetine after initial nonresponse may benefit some patients and should be a possible treatment consideration. Given the small sample size, further investigation is warranted. Fluoxetine also appeared to be well tolerated across all three dosages. The group that received dosage escalations up to 40–60 mg/day did not have an increased number or severity of side effects, and the events reported did not significantly differ from those reported by the group who continued taking 20 mg/day.

In a double-blind placebo-controlled study, Emslie et al. (2004) compared fluoxetine with placebo for prevention of relapse in youth with a DSM-IV diagnosis of MDD using similar inclusion/exclusion criteria to those used in the Emslie et al. (2002) study. The purpose of the 2004 study was to examine the potential long-term benefit of fluoxetine in youth with depression. At fluoxetine dosages of 20–60 mg/day versus placebo, only those who had a CDRS-R score of ≤28 at week 19 were then admitted to the relapse prevention phase of this study. Seventy-five responders were eligible to enter this relapse prevention portion of study based on the response criteria (40 fluoxetine responders, 35 pill placebo responders). The 40 fluoxetine responders were once again randomly assigned into one of two groups: those continuing their previous treatment regimen ($n=20$) and those who then received placebo ($n=20$). The placebo responders were maintained on placebo during this arm of the study. Relapse was defined as a CDRS-R score of ≥40 along with a 2-week history of worsening symptoms as assessed by a child psychiatrist. The relapse rate was longer in the fluoxetine group that continued taking active drug than in the group that was rerandomized to placebo (181 days vs. 71 days, $P<0.046$). The relapse rate after 32 weeks was 34% for the group that continued taking fluoxetine versus 60% for the group that switched to placebo. The relapse rate for the group maintained on placebo was only 17%, suggesting that other factors (attention to the factors exacerbating the depression, support from the study, or sustained placebo effect) may have been beneficial in addressing the depression. No serious side effects were reported after the 32-week relapse prevention phase (total study time was 51 weeks). The group that switched from fluoxetine to placebo did not exhibit any discontinuation symptoms. Furthermore, long-term fluoxetine appeared well tolerated. There were no statistically significant differences between groups for vital signs, weight, or other side effects solicited in a questionnaire. Four patients in this phase had suicidal ideation or self-harm behaviors (2 in placebo group, 1 in fluoxetine to fluoxetine group, 1 in fluoxetine to placebo group). There was a trend difference (P=0.065) in height change across the three groups (fluoxetine to fluoxetine group=1.1±2.1 cm; fluoxetine to placebo group=2.4±2.4 cm; placebo to placebo group= 2.1 ±2.7 cm), suggesting that youth who take fluoxetine over a 51-week period may have slower height growth. Similar results have been found in other antidepressant trials (Weintrob et al. 2002). More evaluation regarding the association between antidepressants and growth needs to be done, but these findings suggest that clinicians should monitor the height of children and adolescents who take these agents. Taken together, the study supports long-term efficacy of fluoxetine in youth with MDD who were initial responders.

In light of the FDA scrutiny of suicidality in children using antidepressants and the subsequent black box warning label, the NIMH funded TADS. (The studies previously described in this section were privately funded.) The TADS team consisted of multiple sites with expertise in treating pediatric depression. Unlike previous studies, the TADS study attempted to minimize the exclusionary criteria and included children with comorbid diagnoses (Treatment for Adolescents With Depression Study Team 2003). In addition, the sample consisted of youth with moderate to severe depression as defined by scores on the Clinical Global Impression Severity Scale (CGI-S) and CDRS-R. Furthermore, the TADS study was limited to adolescents (ages 12–17 years).

The initial TADS study was a multicenter project that evaluated four types of treatment over a 12-week period (March et al. 2004). Patients were randomly assigned to one of four treatment groups: 1) fluoxetine alone (10–40 mg/day), 2) CBT alone, 3) CBT plus fluoxetine (10–40 mg/day), or 4) a pill placebo. Fluoxetine and placebo alone were administered double-blind, whereas CBT and CBT plus fluoxetine were administered unblinded. A total of 439 children in outpatient settings who met DSM-IV criteria for MDD participated in the study. The mean baseline CDRS-R score was 76. Using a CGI-I score of "much" or "very much" improved, the TADS study found at endpoint that the response rate to fluoxetine plus CBT was 71%, fluoxetine alone was 61%, CBT alone was 43% and placebo was 35%. Head-to-head comparison on the CDRS-R showed that fluoxetine plus CBT or fluoxetine alone resulted in a significant decrease in symptoms compared with placebo (P=0.001 and 0.002, respectively). In sharp contrast, CBT alone was not superior to placebo (P=0.97). Furthermore, fluoxetine plus CBT was superior to CBT alone (P=0.001) but not to fluoxetine alone (P=0.13). These findings suggest a more rapid rate of improvement in the acute phase of treatment using a combination of fluoxetine plus CBT when compared with fluoxetine alone. Suicidal ideation was reduced across all treatment groups, but suicidal events were most prevalent in the fluoxetine alone group (11.9%) compared with the fluoxetine plus CBT (8.4%), CBT alone (4.5%), or placebo (5.4%) groups. These findings are consistent with other findings of suicidality in patients who receive antidepressants (Hammad et al. 2006). Of note, the finding of a lower risk of suicidal events in the fluoxetine plus CBT group than in the fluoxetine alone group, suggests that the combined intervention approach may reduce the risk of suicidality. Headache was the only side effect that occurred (10%), although there was no statistical difference between all groups, with the exception of the CBT alone group, which had a lower rate of headaches when compared with the fluoxetine groups. The other side effects commonly reported were sedation (2.8%), upper abdominal pain (5.5%), and insomnia (4.7%) in the fluoxetine group. Taken together, combined fluoxetine plus CBT appears to be well tolerated and the treatment of choice for MDD in adolescents.

Curry et al. (2006) examined predictors and moderators of acute treatment response. Adolescents younger than 16 years had a more robust improvement at end point than adolescents 16 years and older. Other predictors of improvement included better overall baseline function as measured by the Children's Global Assessment Scale (CGAS) score at study entry, shorter duration of an MDD episode (<40 weeks), fewer melancholic features of depression at baseline, fewer comorbid disorders, and no comorbid anxiety disorders. Using a self-report assessment, the Suicidal Ideation Questionnaire—Junior (SIQ-Jr), adolescents with less suicidal ideation at baseline or throughout the study, less hopelessness, and higher expectations for improvement were more likely to respond to any intervention (either fluoxetine, CBT, fluoxetine and CBT, or placebo and psychosocial intervention). These findings suggest that younger, higher functioning patients have a better rate of response to fluoxetine and that early identification and treatment of MDD improves the chances for remission.

Following the acute phase of the TADS study, there was an unblinded follow-up phase lasting 24 weeks (6 weeks of continuation and 18 weeks of maintenance), for a total study duration of 36 weeks for all treatment groups (March et al. 2007b). The authors excluded the placebo group from the follow-up phase analyses. At week 18, the rates of response were 73% for fluoxetine plus CBT, 62% for fluoxetine alone, and 65% for CBT alone. By week 36, the response rates were 86% for fluoxetine plus CBT, 81% for fluoxetine alone, and 81% for CBT alone. Suicidal events overall were more common in the fluoxetine group (14.7%) than in the fluoxetine plus CBT group (8.4%) or CBT group (6.3%). These findings at 36 weeks extend findings from the 12-week acute trial TADS study, further indicating that suicidal ideation and/or events are more likely in adolescents who are treated with fluoxetine alone. Furthermore, CBT may mediate some of that risk, possibly either by facilitating the response to lower dosages of fluoxetine (mean=28 mg/day in the combination group vs. 32 mg/day in the fluoxetine monotherapy group) or by preventing progression of suicidal ideation to attempt by improving coping strategies and family/systems stressors. In addition, although all three treatment groups showed similar response rates after 36 weeks, the findings after 12 and 24 weeks suggest that fluoxetine may shorten the response rate to CBT for depression.

In another TADS study, Kratochvil et al. (2006) assessed sustained response during acute (12 weeks), continuation (18 weeks), and maintenance (36 weeks) therapy across all three treatment groups relative to placebo. Sustained response was defined as two consecutive ratings of a full response (CGI-I score of ≤2) in assessments 6 weeks apart. In the acute phase, fluoxetine and fluoxetine plus CBT were superior to CBT alone for a sustained response. Also, of the 39% of patients who had not achieved a sustained response in the acute phase (at 12 weeks), 80% of the fluoxetine plus CBT, 61.5% of the fluoxetine alone, and 77.3% of the CBT alone patients achieved sustained response by the 36-week time point. Of the 61% of patients who were able to achieve a sustained response in the acute phase, CBT patients were more likely than the fluoxetine patients to maintain the benefits through week 36 (96.9% vs. 74.1%, P=0.007). Therefore, although all treatment modalities were found to be efficacious, CBT may have the slowest effect in treating depression but may have the lowest chance for relapse, especially in those youth who have an early sustained response to this therapy modality.

Emslie et al. (2008) examined remission and relapse in children and adolescents ages 7–18 years with depression in a single-site double-blind study funded by NIMH. Subjects were outpatients with a DSM-IV diagnosis of MDD. Symptom severity criteria for enrollment were similar to those in the TADS study (CDRS-R ≥40 vs. 45 in the TADS study). Subjects were initially given open-label fluoxetine 10 mg/day for 1 week, and the dosage was then titrated up to 20 mg/day. The dosage could be increased to 30–40 mg/day at the discretion of the clinical team, or reduced to 10 mg/day if side effects were not tolerated. Subjects were allowed to proceed in the continuation phase if remission was achieved, as defined by a CGI-S score of 1 or 2, or a decrease of ≥50% on their CDRS-R score, after 12 weeks of open-label treatment. A total of 102 youth were eligible and participated in the double-blind continuation phase of the study. Half were randomly assigned to receive fluoxetine (continuation of fluoxetine), and half were randomly assigned to receive placebo (crossover from fluoxetine to placebo) over a 6-month period.

Relapse was defined as a CDRS-R score ≥40 accompanied by worsening depressive symptoms for at least 2 weeks or, alternatively, clinician determination that there was significant clinical deterioration to warrant intervention to prevent an inevitable relapse. Relapse rates were higher in the placebo group (69.2%) than in the fluoxetine group (42.0%) (P=0.009). For the placebo group, the median time to relapse was 8 weeks after discontinuation of fluoxetine. For the fluoxetine group, the median time to relapse was >24 weeks. The relapse rates were equal for children and adolescents and for males and females. Although the majority of subjects were first-episode depressed patients, there was a high relapse rate after fluoxetine discontinuation. Therefore, the findings support the notion that continued use of fluoxetine is required even after remission is achieved, and that the adult guidelines of waiting 6–9 months before tapering treatment are also warranted in children and adolescents (Emslie et al. 2008).

Kennard et al. (2008) examined relapse in 46 patients (ages 11–18 years) who had responded to acute 12-week treatment of fluoxetine. Entry criteria followed the same protocol as in the Emslie et al. (2008) study. Patients were randomly assigned to receive either fluoxetine continuation or fluoxetine plus CBT for 6 months. Relapse was defined as a CDRS-R score ≥40 with an associated 2-week history of worsening depressive symptoms or a clinician-noted significant deterioration that would suggest relapse if intervention was not given. After the subjects spent 36 weeks in the continuation phase, the estimated probabilities of relapse were 37% in the fluoxetine group and 15% in the fluoxetine plus CBT group. Adolescents who did not receive adjunctive CBT therapy were eight times more likely to relapse. The findings in the fluoxetine group showed relapse rates similar to those in the Emslie et al. (2008) study previously described (42% relapse rate at 36 weeks). These findings support the use of CBT during the continuation phase of fluoxetine treatment to further reduce the risk of relapse.

Epidemiological studies in youth with MDD show that most recover within 1–2 years, and subsequently approximately 50% relapse after treatment with either pharmacotherapy or psychosocial interventions. As described previously, the studies conducted by Emslie and colleagues and the TADS team suggest that MDD is a chronic illness that can spontaneously remit even after the course of successful treatment. Therefore, the TADS team conducted a 1-year naturalistic follow-up after discontinuation of the 36-week TADS study (March et al. 2009). No between-group differences were found regarding study completion rates (42.2%–47.7%). Over the course of 1-year post-TADS interventions, the benefits continued in all measures of depression and suicidality. These findings differ from previous epidemiological and short-term treatment studies that showed high rates of relapse. Therefore, March et al. suggest that longer-term treatments (36 weeks) may reduce the risk of future relapse. Close to one-third of patients in either fluoxetine-treated group (i.e., the group receiving fluoxetine and the group receiving both fluoxetine and CBT) relapsed after 1 year. Taken together, long-term treatment with fluoxetine is superior to short-term treatment, but there continues to be a risk of relapse and suicidality.

Escitalopram

Escitalopram recently received an indication for MDD in adolescents 12–17 years of age. Wagner et al. (2006) conducted the first randomized, double-blind, placebo-controlled trial of escitalopram in both children and adolescents (ages 6–17 years). The study was funded by Forest Laboratories. The 8-week trial randomly assigned 264 patients to receive either escitalopram (10–20 mg/day) or placebo. The primary efficacy measure was mean change from baseline in the CDRS-R score. Overall, escitalopram was not superior to placebo. However, a post hoc analysis of adolescents alone (ages 12–17) did show that escitalopram significantly improved depression when compared with placebo (P=0.047). Headache and abdominal pain were the most common side effects reported on the side-effects questionnaire, but they did not occur significantly more often than with placebo. There were three potential suicide or self-injurious events, although they were not characterized as serious events: one patient (self-inflicted injury) was taking escitalopram, and the other two (possible overdose and self-inflicted injury) were given placebo. These findings suggest that escitalopram is well tolerated and may be more effective in adolescents than in children.

A second multisite controlled trial of escitalopram for MDD was conducted in adolescents only (ages 12–17 years) by Emslie et al. (2009) and supported by Forest Laboratories. Three hundred sixteen patients were randomly assigned to receive escitalopram (10–20 mg/day) or placebo. Efficacy was assessed using the change in CDRS-R score from baseline. Escitalopram produced greater improvement in depressive symptoms than did placebo (P=0.022). Using CGI-I scores ≤2 to define response, escitalopram had a 64.3% response rate compared to a placebo rate of 52.9% (P=0.03). The most common side effects reported were headache, insomnia, and nausea, although none occurred significantly more often with escitalopram than with placebo. Suicidal ideation and/or self-injurious behaviors were observed in both groups (six in each group), and one serious adverse event occurred per group. Despite the high placebo response, escitalopram was shown to be superior to placebo in this study.

Taken together, the two studies support the use of escitalopram to safely treat the acute phase of MDD in adolescents.

Paroxetine

Three controlled paroxetine studies have been published to date. Keller et al. (2001) recruited 275 adolescents (ages 13–17) with MDD for an 8-week trial of paroxetine (20–40 mg/day), imipramine (200–300 mg/day), or placebo. The group used the Hamilton Rating Scale for Depression (Ham-D) score of ≤8 or ≥50% reduction from Ham-D baseline score as measures of efficacy. Sixty-three percent of patients taking paroxetine, 50% of patients taking imipramine, and 46% of patients given placebo responded based on Ham-D scores. Paroxetine was found to be superior to placebo ($P=0.02$), but imipramine was not ($P=0.57$). Somnolence was found in 17.2% of patients taking paroxetine, which was significantly different from the rate for patients given placebo.

A multicenter international controlled study was conducted with 286 adolescents (ages 13–18) diagnosed with MDD (Berard et al. 2006). Patients were given placebo or paroxetine (20–40 mg/day). Efficacy was defined by a ≥50% improvement from the baseline score on the Montgomery-Åsberg Depression Rating Scale (MADRS). Response rates were high for both groups (paroxetine 60.5%, placebo 58.2%) and not significantly different. Paroxetine was generally well tolerated.

Emslie et al. (2006) assessed the efficacy and tolerability of paroxetine in both children and adolescents (ages 7–17 years) with MDD. (This is the only one of the three paroxetine trials to assess preadolescents.) In this multicenter, double-blind controlled trial, patients took paroxetine (10–50 mg/day) or placebo for 8 weeks. A total of 149 youth completed the trial. On the basis of changes in the CDRS-R score from baseline and CGI-I scores, both groups improved, but there were no significant differences between the paroxetine group and the placebo group. Of note, patients taking paroxetine exhibited increased cough (5.9%), dyspepsia (5.9%), vomiting (5.9%), and dizziness (5%) from baseline compared with patients receiving placebo. Suicidal ideation or behaviors was 1.9% in the paroxetine group versus 1% in the placebo group. The side effects were more common in children than adolescents.

According to the combined findings from these three studies, paroxetine may not be efficacious in treating MDD in children and adolescents and is not recommended for use in youth at this time.

Sertraline

Wagner et al. (2003a) published pooled analyses of two international multicenter, randomized, double-blind, placebo-controlled trials of sertraline for MDD in youth. This study was supported by Pfizer. A total of 376 children and adolescents ages 6–17 years participated. They were randomly assigned to receive either sertraline (50–200 mg/day) or placebo over a 10-week trial. Effectiveness was defined by a CDRS-R score decrease of ≥40% from baseline. The patients who received sertraline had a 69% response rate, which separated out from placebo (59%, P=0.05). Sertraline was generally well tolerated. Adverse events in at least 5% of the sertraline group and at least double that percentage of the placebo group included diarrhea, vomiting, anorexia, and agitation. These findings support the use of sertraline in treating the acute phase of MDD in both children and adolescents.

The findings were further extended by a national funding source program in Australia. The Time for a Future adolescent depression program aimed to evaluate sertraline, CBT, and their combination in treatment of depression in adolescents (Melvin et al. 2006). Seventy-three adolescents (ages 12 and 18 years) were randomly assigned to receive sertraline monotherapy, CBT monotherapy, or a combination. All three treatments were found to be equally efficacious, and the combination of sertraline plus CBT was not found to be superior to the monotherapy groups. The patients had no serious adverse events, and no patients required treatment change or discontinuation due to suicidality. The lack of a comparison placebo group is a large drawback to this study. Nevertheless, these findings further support the initial study done by Wagner et al. (2003a), indicating that sertraline may be effective in treating youth with depression.

An open-label maintenance study for sertraline in adolescents ages 13–19 with MDD was conducted in Canada and funded by the Canadian Institutes of Health Research (Cheung et al. 2008). The responders (defined by Ham-D score <9 and >50% reduction in baseline Ham-D score) from the acute 12-week trial entered the continuation phase (24 weeks). Those who maintained a response during the continuation phase were rerandomized either to continued sertraline or to placebo for an additional 52 weeks. Twenty-two subjects participated in this phase of the study. Of the patients taking sertraline, 38% remained well, compared with 0% of patients rerandomized to placebo. Although the sample size was too small to detect a significant difference, the findings suggest a possible benefit to using sertraline in the maintenance phase. Caution is advised in interpreting these findings because the medications were given nonblinded, although the results support further investigation. Compared with placebo, sertraline had no significant long-term side effects.

Citalopram

Wagner et al. (2004b) conducted an 8-week randomized placebo-controlled trial, funded by Forest Pharmaceuticals, of citalopram for MDD in both children and adolescents (ages 7–17 years). A total of 174 patients were randomized to either citalopram (20–40 mg/day) or placebo. Efficacy was defined by a CDRS-R score of ≤28. At week 8, the response rate was significantly higher in the citalopram group (36%) than in the placebo group (24%) (P=0.05). Citalopram was generally well tolerated, with the most common and significant side effects reported being rhinitis, nausea, and abdominal pain compared with placebo.

Citalopram was also studied in adolescents with MDD in a European multicenter controlled trial funded by H. Lundbeck (von Knorring et al. 2006). The 244 inpatient and outpatient adolescents (ages 13–18 years) were randomly assigned to receive either citalopram (10–40 mg/day) or placebo. The response rate was around 60% in both groups, defined by a MADRS score reduction of ≥50% from baseline or by depression and anhedonia scores ≤2 on the Schedule for Affective Disorders and Schizophrenia for School-Age Children: Present Episode (K-SADS-P).

Although the two studies presented yielded mixed findings regarding the use of citalopram, several differences possibly explain the findings. Concomitant psychotropic medications and psychotherapy were allowed but not controlled in the study by von Knorring et al. (2006). Also, the patients in this sample included inpatients, were older in age (implying longer duration of illness), and had higher rates of comorbidity than those in the study by Wagner et al. (2004b). Taken together, the results suggest that further study of the efficacy of citalopram in youth with MDD is warranted.

Fluvoxamine

No controlled studies have been published to support the use of fluvoxamine in children and adolescents with depression.

Venlafaxine

The NIMH-funded Treatment of SSRI-Resistant Depression in Adolescents (TORDIA) trial was a multicenter randomized controlled trial of 334 adolescents (ages 12–18 years) with MDD who had failed to respond to a 2-month initial treatment with an SSRI (Brent et al. 2008). Patients were randomly assigned to receive either a second trial of an SSRI (with or without CBT) or a trial of venlafaxine (with or without CBT) for 12 weeks. The findings were that CBT in combination with a switch to a different SSRI or venlafaxine was effective (54.8% response rate), based on improvement in the CDRS-R score of ≥50% or a CGI-I score ≤2. Venlafaxine was not superior to switching to another SSRI and was less well tolerated. Significant increases in diastolic blood pressure and pulse, as well as more frequent skin problems, occurred in adolescents who switched to venlafaxine rather than another SSRI. No significant effects on suicidal ideation were found between groups. Therefore, if an adolescent fails to respond to the first SSRI antidepressant trial, the findings from the TORDIA study support another trial of an SSRI, weighing risks and benefits.

Bupropion

No controlled studies of bupropion in youth with MDD have been reported. Open-label studies suggest its tolerability and promising effectiveness (Glod et al. 2003), but given the lack of controlled studies, bupropion is not recommended in the first-line treatment of pediatric depression.

Tricyclic Antidepressants

Prior to studies that showed SSRIs to be relatively safe for use in children and adolescents with depression, TCAs were used. Although several controlled studies have been published for the TCAs, all of the findings were negative. A meta-analysis pooling all of the data on TCAs also failed to find any difference between placebo and these agents (Hazell et al. 1995). Given the growing support for some SSRIs in treating pediatric depression, the lack of controlled trials showing efficacy for TCAs, and the less desirable side-effect profile of the TCAs, the use of these agents, particularly as first-line interventions, is not recommended for the treatment of MDD in youth.

Obsessive-Compulsive Disorder

OCD is characterized by obsessions or compulsions that are recurrent and intrusive enough to cause functional impairment. OCD has a prevalence of 0.5% in youth (Reinblatt and Walkup 2005). Several large randomized controlled trials of the treatment of OCD in children have established short-term safety and efficacy of SSRIs. Sertraline, fluoxetine, and fluvoxamine have FDA indications for use in pediatric OCD, and a large controlled trial of paroxetine was published supporting its efficacy as well (Geller et al. 2004). Table 7–3 summarizes the controlled studies of antidepressants for childhood OCD.

Furthermore, a meta-analysis was conducted to compare the efficacy of the antidepressants used to treat pediatric OCD (Geller et al. 2003). A highly significant difference was found between antidepressant and placebo treatment ($P<0.001$) across several OCD measures of efficacy, including the Yale-Brown Obsessive Compulsive Scale—Child Version (CY-BOCS), NIMH Global OCD Scale, and CGI-I scores. Clomipramine was significantly more effective than the other antidepressants on measures of efficacy, and the SSRIs were equally efficacious with each other. Of note, although clomipramine was superior to the SSRIs for treating pediatric OCD, clomipramine (a TCA) has high risk for serious adverse events (anticholinergic and cardiac) and requires more monitoring that may be inconvenient for both the patient and family and the clinician when compared to using an SSRI. For example, regular electrocardiographic and blood level monitoring are required for clomipramine. Therefore, starting with an SSRI is a good first option. Choosing an SSRI should de-

TABLE 7–3. Controlled studies of antidepressants in children and adolescents for obsessive-compulsive disorder

Study	Medication	*N*	Age	Dosage	Duration	Outcome
Flament et al. 1985	Clomipramine	19	7–19	111–171 mg/day	10 weeks	Clomipramine>PBO
Leonard et al. 1989	Clomipramine vs. desipramine	48	10–18	97–203 mg/day	10 weeks	Clomipramine>desipramine
March et al. 1990	Clomipramine vs. desipramine	16	10–18	50–200 mg/day	10 weeks	Clomipramine=desipramine
DeVeaugh-Geiss et al. 1992	Clomipramine	60	10–17	3 mg/kg/day	8 weeks	Clomipramine>PBO
Riddle et al. 1992	Fluoxetine	14	8–15	20 mg/day	8 weeks (20 weeks with crossover)	Fluoxetine>PBO
March et al. 1998	Sertraline	187	6–17	25–200 mg/day	12 weeks	Sertraline>PBO
Geller et al. 2001	Fluoxetine	103	7–17	10–60 mg /day	13 weeks	Fluoxetine>PBO
Riddle et al. 2001	Fluvoxamine	120	8–17	50–200 mg/day	10 weeks	Fluvoxamine>PBO
Liebowitz et al. 2002	Fluoxetine	43	6–18	20–80 mg/day	16 weeks	Fluoxetine>PBO (Child Y-BOCS; NS: NIMH Global, CGI)
Geller et al. 2004	Paroxetine	203	7–17	10–50 mg/day	10 weeks	Paroxetine>PBO

TABLE 7–3. Controlled studies of antidepressants in children and adolescents for obsessive-compulsive disorder *(continued)*

STUDY	MEDICATION	*N*	AGE	DOSAGE	DURATION	OUTCOME
Pediatric OCD Treatment Study Team 2004	Sertraline	112	7–17	25–200 mg/day	12 weeks	Sertraline>PBO Sertraline+CBT>PBO Sertraline+CBT>sertraline
Alaghband-Rad and Hakimshooshtary 2009	Citalopram vs. fluoxetine	29	7–18	20 mg/day 20 mg/day	6 weeks	Citalopram=fluoxetine (Child Y-BOCS); NS (both groups, CGI-S)

Note. CBT=cognitive-behavioral therapy; CGI=Clinical Global Impression scale; CGI-S=Clinical Global Impression—Severity scale; NS=not significant; OCD=obsessive-compulsive disorder; PBO=placebo; Y-BOCS=Yale-Brown Obsessive Compulsive Scale.

pend mainly on matching the desired half-life and side-effect profiles to the individual patient, because all SSRIs appear to be equally efficacious for pediatric OCD. Fewer data are available to support the use of citalopram and escitalopram, but several open-label studies do suggest that they are well tolerated and possibly effective for OCD in youth. Clomipramine may be a consideration for SSRI treatment-resistant pediatric OCD.

No controlled studies have been reported to date that have assessed long-term treatment with antidepressants in pediatric OCD. Two publications of a 52-week open-label extension study of sertraline after a 12-week, double-blind, placebo-controlled study of individuals ages 6–18 years reported continued improvement in OCD symptoms, although the rate of improvement slowed over time (Cook et al. 2001; Wagner et al. 2003b). In this extension study, after completion of the controlled 12-week trial, all subjects either continued or initiated (if given placebo) sertraline at extension study entry. Cook et al. (2001) reported that 85% of initial sertraline responders from the acute controlled study phase maintained a response in the extension phase. Also, of those who had not initially responded to the antidepressant, an additional 43% responded in the extension trial. Wagner et al. (2003b) reported that 47% of patients achieved full remission (defined as a CY-BOCS score ≤8); partial remission (defined as a CY-BOCS score >8 and ≤15) was achieved in an additional 31% of patients.

No controlled studies have assessed discontinuation of antidepressants in pediatric OCD. Given that OCD is a chronic disease with a likely high remission response and relapse rate in long-term treatment, great caution should be used when considering discontinuation of active treatment, which should occur only after OCD symptoms are manageable for at least 9–18 months. Summer months may be a better time to taper medications to minimize functional impairment.

Anxiety

Anxiety disorders in children and adolescents have a prevalence of 6%–20%, based on several large-scale epidemiological studies (Connolly and Bernstein 2007). Anxiety disorders in youth are associated with a 3 times greater risk of having anxiety disorders in adulthood. Furthermore, an untreated anxiety disorder increases the risk of MDD, substance use disorders, and educational issues in later years. Social and self-esteem problems can impact future relationships. Therefore, early detection and treatment of anxiety disorders in children and adolescents are imperative.

The multisite Child/Adolescent Anxiety Multimodal Study (CAMS) is a recently completed large (*N*=448) randomized placebo-controlled trial funded by NIMH, and its study design was recently published (Compton et al. 2010). The aims are to compare sertraline, CBT, and the combination of sertraline plus

CBT against placebo for the treatment of separation anxiety disorder, generalized anxiety disorder, and social phobia in both children and adolescents. When the data on safety and efficacy are published, CAMS will likely set the treatment standard for childhood anxiety disorders.

Until evidence is available to compare psychotherapeutic and psychopharmacological management of childhood anxiety disorders, the American Academy of Child and Adolescent Psychiatry (AACAP) practice parameter (Connolly and Bernstein 2007) should be used as a guide. The work group recommends that antidepressants be used in children with moderate to severe anxiety disorders or those who have had no or partial response to initial psychotherapy treatment. The recommendation is that antidepressants, specifically SSRIs, be used only in combination with psychotherapy.

The controlled clinical trials that have examined the safety and efficacy of SSRIs and TCAs in selective mutism, social phobia, separation anxiety disorder, and generalized anxiety disorder are featured in Table 7–4. Although the studies' efficacy results were mixed, SSRIs can be considered in certain situations, as mentioned in the previous paragraph. They are generally well tolerated in childhood anxiety disorders. The most common side effects that have been reported include gastrointestinal distress, headache, increased motor activity, and insomnia. In addition, children and adolescents with anxiety and their parents or guardians (in terms of reporting) are often more sensitive to real or perceived side effects to medications than are children and families who do not have anxiety disorders. SSRIs may also be beneficial in treating childhood panic disorder, although no controlled studies have been published (Masi et al. 2006).

Results from controlled studies suggest that extended-release venlafaxine is safe and effective in the treatment of both social phobia and generalized anxiety disorder (March et al. 2007a; Rynn et al. 2007). The use of this extended-release SNRI, when compared with SSRIs, is limited by less favorable side effects and the potential for withdrawal symptoms.

No controlled trials have assessed the long-term safety and efficacy of antidepressants in childhood anxiety disorders. At present, the AACAP practice parameter (Connolly and Bernstein 2007) recommends that clinicians consider tapering the antidepressant after 1 year of stability in patients who have symptom remission or in patients in whom functional impairment is achieved.

Attention-Deficit/Hyperactivity Disorder

ADHD is one of the most common childhood psychiatric diagnoses. Epidemiological studies estimate that the prevalence of ADHD is 6.7%–10% (Pliszka 2007). Efficacy has been firmly established to support the use of psychostimulants for ADHD, and these medications remain the mainstay treatment. In select cases, however, atomoxetine, an FDA-approved SNRI may be more ben-

TABLE 7–4. Controlled studies of antidepressants in children and adolescents for anxiety disorders

Study	Diagnosis	Medication	*N* (years)	Age	Dose (mg/day)	Outcome
Gittleman-Klein and Klein 1971	School phobia	Imipramine	35	6–14	100–200	Imipramine>PBO
Berney et al. 1981	School refusal	Clomipramine	51	9–14	40–75	NS
Klein et al. 1992	SAD	Imipramine	21	6–15	75–275	NS
Black and Uhde 1994	Selective mutism with social phobia/ avoidant disorder	Fluoxetine	15	6–11	12–27	Fluoxetine>PBO
RUPP Anxiety Study Group 2001	Social phobia, SAD, GAD	Fluvoxamine	128	6–17	50–300	Fluvoxamine>PBO
Rynn et al. 2001	GAD	Sertraline	22	5–17	50	Sertraline>PBO
Birmaher et al. 2003	GAD, social phobia, SAD	Fluoxetine	74	7–17	20	Fluoxetine> PBO (NS)
Wagner et al. 2004a	Social phobia	Paroxetine	322	8–17	10–50	Paroxetine>PBO
Rynn et al. 2007	GAD	Venlafaxine ER	320	6–17	37.5–225	Venlafaxine ER> PBO
March et al. 2007a	Social phobia	Venlafaxine ER	219	8–17	37.5–225	Venlafaxine ER>PBO

Note. ER=extended release; GAD=generalized anxiety disorder; NS=not significant; PBO=placebo; RUPP=Research Unit on Pediatric Psychopharmacology; SAD=social anxiety disorder.

eficial for children and adolescents who have ADHD. Atomoxetine has demonstrated efficacy over placebo in both children and adolescents with ADHD (Michelson et al. 2001, 2002), although one head-to-head study did not demonstrate superiority of this agent to psychostimulants.

Unlike the psychostimulants, atomoxetine is not a Drug Enforcement Agency (DEA) Schedule II controlled substance. Therefore, atomoxetine may be preferred for youth who have comorbid substance use or abuse. In addition, due to its more benign side-effect profile relative to appetite and sleep disturbances, atomoxetine may be used to avoid the potential side effects associated with psychostimulants (potential vital sign changes, decreases in height and weight velocity, insomnia, tics).

Atomoxetine has also been studied in the treatment of patients with ADHD and comorbid anxiety disorders. Geller et al. (2007) randomly assigned 176 patients (ages 8–17 years) with ADHD and anxiety (social anxiety disorder, generalized anxiety disorder, or social phobia) in a 12-week, double-blind, placebo-controlled study of atomoxetine. Atomoxetine was generally well tolerated and was superior to placebo in reducing the symptoms of ADHD, anxiety, and overall global functioning. Therefore, atomoxetine may be a useful alternative to a psychostimulant plus SSRI in the management of youth with comorbid ADHD and anxiety.

The most common side effects from atomoxetine include gastrointestinal distress, sedation, and decreased appetite. Although atomoxetine is generally well tolerated, cases of atomoxetine-induced liver injury have been reported to the FDA. A boldfaced warning appears on the label of atomoxetine regarding this potential risk, and therefore monitoring precautions are advised.

Bupropion and TCAs have also been commonly prescribed for ADHD, although they have not received FDA approval. Given the relative lack of recent controlled trials and the strong evidence to support psychostimulants (or atomoxetine), the AACAP practice parameter (Connolly and Bernstein 2007) suggests that a careful review of the diagnosis of ADHD and/or behavioral therapies may be a better next-step option before considering bupropion or TCAs.

Substance Use Disorders

Adolescents with substance use disorders (SUDs) have higher rates of comorbid depression than do adolescents without substance abuse problems. In turn, depression is associated with more active substance use, worse substance use treatment outcomes, and higher substance use relapse rates. Despite the high comorbidity of depression and substance use disorders and the worsening prognosis for adolescents diagnosed with both, few studies have been conducted to assess safety and efficacy of pharmacotherapies. Clinically, physicians are often less likely to prescribe antidepressants for depression when youth have active SUDs and are referred first for substance treatment.

Riggs et al. (2007) explored the effect of fluoxetine compared with placebo in a randomized, double-blind, placebo-controlled trial of adolescents with comorbid MDD (current), SUD, and conduct disorder who were receiving concomitant CBT related to their SUD. The study, funded by the National Institute on Drug Abuse, was conducted for 16 weeks at a single site, with the fluoxetine group receiving 20 mg/day. To date, this is the only controlled trial examining the safety and efficacy of antidepressants in the treatment of depression in adolescents with comorbid SUDs. Fluoxetine was very well tolerated, without significant adverse events compared to the placebo group. The study had mixed results on fluoxetine's effect on depressive symptoms. Using a CDRS-R score ≤28 as a response, the researchers found that the fluoxetine group was trending toward superiority over placebo (69.8% and 52.4% response rates, respectively); however, when a CGI-I score of ≤2 was used as a measure of efficacy, the response rates of the groups were not significant (76% and 67%, respectively). On measures of substance use and conduct disorder symptoms, no significant effect was found for fluoxetine or placebo. Although the CBT was focused on the SUD, the placebo group's depressive symptoms showed a larger than expected improvement. Taken together, the results of this study suggest that using fluoxetine in youth with comorbid MDD, SUD, and conduct disorder is a safe treatment for the acute phase. On the other hand, given the mixed findings regarding fluoxetine's benefits on depression and the negative findings regarding its impact on substance use and conduct disorder, using CBT alone may be an important consideration.

Eating Disorders

Fluoxetine has FDA approval for treatment of adults with bulimia nervosa, and at a target dosage of 60 mg/day, it has been shown to decrease bingeing and vomiting. In youth, the only pilot study published to date was an 8-week open-label study of children ages 12 years and older (Kotler et al. 2003). Fluoxetine at 60 mg/day was generally well tolerated and exhibited reductions in bingeing and purging (50% "improved," 20% "much improved"). These promising results support the need for more controlled studies in youth with bulimia nervosa.

Posttraumatic Stress Disorder

An NIMH-funded pilot controlled trial of sertraline was conducted by Cohen et al. (2007) in children and adolescents with posttraumatic stress disorder (PTSD) who were receiving concomitant trauma-focused CBT. Twenty-four youth (ages 10–17 years) were randomly assigned to receive either sertraline (50–200 mg/day) or placebo for 12 weeks. Medication was started at 25 mg/day for 3 days, with instructions to increase to 50 mg/day for the next 2 weeks. In subjects who were not significantly improved, the dosage was increased to 100 mg/day for another 2 weeks. Dose titration continued up to a maximum dosage of 200 mg/day. Both groups improved significantly and equivalently not only for PTSD symptoms, but also for symptoms of depression, anxiety, and general behavior problems. Despite the small sample size, the findings do not support any additional benefit to adding sertraline to trauma-focused CBT for youth with PTSD. More studies are necessary to make further conclusions.

Insomnia

Although sleep disturbance affects about 11% of children and adolescents, and up to 75% of youth with psychiatric or neurodevelopmental disorders, very limited data are available on the safety and efficacy of medications used (Owens et al. 2005). Given the paucity of data, consensus panels consisting of multidisciplinary treaters have formed opinions on the use of medications in children with insomnia (Owens and Moturi 2009). Although behavioral interventions are the first-line treatment for properly diagnosed insomnia, medications are commonly used. Especially in the psychiatric population, antidepressants with a favorable sedating profile have been used to treat insomnia. Trazodone has sedative-hypnotic properties when prescribed at low dosages (25–50 mg), whereas at higher dosages, it has more antidepressant properties. One serious but rare side effect is priapism. Like trazodone, mirtazapine has histamine (H_1) receptor antagonistic properties. Mirtazapine is dosed at 15 or 30 mg at bedtime and may reduce sleep onset time. Both trazodone and mirtazapine can cause excessive daytime sleepiness.

Prior to the popularity of SSRIs, TCAs were prescribed to youth because of the sedating profile of this class of drugs. However, because of their risk of cardiotoxicity and anticholinergic properties, TCAs are not advised for use in pediatric insomnia.

Suicide Risk and Antidepressants

Suicidal ideation and behavior are common features of depression in youth. In fact, 60% of children with a depressive disorder have suicidal ideation, and about 30% will make a suicide attempt (Birmaher et al. 2007). Given the significant morbidity and mortality associated with depression in youth, several multisite clinical trials sponsored by NIMH have been conducted, as described in previous sections of this chapter.

In 2004, the U.S. Food and Drug Administration issued a black box warning on all antidepressant medications for patients under age 18. Then in 2006, the warning was extended up to age 24. The warning states that antidepressants may be associated with an increase in the risk of suicidal thinking and behavior in youth with MDD and other psychiatric disorders. The warning was based on analysis of pooled data from nine placebo-controlled antidepressant trials. Of note, the warning did not state that antidepressants cause suicide. In this pooled data analysis of the acute phase trials (4–6 weeks in duration), the risk of suicidal thinking or behavior was found to be 4% for patients taking antidepressants versus 2% for those given placebo. Of note, there were no completed suicides (Hammad et al. 2006). In addition to cautioning about suicidal ideation or behavior, the black box warning recommends that children and adolescents should be closely monitored for any worsening depressive symptoms or unusual changes in behavior, such as sleeplessness, agitation, or withdrawal from normal social situations. Weekly monitoring is especially recommended during the first month of treatment, when the risk may be greatest for these adverse reactions (U.S. Food and Drug Administration 2004).

Suicidal ideation and behaviors in general are linked to depression, a history of previous suicide attempts, psychosis, SUDs, sleep problems, and comorbid anxiety or disruptive behavior disorders (Bridge et al. 2006). Given the complex interplay of multiple risk factors, depression, and antidepressant treatment, systematic and sophisticated studies to assess the specific risk of antidepressants are necessary.

The TADS study was funded by NIMH to evaluate fluoxetine and CBT during the acute phase of treatment, the remission phase, and the relapse phase in adolescents (March et al. 2007b). Clinical measures included adverse events, such as suicidal ideation and behavior. The group sought to examine whether suicidal ideation or suicide attempts 1) occur early in treatment, 2) have an association with activation, and 3) can be predicted by assessment of risk factors (Vitiello et al. 2009). Suicidal ideation was assessed using self-report measures (SIQ-Jr and the Adolescent Depression Scale [ADS]) and clinician measures (CDRS-R). Suicidal events were coded using the Columbia Classification Algorithm of Suicidal Assessment, a robust tool to differentiate actual suicidal ideation, attempts, or preparatory acts from acts that did not imply intent (i.e., suicidal gestures for attention seeking). After 36 weeks, 10% of adolescents presented with one or more suicidal events. The number of suicidal ideation events was 23, and the number of suicide attempts was 21. There were no completed suicides. The incidence did not differ by gender, race/ethnicity, or age. The total number of suicidal events in the fluoxetine treatment group (14.7%) was higher than in the CBT group (6.3%, $P<0.05$), which was not different from the combined treatment group (8.4%), while the combined treatment and fluoxetine groups did not significantly differ from each other. Of note, suicidal ideation decreased with treatment in all groups. Although the investigators expected an early suicidal event response secondary to fluoxetine, the time to suicidal event was variable, and no relationship was found between antidepressant (SSRI) treatment and earlier suicidal events. Furthermore, the group sought to see if activation was related to the early events, and those results were negative. There was no evidence of increased agitation, irritability, or insomnia to suggest that activation was the mechanism of suicidal events secondary to antidepressant treatment. The TADS study is limited in that the fluoxetine dosage stayed fixed at 10 mg/day in the early stages of treatment, when activation is thought to occur.

The majority of adolescents who went on to have a suicidal event in the TADS study were still clinically depressed at the time of the suicidal event, showed minimal improvement, and reported an interpersonal stressor immediately prior to the suicidal event. Therefore, rather than activation, continued depression with limited response to the medication intervention and acute interpersonal conflict could explain the context for adolescents who have suicidal ideation or behaviors.

The pretreatment self-report scores of the SIQ-Jr and ADS, but not the clinician-rated CDRS-R scores, were associated with subsequent suicidal events but did not appear to have significant sensitivity or specificity. Nevertheless, adolescents appear to be more likely to report suicidal ideation in a self-report questionnaire than in interactions with a clinician.

Several clinical conclusions from the TADS study relate to suicidality and antidepressants: 1) adolescents with depression who are suicidal at baseline are more likely to have suicidal events during treatment, 2) self-report tools to assess suicidality may be an important adjunct to the clinical interview, 3) the risk for suicidal ideation or behaviors persists past the first month of treatment, 4) adolescents most at risk include those who are still significantly depressed and have minimal improvement from treatment, and 5) suicidality does not appear to be explained by SSRI-induced activation.

The FDA advisory and subsequent black box warning may have inadvertently created reductions in rates of diagnosis and treatment of depression, and subsequently increased suicide rates in children and adolescents. Libby et al. (2007) analyzed data from a large national pediatric cohort (PharMetric Patient-Centric Database) from 1997 to 2005. The data were collected from more than 85 managed care plans nationally, and the demographic data did not differ statistically from the 2000 U.S. Census data. From 1999 to 2004, the rate of new episodes of depression in youth increased steadily, but in 2005, after the FDA advisory was issued, the rate dramatically dropped (65%–71% less than the predicted rate). Another unintended effect of the FDA advisory was that antidepressant prescriptions were filled less frequently by patients and families (a 58% reduction for SSRIs). These findings were further extended to the year 2007 by Libby et al. (2009), who also found that there was no compensatory increase in psychotherapy intervention for children and adolescents. Gibbons et al. (2005) examined data from both the United States (IMS Health database and U.S. Centers for Disease Control and Prevention) and the Netherlands (Central Bureau of Statistics). There were decreases in the rates of SSRI prescriptions in youth after the U.S. and European regulatory drug agencies issued their warnings of the potential risk of suicide with antidepressants. Prior to the FDA and European warnings, from 1998 to 2003, there was a 91% increase in SSRI prescription rate in youth and a 33% decrease in suicide rate in the United States, and a 120% increase in SSRI prescription rate and a 31% decrease in suicide rate in the Netherlands. After the FDA and European warnings, the United States had a 14% increase in suicide rate in 2004 and the Netherlands had a 49% increase in suicide rate between 2003 and 2005. These findings are in sharp contrast to the FDA's warning that there may be an association between antidepressants and suicide.

Furthermore, the FDA's meta-analysis of the suicide data that subsequently led to the black box warning had some limitations (Hammad et al. 2006). As described previously in this section, there were no completed suicides. In addition, suicidal ideation and attempts were measured by single items on the Ham-D and CDRS-R rather than rating scales specific to suicide, which better elicit suicidal intent and severity of the suicidal ideation.

Given the unintended decrease in diagnosis and treatment of depression in youth and the subsequent increases in completed suicides since the FDA advisory, more awareness of both depression and suicide needs to be communicated to all health providers treating children and adolescents. Although increased monitoring and assessment of the risk-benefit ratio is vital before an antidepressant is prescribed, the FDA advisory is not meant to deter active treatment when medically indicated. In fact, recent large-scale epidemiological studies demonstrate that withholding treatment may have detrimental effects.

KEY CLINICAL CONCEPTS

- A comprehensive diagnostic assessment and multimodal treatment planning process that is youth driven and parent guided is imperative before an antidepressant is prescribed for a child or adolescent.

- In young patients with an anxiety or depressive disorder, the clinician should consider a course of psychotherapy (CBT) prior to starting an antidepressant.
- The diagnosis, side effects, and monitoring strategies must be reviewed carefully with both the youth and parent or guardian.
- Few antidepressants have FDA indications for children and adolescents, but good safety and efficacy data may be available to support off-label prescription of antidepressants with a thorough assent/consent process.
- Although SSRIs are generally well tolerated, all antidepressants should be started at low dosages and titrated slowly because children are more vulnerable to side effects.
- Ongoing monitoring of antidepressant treatment and side effects (with special attention to suicidal ideation or behaviors and activation) should occur weekly for the first month of treatment, biweekly for the next month, then monthly thereafter.

References

Alaghband-Rad J, Hakimshooshtary M: A randomized controlled clinical trial of citalopram versus fluoxetine in children and adolescents with obsessive-compulsive disorder (OCD). Eur Child Adolesc Psychiatry 18:131–135, 2009

American Psychiatric Association: Quick Reference to the Diagnostic Criteria From DSM-III. Washington, DC, American Psychiatric Association, 1980

American Psychiatric Association: Diagnostic Criteria From DSM-IV. Washington, DC, American Psychiatric Association, 1994

Berard R, Fong R, Carpenter DJ, et al: An international, multicenter, placebo-controlled trial of paroxetine in adolescents with major depressive disorder. J Child Adolesc Psychopharmacol 16:59–75, 2006

Berney T, Kolvin I, Bhate SR, et al: School phobia: a therapeutic trial with clomipramine and short-term outcome. Br J Psychiatry 138:110–118, 1981

Birmaher B, Axelson DA, Monk K, et al: Fluoxetine for the treatment of childhood anxiety disorders. J Am Acad Child Adolesc Psychiatry 42:415–423, 2003

Birmaher B, Brent D, Bernet W, et al: Practice parameter for the assessment and treatment of children and adolescents with depressive disorders. J Am Acad Child Adolesc Psychiatry 46:1503–1526, 2007

Black B, Uhde TW: Treatment of elective mutism with fluoxetine: a double-blind, placebo-controlled study. J Am Acad Child Adolesc Psychiatry 33:1000–1006, 1994

Brent D, Emslie G, Clarke G, et al: Switching to another SSRI or to venlafaxine with or without cognitive behavioral therapy for adolescents with SSRI-resistant depression: the TORDIA randomized controlled trial. JAMA 299:901–913, 2008

Bridge JA, Goldstein TR, Brent DA: Adolescent suicide and suicidal behavior. J Child Psychol Psychiatry 47:372–394, 2006

Cheung A, Kusumakar V, Kutcher S, et al: Maintenance study for adolescent depression. J Child Adolesc Psychopharmacol 18:389–394, 2008

Cohen JA, Mannarino AP, Perel JM, et al: A pilot randomized controlled trial of combined trauma-focused CBT and sertraline for childhood PTSD symptoms. J Am Acad Child Adolesc Psychiatry 46:811–819, 2007

Compton SN, Walkup JT, Albano AM, et al: Child/Adolescent Anxiety Multimodal Study (CAMS): rationale, design, and methods. Child Adolesc Psychiatry Ment Health 4:1, 2010

Connolly SD, Bernstein GA: Practice parameter for the assessment and treatment of children and adolescents with anxiety disorders. J Am Acad Child Adolesc Psychiatry 46:267–283, 2007

Cook EH, Wagner KD, March JS, et al: Long-term sertraline treatment of children and adolescents with obsessive-compulsive disorder. J Am Acad Child Adolesc Psychiatry 40:1175–1181, 2001

Curry J, Rohde P, Simons A, et al: Predictors and moderators of acute outcome in the Treatment for Adolescents with Depression Study (TADS). J Am Acad Child Adolesc Psychiatry 45:1427–1439, 2006

DeVeaugh-Geiss J, Moroz G, Biederman J, et al: Clomipramine hydrochloride in childhood and adolescent obsessive-compulsive disorder: a multicenter trial. J Am Acad Child Adolesc Psychiatry 31:45–49, 1992

Emslie GJ, Rush AJ, Weinberg WA, et al: A double-blind, randomized, placebo-controlled trial of fluoxetine in children and adolescents with depression. Arch Gen Psychiatry 54:1031–1037, 1997

Emslie GJ, Heiligenstein JH, Wagner KD, et al: Fluoxetine for acute treatment of depression in children and adolescents: a placebo-controlled, randomized clinical trial. J Am Acad Child Adolesc Psychiatry 41:1205–1215, 2002

Emslie GJ, Heiligenstein JH, Hoog SL, et al: Fluoxetine treatment for prevention of relapse of depression in children and adolescents: a double-blind, placebo-controlled study. J Am Acad Child Adolesc Psychiatry 43:1397–1405, 2004

Emslie GJ, Wagner KD, Kutcher S, et al: Paroxetine treatment in children and adolescents with major depressive disorder: a randomized, multicenter, double-blind, placebo-controlled trial. J Am Acad Child Adolesc Psychiatry 45:709–719, 2006

Emslie GJ, Kennard BD, Mayes TL, et al: Fluoxetine versus placebo in preventing relapse of major depression in children and adolescents. Am J Psychiatry 165:459–467, 2008

Emslie GJ, Ventura D, Korotzer A, et al: Escitalopram in the treatment of adolescent depression: a randomized placebo-controlled multisite trial. J Am Acad Child Adolesc Psychiatry 48:721–729, 2009

Flament MF, Rapoport JL, Berg CJ, et al: Clomipramine treatment of childhood obsessive-compulsive disorder: a double-blind controlled study. Arch Gen Psychiatry 42:977–983, 1985

Geller DA, Hoog SL, Heiligenstein JH, et al: Fluoxetine treatment for obsessive-compulsive disorder in children and adolescents: a placebo-controlled clinical trial. J Am Acad Child Adolesc Psychiatry 40:773–779, 2001

Geller DA, Biederman J, Stewart SE, et al: Which SSRI? A meta-analysis of pharmacotherapy trials in pediatric obsessive-compulsive disorder. Am J Psychiatry 160:1919–1928, 2003

Geller DA, Wagner KD, Emslie G, et al: Paroxetine treatment in children and adolescents with obsessive-compulsive disorder: a randomized, multicenter, double-blind, placebo-controlled trial. J Am Acad Child Adolesc Psychiatry 43:1387–1396, 2004

Geller D, Donnelly C, Lopez F, et al: Atomoxetine treatment for pediatric patients with attention-deficit/hyperactivity disorder with comorbid anxiety disorder. J Am Acad Child Adolesc Psychiatry 46:1119–1127, 2007

Gibbons RD, Hur K, Bhaumik DK, et al: The relationship between antidepressant medication use and rate of suicide. Arch Gen Psychiatry 62:165–172, 2005

Gittelman-Klein R, Klein DF: Controlled imipramine treatment of school phobia. Arch Gen Psychiatry 25:204–207, 1971

Glod CA, Lynch A, Flynn E, et al: Open trial of bupropion SR in adolescent major depression. J Child Adolesc Psychiatr Nurs 16:123–130, 2003

Guy W: ECDEU Assessment Manual for Psychopharmacology, 2nd Edition. Washington, DC: U.S. Government Printing Office, 1976

Hammad TA, Laughren T, Racoosin J: Suicidality in pediatric patients treated with antidepressant drugs. Arch Gen Psychiatry 63:332–339, 2006

Hazell P, O'Connell D, Heathcote D, et al: Efficacy of tricyclic drugs in treating child and adolescent depression: a meta-analysis. BMJ 310:897–901, 1995

Heiligenstein JH, Hoog SL, Wagner KD, et al: Fluoxetine 40–60 mg versus fluoxetine 20 mg in the treatment of children and adolescents with a less-than-complete response to nine-week treatment with fluoxetine 10–20 mg: a pilot study. J Child Adolesc Psychopharmacol 16:207–217, 2006

Keller MB, Ryan ND, Strober M, et al: Efficacy of paroxetine in the treatment of adolescent major depression: a randomized, controlled trial. J Am Acad Child Adolesc Psychiatry 40:762–772, 2001

Kennard BD, Emslie GJ, Mayes TL, et al: Cognitive-behavioral therapy to prevent relapse in pediatric responders to pharmacotherapy for major depressive disorder. J Am Acad Child Adolesc Psychiatry 47:1395–1404, 2008

Klein RG, Koplewicz HS, Kanner A: Imipramine treatment of children with separation anxiety disorder. J Am Acad Child Adolesc Psychiatry 31:21–28, 1992

Kotler LA, Devlin MJ, Davies M, et al: An open trial of fluoxetine for adolescents with bulimia nervosa. J Child Adolesc Psychopharmacol 13:329–335, 2003

Kratochvil C, Emslie G, Silva S, et al; TADS Team: Acute time to response in the Treatment for Adolescents with Depression Study (TADS). J Am Acad Child Adolesc Psychiatry 45:1412–1418, 2006

Leonard HL, Swedo SE, Rapoport JL, et al: Treatment of obsessive-compulsive disorder with clomipramine and desipramine in children and adolescents: a double-blind crossover comparison. Arch Gen Psychiatry 46:1088–1092, 1989

Libby AM, Brent DA, Morrato EH, et al: Decline in treatment of pediatric depression after FDA advisory on risk of suicidality with SSRIs. Am J Psychiatry 164:884–891, 2007

Libby AM, Orton HD, Valuck RJ: Persisting decline in depression treatment after FDA warnings. Arch Gen Psychiatry 66:633–639, 2009

Liebowitz MR, Turner SM, Piacentini J, et al: Fluoxetine in children and adolescents with OCD: a placebo-controlled trial. J Am Acad Child Adolesc Psychiatry 41:1431–1438, 2002

March JS, Johnston H, Jefferson JW, et al: Do subtle neurological impairments predict treatment resistance to clomipramine in children and adolescents with obsessive-compulsive disorder? J Child Adolesc Psychopharmacol 1:133–140, 1990

March JS, Biederman J, Wolkow R, et al: Sertraline in children and adolescents with obsessive-compulsive disorder: a multicenter randomized controlled trial. JAMA 280:1752–1756, 1998

March J, Silva S, Petrycki S, et al: Fluoxetine, cognitive-behavioral therapy, and their combination for adolescents with depression: Treatment for Adolescents With Depression Study (TADS) randomized controlled trial. JAMA 292:807–820, 2004

March JS, Entusah AR, Rynn M, et al: A randomized controlled trial of venlafaxine ER versus placebo in pediatric social anxiety disorder. Biol Psychiatry 62:1149–1154, 2007a

March JS, Silva S, Petrycki S, et al: The Treatment for Adolescents With Depression Study (TADS): long-term effectiveness and safety outcomes. Arch Gen Psychiatry 64:1132–1144, 2007b

March JS, Silva S, Curry J, et al: The Treatment for Adolescents With Depression Study (TADS): outcomes over 1 year of naturalistic follow-up. Am J Psychiatry 166:1141–1149, 2009

Martin A, Volkmar FR (eds.): Lewis's Child and Adolescent Psychiatry: A Comprehensive Textbook. Philadelphia, PA, Lippincott Williams & Wilkins, 2007

Masi G, Pari C, Millepiedi S: Pharmacological treatment options for panic disorder in children and adolescents. Expert Opin Pharmacother 7:545–554, 2006

Melvin GA, Tonge BJ, King NJ, et al: A comparison of cognitive-behavioral therapy, sertraline, and their combination for adolescent depression. J Am Acad Child Adolesc Psychiatry 45:1151–1161, 2006

Michelson D, Faries D, Wernicke J, et al: Atomoxetine in the treatment of children and adolescents with attention-deficit/hyperactivity disorder: a randomized, placebo-controlled, dose-response study. Pediatrics 108:E83, 2001

Michelson D, Allen AJ, Busner J, et al: Once-daily atomoxetine treatment for children and adolescents with attention deficit hyperactivity disorder: a randomized, placebo-controlled study. Am J Psychiatry 159:1896–1901, 2002

Owens JA, Moturi S: Pharmacologic treatment of pediatric insomnia. Child Adolesc Psychiatr Clin N Am 18:1001–1016, 2009

Owens JA, Babcock D, Blumer J, et al: The use of pharmacotherapy in the treatment of pediatric insomnia in primary care: rational approaches: a consensus meeting summary. J Clin Sleep Med 1:49–59, 2005

Pediatric OCD Treatment Study Team: Cognitive-behavior therapy, sertraline, and their combination for children and adolescents with obsessive-compulsive disorder: the Pediatric OCD Treatment Study (POTS) randomized controlled trial. JAMA 292:1969–1976, 2004

Pliszka S: Practice parameter for the assessment and treatment of children and adolescents with attention-deficit/hyperactivity disorder. J Am Acad Child Adolesc Psychiatry 46:894–921, 2007

Poznanski EO, Grossman JA, Buchsbaum Y, et al: Preliminary studies of the reliability and validity of the children's depression rating scale. J Am Acad Child Psychiatry 23:191–197, 1984

Reinblatt SP, Walkup JT: Psychopharmacologic treatment of pediatric anxiety disorders. Child Adolesc Psychiatr Clin N Am 14:877–908, x, 2005

Research Unit on Pediatric Psychopharmacology Anxiety Study Group: Fluvoxamine for the treatment of anxiety disorders in children and adolescents. The Research Unit on Pediatric Psychopharmacology Anxiety Study Group. N Engl J Med 344:1279–1285, 2001

Riddle MA, Scahill L, King RA, et al: Double-blind, crossover trial of fluoxetine and placebo in children and adolescents with obsessive-compulsive disorder. J Am Acad Child Adolesc Psychiatry 31:1062–1069, 1992

Riddle MA, Reeve EA, Yaryura-Tobias JA, et al: Fluvoxamine for children and adolescents with obsessive-compulsive disorder: a randomized, controlled, multicenter trial. J Am Acad Child Adolesc Psychiatry 40:222–229, 2001

Riggs SA, Sahl G, Greenwald E, et al: Family environment and adult attachment as predictors of psychopathology and personality dysfunction among inpatient abuse survivors. Violence Vict 22:577–600, 2007

Rynn MA, Siqueland L, Rickels K: Placebo-controlled trial of sertraline in the treatment of children with generalized anxiety disorder. Am J Psychiatry 158:2008–2014, 2001

Rynn MA, Riddle MA, Yeung PP, et al: Efficacy and safety of extended-release venlafaxine in the treatment of generalized anxiety disorder in children and adolescents: two placebo-controlled trials. Am J Psychiatry 164:290–300, 2007

Safer DJ, Zito JM: Treatment-emergent adverse events from selective serotonin reuptake inhibitors by age group: children versus adolescents. J Child Adolesc Psychopharmacol 16:159–169, 2006

Simeon JG, Dinicola VF, Ferguson HB, et al: Adolescent depression: a placebo-controlled fluoxetine treatment study and follow-up. Prog Neuropsychopharmacol Biol Psychiatry 14:791–795, 1990

Son SE, Kirchner JT: Depression in children and adolescents. Am Fam Physician 62:2297–2308, 2311–2312, 2000

Treatment for Adolescents With Depression Study Team: Treatment for Adolescents With Depression Study (TADS): rationale, design, and methods. J Am Acad Child Adolesc Psychiatry 42:531–542, 2003

U.S. Food and Drug Administration: Advisory on antidepressants. FDA Consum 38:4, 2004

Vitiello B, Silva SG, Rohde P, et al: Suicidal events in the Treatment for Adolescents With Depression Study (TADS). J Clin Psychiatry 70:741–747, 2009

von Knorring AL, Olsson GI, Thomsen PH, et al: A randomized, double-blind, placebo-controlled study of citalopram in adolescents with major depressive disorder. J Clin Psychopharmacol 26:311–315, 2006

Wagner KD, Ambrosini P, Rynn M, et al: Efficacy of sertraline in the treatment of children and adolescents with major depressive disorder: two randomized controlled trials. JAMA 290:1033–1041, 2003a

Wagner KD, Cook EH, Chung H, et al: Remission status after long-term sertraline treatment of pediatric obsessive-compulsive disorder. J Child Adolesc Psychopharmacol 13 Suppl 1:S53–60, 2003b

Wagner KD, Berard R, Stein MB, et al: A multicenter, randomized, double-blind, placebo-controlled trial of paroxetine in children and adolescents with social anxiety disorder. Arch Gen Psychiatry 61:1153–1162, 2004a

Wagner KD, Robb AS, Findling RL, et al: A randomized, placebo-controlled trial of citalopram for the treatment of major depression in children and adolescents. Am J Psychiatry 161:1079–1083, 2004b

Wagner KD, Jonas J, Findling RL, et al: A double-blind, randomized, placebo-controlled trial of escitalopram in the treatment of pediatric depression. J Am Acad Child Adolesc Psychiatry 45:280–288, 2006

Weintrob N, Cohen D, Klipper-Aurbach Y, et al: Decreased growth during therapy with selective serotonin reuptake inhibitors. Arch Pediatr Adolesc Med 156:696–701, 2002

Weller EB, Weller RA: Clinical aspects of childhood depression. Pediatr Ann 15:843–847, 1986

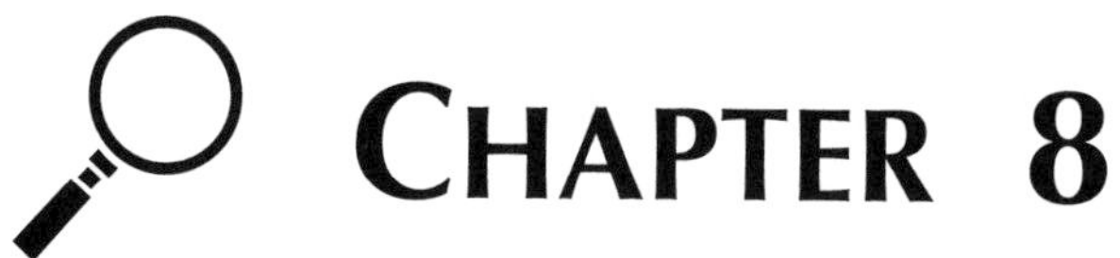

CHAPTER 8

Use of Antidepressants in Geriatric Patients

Benjamin Liptzin, M.D.
Cassandra Hobgood, M.D.

APPROPRIATE use of antidepressant medications in older patients requires the clinician to understand what makes older persons, especially older depressed persons, different from younger persons. Great variability and heterogeneity exist among older persons. A 60-year-old, if healthy, can be indistinguishable from a 40-year-old, but a 60-year-old who has experienced a stroke or myocardial infarction or is in the early stages of Alzheimer's disease can be more like a frail 90-year-old. Some physiological and psychosocial changes that occur as individuals age affect their susceptibility to depression and their response to treatment.

Age-Associated Changes

Although there is great variability across individuals as they age, in general, older individuals are more likely to experience medical problems and to be taking medications to treat those problems. These medical problems can also cause frailty and a reduction in activity or a decrease in the enjoyment of activities. Medical difficulties can lead to worries about the future and about how much time is left to live. Changes in vision and hearing may further reduce activities that were previously enjoyed. Physical changes that restrict driving reduce social contact or activity and can cause a loss of self-esteem. Older persons are more likely to have experienced the illness or death of loved ones, which can lead to normal or pathological grief reactions and to a loss of social support or loss of a companion or sexual partner. Older persons who were gainfully employed may work less or retire completely, which may reduce their income, their social contacts, and the self-esteem that comes from working. Conversely, many older people may outlive their pensions (or a company that was expected to provide the pension) and continue working into their 70s or 80s out of necessity. All of these possible changes can decrease the quality of life and lead to a decreased mood.

Despite all the changes that are common in elderly people, most older persons rate their health as good despite some health problems or activity limitations. Most older persons also learn to cope with and accept the losses that are common with aging. Thanks to Social Security, Medicare, and other programs, elderly people have a lower rate of poverty than younger people. Although some individuals complain that the "golden years" can be challenging, most in the current elderly cohort had some experience with the Great Depression of the 1930s and the stresses of World War II. Most, therefore, experience their lives as much better than their parents' lives and better than they expected for themselves.

Depression in Elderly Persons

Depression in older persons may differ in important respects from that in younger persons. Older persons may be more likely than younger persons to present to their primary care physician complaining of physical symptoms rather than sadness or depression. The physician needs to be alert to the possibility that the complaints could represent a "masked depression." A beneficial practice is to use a standardized symptom rating scale that has been specifically designed for use in older patients (e.g., Yesavage et al. 1982).

The older patient may also have comorbid illnesses or be taking medications that could explain depressive symptoms such as lack of energy (e.g., anemia, hypothyroidism, effects from β-blockers), lack of interest, difficulty sleeping (e.g., pain, breathing difficulty), loss of appetite (e.g., gastrointestinal problems), or difficulty concentrating (e.g., dementia, effects of medication). The presence of comorbid medical conditions can reduce the effectiveness of antidepressant treatment, leading to lower rates of depression symptom improvement and higher rates of relapse (Iosifescu et al. 2004). Patients may also present with cognitive complaints and be concerned that these problems might indicate the beginning of a dementing illness. They may have suffered a recent loss and be sad as a result of their grief. They may be sleeping poorly because of nocturia, loss of their usual partner in bed, or disruption of their sleep cycle due to staying up late and sleeping late in the morning. Poor sleep can lead to decreased activity, which can lead to a decreased mood, which might then worsen the sleep disturbance. Lack of interest may be due to boredom in elderly patients, if they no longer have their regular job or scheduled activities. Apathy may be difficult to distinguish from clinical depression (Lenze et al. 2009).

Because of the variety of possible contributors to depression, a careful medical workup is necessary to rule out physical causes for the symptoms of depression. This workup should include a careful history that includes questions about recent medication changes. Appropriate laboratory studies, including a brain imaging study, should also be considered.

Case Examples

A 78-year-old woman presented to a psychiatrist with depression characterized by loss of appetite, decreased energy, and decreased interest. History revealed that these symptoms had started soon after she began taking cimetidine for reflux. When the medication was stopped, the symptoms disappeared.

A 63-year-old physician was admitted to a psychiatric unit because of "severe depression." For months she had hardly gotten out of bed and could no longer work or take care of her house. On admission, she was noted to have lost her sense of smell. A computed tomography (CT) scan confirmed the presence of an olfactory meningioma, and the patient underwent a neurosurgical resection. In the recovery room, her family noted that her "depression" had disappeared and that she was back to her usual self.

A 78-year-old woman was admitted to a psychiatric unit because of significant weight loss. Despite an extensive workup, no medical explanation was found. The patient appeared to be quite depressed, with little energy or interest. She had no appetite and complained that she just didn't feel like eating. An abdominal CT scan was repeated and revealed a carcinoma of the head of the pancreas.

When patients present with depressive symptoms after loss of a spouse, the differential between major depression and normal bereavement needs to be clarified. Normal bereavement generally lasts no more than 6 months and rarely leads to profound loss of appetite, weight loss, and withdrawal from all pleasurable activities. An 83-year-old patient seemed to understand the difference: "I expected to feel sad after my husband died, but this has gone on too long and I should have resumed some of my activities by now. I lost both my parents and have lost several siblings and close friends and never was this bad." She was treated with an antidepressant, and her mood, energy, and interest improved dramatically and she started baking cookies for her granddaughter.

Older patients who present with cognitive impairment are often assumed to have dementia due to a neurodegenerative or vascular process. In fact, in many cases, these patients have "pseudodementia," or what is now called the "dementia syndrome of depression." Such patients usually show other symptoms of depression and do not make much effort on cognitive testing. In contrast, patients with dementia will try hard on testing but simply lack the cognitive capacity to answer questions correctly. Some patients with dementia may also present with a comorbid depression that can respond to treatment. Depression may be evident if an abrupt decline has occurred in a patient's functioning, including his or her interest and activity level, that cannot be explained by a worsening of the dementia. Executive dysfunction is common in late-life depression and predicts slow, poor, and unstable response to antidepressants (Alexopoulos et al. 2005).

Epidemiology of Depression in the Elderly

Until 25 years ago, most textbook descriptions suggested that depression was known to be more common in elderly people. That increased occurrence was thought to be due to all the "depressing" changes that happen with aging, as was described earlier in the section "Age-Associated Changes." For many years, the rate of completed suicide has been higher among elderly people than among younger people, largely because older white men who attempt suicide do it through violent means such as shooting or hanging (Conwell and Thompson 2008). The rate of attempted suicide, however, is highest among younger women. The Epidemiological Catchment Area study found that the rate of major depression in their community survey was lower among older persons than younger persons (Regier et al. 1988). The prevalence of major depression in individuals over age 65 living in the community is estimated to be around 5% (Gallo and Lebowitz 1999); however, the methodology and conclusions of that study have been questioned because the rate of depression is higher among hospitalized elderly or those in nursing homes and inclusion of those individuals would raise the overall depression rate. Other studies have shown that the prevalence of depressive symptoms is higher among elderly people even if major depression is not more common. It is easy to either miss symptoms of depression in an older person or dismiss them as an expected part of getting older.

Drug Prescribing in Elderly Patients

Physiological changes that occur with aging (Table 8–1) suggest some general rules about prescribing for elderly people (summarized in Table 8–2). Because older patients are more likely to have underlying medical problems or to be taking medications that could be causing their symptoms, a careful medical history is essential and may lead to a medical workup and treatment of identified medical problems. If the patient is dealing with loss of a spouse, a lack of activity or social supports, or other psychosocial stresses, psychotherapy may be the appropriate treatment (Areàn et al. 2010). Older patients may be more willing to take an antidepressant than in previous years, as indicated by a 2006 survey that found that 98% of individuals over age 55 perceived depression as having a biological cause, compared to only 73% in 1996 (Blumner and Marcus 2009). Although much of the literature is from clinical trials of antidepressants in patients who fit neatly into a DSM-IV category of major depression (American Psychiatric Association 1994), in the real world patients present with comorbidity from medical conditions, concomitant medications, or psychosocial situations that may explain some of their symptoms.

The treating clinician and the patient should clearly understand what the prescribed medication is designed to help so that both can know whether it is working and should be continued or whether it is ineffective and should be stopped. Some patients may be unable or unwilling to take the medication as prescribed because of cognitive difficulties, physical problems such as arthritis or hemiparesis, or financial limitations that force them to choose between medication and other necessities of life. Data from a Prevention of Suicide in Primary Care Elderly: Collaborative Trial (PROSPECT) study demonstrated that care management in older depressed primary care patients can maintain high utilization of treatment for depression and thereby reduce suicidal ideation and improve the outcomes for patients with major depression over 2 years (Alexopoulos et al. 2009). A study from the Improving Mood-Promoting Access

TABLE 8–1. Physiological changes in elderly patients associated with altered pharmacokinetics and drug response

PHYSIOLOGICAL FUNCTION	EFFECTS OF AGING CHANGES
Absorption	Aging has no significant effect. Acid secretion, GI perfusion, and membrane transport may delay or decrease absorption, but GI transit time is prolonged and increases absorption, so there is no net change. Antacids, high-fiber supplements, and cholestyramine may significantly diminish absorption.
Volume of distribution	Aging affects dosing of lithium and lipid-soluble psychotropics. Lean body mass and total body water are decreased and fat tissue increases, resulting in a lower volume of distribution for water-soluble drugs and an increased volume of distribution for lipid-soluble drugs. Lithium is water soluble, and the same oral dose in older patients can lead to higher blood levels. Psychotropics that are lipid soluble will have a longer half-life and drug accumulation.
Protein binding	Aging has no effect.
Serum albumin	Reductions in serum albumin with aging or with malnutrition may lead to increased free concentration of drugs in plasma, but this increase is not usually clinically significant.
Renal clearance	Decreases with aging may increase blood levels of lithium or other drugs/ metabolites excreted by the kidney.
Hepatic metabolism	Reductions in hepatic mass and blood flow with aging cause greater interindividual differences. Drug interactions may also affect metabolism and lead to longer half-lives and plasma levels.
Altered receptor sensitivity	Increased receptor sensitivity with aging means that drugs should be given in lower dosages.

Note. GI=gastrointestinal.

TABLE 8–2. Principles of drug prescribing for elderly patients

1. Before prescribing any medication, look for a medical or other cause for the patient's symptoms.
2. Consider whether psychosocial interventions or psychotherapy should be tried before prescribing medication.
3. Clearly identify the target symptoms to be treated and monitored.
4. Evaluate the patient's ability to take medication as prescribed, simplify the regimen to once-daily or at most twice-daily dosing, and encourage use of a pill box as a reminder.
5. Review any previous response to medications by the patient and first-degree relatives.
6. Start with a low initial dose.
7. Increase slowly as needed and tolerated to reduce the target symptoms.
8. Although lower doses are usually effective, do not hesitate to use a full adult dose if the patient tolerates it.
9. In addition to prescribing medication, provide appropriate psychotherapy or other psychosocial interventions and optimize the patient's medical conditions.
10. After the patient responds, consider how long to continue the medication.
11. Consider electroconvulsive therapy if the patient is psychotic, is refusing oral medication, or is not responding.

to Collaborative Treatment (IMPACT) collaborative care management program had previously demonstrated improved outcomes of depression through care management over a 1-year period (Unutzer et al. 2002). Care management is particularly important because patients 65 and older were less likely to receive guideline-concordant follow-up visits than were younger patients (Chen et al. 2010). A patient's or family member's previous response to a medication can help in medication selection.

Because of the changes in pharmacokinetics and pharmacodynamics that occur with aging (see Table 8–1), pharmaceutical treatment for elderly patients should be started at a low dosage. The patient not only might respond to a low dosage but also might have a serious adverse reaction if the initial dosage is too high. For example, a medication that can cause orthostatic hypotension might be tolerated in a younger patient, but in an older patient, the medication may lead to a fall. Hanlon et al. (2009) reported that higher total daily doses of central nervous system medications (including antidepressants) were associated with recurrent falls. Furthermore, a fall is more likely to lead to a broken hip in an older person. Also, medication increases should be slow and carefully monitored for tolerability. In an inpatient setting, these slow adjustments can lead to longer stays for older compared to younger patients. Given interindividual variability, some patients may require full adult dosages of medication despite their age; as long as they are tolerating the medication, that dosing is not a problem. Stopping a medication that is no longer needed for maintenance treatment to prevent relapse or a recurrence is a good idea for patients of any age. However, it is particularly important for older patients who are more likely to be taking multiple medications or have other medical comorbidity that puts them at risk of drug-disease or drug-drug interactions. Stopping a medication will also reduce their financial burden.

Even if medication is prescribed, the patient may also need psychotherapy or other psychosocial intervention. Depression is a recurrent illness, and a controlled maintenance trial found that 65% of elderly patients with major depression remained in remission over 24 months while treated with paroxetine and monthly psychotherapy compared with only 32% who received placebo and psychotherapy (Reynolds et al. 2006).

Evidence Base for Antidepressant Treatment in Elderly Patients

The clinical strategies used to treat older depressed patients are largely extrapolated from studies in younger patients. In fact, although the newest edition of the practice guideline for the treatment of major depression published by the American Psychiatric Association (2010) has a section on older age, the guideline concludes, "Once the patient has been thoroughly assessed, the treatment considerations for depressed geriatric patients are essentially the same as for younger patients." Many clinical trials specifically excluded geriatric patients because of their age or medical comorbidity or concomitant medication use. Even when older patients were included, they generally were represented in small numbers or at ages 55–65; no conclusions could be drawn about their differences from younger patients, and the results could not be generalized to a very old, frail, medically compromised geriatric patient. Steinmetz et al. (2005) pointed out that only 28% of the package inserts for the medications most commonly prescribed for older patients have specific dosing recommendations.

Perhaps the largest real-world clinical trial for patients with depression, the National Institute of Mental Health's Sequenced Treatment Alternatives to Relieve Depression (STAR*D; Gaynes et al. 2009), enrolled patients up to age 75 but provided little or no advice about strategies for specifically treating geriatric patients. Furthermore, most clinical trials are conducted in outpatient psychiatric settings, although most depressed patients, especially older ones, are treated in primary care offices. The IMPACT and PROSPECT studies are valuable because they were done in primary care practices (Alexopoulos et al. 2009; Unutzer et al. 2002).

Nevertheless, with the development of geriatric psychiatry, many clinical trials focusing on elderly patients have been done in the last 20 years. Mulsant and Pollock (2010) have summarized the published randomized controlled trials (RCTs) of selective serotonin reuptake inhibitors (SSRIs) for acute treatment of geriatric depression. These RCTs included 7 trials of citalopram with a total of 1,343 participants, 1 of escitalopram with 517 participants, 13 of fluoxetine with 2,092 participants, 4 of fluvoxamine with 278 participants, 8 of paroxetine with 1,444 participants, and 10 of sertraline with 1,817 participants. Similarly, there have been 2 geriatric trials of bupropion with 163 participants, 2 of duloxetine with 610 participants, 2 of mirtazapine with 370 participants, and 7 of venlafaxine with 921 participants. These studies are described in the later sections on individual drugs.

Dosage, Side Effects, and Choice of Drugs

No perfect antidepressant exists that works quickly, is effective in a wide spectrum of cases, and produces no side effects. Table 8–3 lists the antidepressants available and the usual dosage range for elderly patients. Some patients may not tolerate even the lower end of the dosage range listed, whereas other patients may be able to tolerate a dosage above the higher end that is normally required for a full response.

Table 8–4 lists the usual side effects of antidepressants. Some of these side effects are more bothersome or worrisome in elderly patients. The tricyclic antidepressants (TCAs) fell out of favor because of their anticholinergic side effects. Dry mouth may make dentures fit less well. Constipation is already a problem for many older patients. Urinary retention is more likely in older men with an enlarged prostate than in younger men. Orthostatic hypotension is more likely to lead to a fall in an older patient, and a fall is more likely to lead to a hip fracture. Older patients are more likely to have narrow-angle glaucoma and are at risk of increased intraocular pressure. Older patients are also at greater risk of developing full-blown anticholinergic delirium. SSRIs or serotonin-norepinephrine reuptake inhibitors (SNRIs) can cause nausea, reflux, or

TABLE 8–3. Antidepressants and usual dosage ranges in elderly patients

ANTIDEPRESSANT	DOSAGE RANGE (MG/DAY)
Selective serotonin reuptake inhibitors	
Citalopram	10–40
Escitalopram	10–20
Fluoxetine	5–20
Fluvoxamine	50–200
Paroxetine	10–30
Sertraline	12.5–100
Serotonin-norepinephrine reuptake inhibitors	
Desvenlafaxine	50–100
Duloxetine	20–40
Venlafaxine	25–150
Tricyclic antidepressants	
Amitriptyline	10–50
Desipramine	10–100
Doxepin	10–100
Imipramine	10–100
Nortriptyline	10–50
Monoamine oxidase inhibitors	
Phenelzine	15–60
Tranylcypromine	10–40
Psychostimulants	
Methylphenidate	2.5–20
Others	
Bupropion	50–300
Mirtazapine	7.5–60
Trazodone	25–200

diarrhea, which can be more problematic in a frail elder. The more sedating antidepressants such as trazodone or mirtazapine may make older patients too sleepy the next day, putting them at risk of falls and further reducing their activity.

TABLE 8–4. Side effects of antidepressants

Drug class	Possible side effects
Selective serotonin reuptake inhibitors	Loss of appetite, nausea, diarrhea, increased sweating, salivation, sexual dysfunction, SIADH, anxiety, restlessness, insomnia
Serotonin-norepinephrine reuptake inhibitors	Nausea, dizziness, anxiety, insomnia, hypertension, dry mouth, constipation
Tricyclic antidepressants	Sedation, dry mouth, constipation, urinary retention, blurred vision, tachycardia, confusion, disorientation, orthostatic hypotension, cardiac conduction delays
Monoamine oxidase inhibitors	Orthostatic hypotension, hypertensive crisis from dietary indiscretion
Stimulants	Tachycardia, hypertension, insomnia, restlessness, cardiac arrhythmias, seizures
Others	
Bupropion	Seizures, anxiety, agitation, restlessness
Mirtazapine	Sedation, weight gain, neutropenia
Trazodone	Sedation, priapism

Note. SIADH=syndrome of inappropriate antidiuretic hormone secretion.

Case Examples

An 83-year-old man was seen by his primary care physician because he was depressed after allowing himself to be swindled. He began taking amitriptyline 25 mg/day. The family noted that over the next several days, the patient became disoriented and was talking to the plants in his living room and urinating on the floor. His delirium cleared when the medication was stopped.

A 78-year-old woman was diagnosed with depression and given nortriptyline 10 mg/day. At that dosage, her blood pressure dropped to 60/20 when she tried to stand but instead fell to the floor. Fortunately, she did not suffer any injury.

An 83-year-old woman with depression began taking fluoxetine. Her family noted that she was eating less and complaining of stomach discomfort and diarrhea. These symptoms disappeared when the medication was stopped.

Little efficacy evidence is available to support the use of one particular drug or class over another. In a Cochrane review, Mottram et al. (2006) looked at 29 RCTs and did not find any differences in efficacy when comparing classes of antidepressants, although the authors noted that the trials contained relatively small numbers of patients so that a difference might not have been detected even if present. Nelson et al. (2008) reviewed 10 RCTs of second-generation antidepressants in late-life depression and concluded that the benefits found during acute treatment were modest and variable. Usually, therefore, the side-effect profile determines the choice of drug. Mottram et al. (2006) suggested that patients treated with TCAs had a higher withdrawal rate due to side effects. Alexopoulos et al. (2001) summarized the consensus guidelines developed by a panel of experts in geriatric psychiatry. They recommended an SSRI as the first-line treatment for late-life depression based on ease of use, safety, and generally good tolerability. TCAs are generally used as second- or third-line treatments in older patients because of their side effects. Similarly, monoamine oxidase inhibitors (MAOIs) are reserved for patients with treatment-resistant depression (or those who responded to an MAOI earlier in life) because of the risk of hypertension, which could increase the risk of a stroke, or hypotension, which increases the risk of a fall and possible fracture. The dietary restrictions necessary for preventing hypertensive crises and some concern over possible legal exposure have also limited the use of MAOIs, especially in the United States.

Cost is another consideration in drug selection, especially for older patients on fixed incomes. Of the drugs listed in Table 8–3, generics are available for all except desvenlafaxine, escitalopram, and duloxetine. A prudent practice is to initiate treatment with a generic drug and consider one of the others if the patient fails to respond.

Studies of Specific Drugs in Elderly Patients

In this section, we summarize the evidence for several antidepressants from different classes. Readers looking for a more exhaustive summary can refer to Mulsant and Pollock (2010) or to an earlier Cochrane review by Mottram et al. (2006).

Citalopram

Citalopram is the SSRI that was chosen as the first treatment option in the STAR*D trial of depression in patients of all ages. Citalopram was also used as the first step in the algorithm for treating elderly depressed patients in primary care in the PROSPECT study (Alexopoulos et al. 2009). In trials with older patients, citalopram has been shown to be more efficacious than placebo and as effective as amitriptyline (Rosenberg et al. 2007). More patients taking amitriptyline complain of adverse events, and it is not clear why amitriptyline was chosen as a comparator because it is rarely used in elderly patients. Citalopram has also been shown to be as effective as venlafaxine in geriatric outpatients with major depression (Allard et al. 2004). Tremor was more common in patients taking citalopram, and nausea/vomiting was more common in patients taking venlafaxine.

Paroxetine

Paroxetine is an SSRI that has been studied in elderly patients. It has the advantage of being somewhat sedating so it can help with sleep if taken at night. Like other SSRIs, it has antianxiety activity. However, its use has declined as prescribers have become more aware of significant symptoms of withdrawal, including a flulike illness when the dosage is reduced or the drug is discontinued. Paroxetine also has some anticholinergic activity that can be problematic (see "Dosage, Side Effects, and Choice of Drugs" earlier in this chapter). Rapaport et al. (2003), in a study of controlled-release paroxetine in patients over age 60 who had late-life depression, found that the medication was efficacious and well tolerated. In a landmark study of maintenance treatment, Reynolds et al. (2006) showed that patients 70 and older with major depression who had a response to initial treatment with paroxetine and psychotherapy were less likely to have recurrent depression if they received 2 years of maintenance therapy with paroxetine. Mulsant and Pollock (2010) concluded that paroxetine was more efficacious than placebo and as efficacious as amitriptyline, bupropion, clomipramine, doxepin, fluoxetine, and imipramine. In a study of 24 very old patients with non-major depression in a nursing home, Burrows et al. (2002) found that paroxetine was not clearly superior to placebo and that paroxetine increased the risk of adverse cognitive effects; two patients developed delirium.

Sertraline

Sertraline is an SSRI that has a favorable pharmacokinetic profile and a lower potential for significant drug interactions compared with other SSRIs (Mulsant and Pollock 2010). It has been shown to be more efficacious than placebo and as efficacious as amitriptyline, fluoxetine, fluvoxamine, imipramine, nortriptyline, and venlafaxine. Lyketsos et al. (2003) reported on its use in depression of patients with Alzheimer's disease.

Duloxetine

Duloxetine is an SNRI that has been shown to be effective for the treatment of major depression in older patients (Nelson et al. 2005). Raskin et al. (2007) studied duloxetine in 311 elderly outpatients with recurrent major depression and reported that duloxetine improved not only depressive symptoms but also cognition and some measures of pain. The drug was safe and well tolerated. In a study of elderly patients with recurrent major depression, Wohlreich et al. (2009) found that compared with placebo, duloxetine significantly reduced depression symptom severity in elderly patients with and without arthritis. The magnitude and time course of depressive symptom improvement did not differ significantly between patients with and without arthritis, although duloxetine did produce significant reduction in several pain measures in patients with comorbid arthritis.

Nortriptyline

Nortriptyline is a TCA and one of the best studied antidepressants in elderly patients. A metabolite of amitriptyline, it has a more favorable side-effect profile with considerably less anticholinergic activity than the parent drug. In a major study of patients ages 59 and older, Reynolds et al. (1999) found that the time to recurrence of a major depressive episode was significantly better in patients who received nortriptyline, interpersonal psychotherapy, or a combination of the two than in patients given placebo. There was also a trend favoring combined therapy over treatment with nortriptyline alone.

Nortriptyline has been found to be effective even in frail, institutionalized elderly with an average age of 85 years (Katz et al. 1990). Unfortunately, 30% of the patients in this study had significant side effects that limited their use of the medication.

For patients who do not respond to or do not tolerate an SSRI or SNRI, nortriptyline is certainly worth trying. Caution should be used, however, because of the risk of anticholinergic side effects. In younger patients, nortriptyline is reported to have a therapeutic window for efficacy; therefore, blood levels are recommended. In practice, however, blood levels are typically obtained only if the patient has not responded to what should be a therapeutic dosage. Such levels may reveal that the patient is a rapid metabolizer and can be safely given a higher dosage. More likely, a low blood level will reveal that the patient has not been taking the drug as prescribed, if at all.

Mirtazapine

Mirtazapine is a newer antidepressant that works differently than SSRIs, SNRIs, or TCAs. In a comparison of mirtazapine and paroxetine in elderly depressed patients, Schatzberg et al. (2002) found that mirtazapine had an earlier onset of action and a better tolerability profile. It has been used to treat depression in frail nursing home patients (Roose et al. 2003). In general, it is used as a second- or third-line agent in older depressed patients who cannot tolerate or have not responded to an SSRI or SNRI. Its other use is in general geriatric practice to increase appetite or promote sleep.

Venlafaxine

Venlafaxine is an SNRI that has been studied in several controlled clinical trials in elderly depressed patients. Mulsant and Pollock (2010) noted that venlafaxine does not inhibit any of the major cytochrome P450 isoenzymes and thus is unlikely to cause clinically significant drug-drug interactions. Its side effects, which are similar to those of SSRIs, include nausea, diarrhea, headaches, excessive sweating, sexual dysfunction, and serotonin syndrome. Like paroxetine, it has been associated with moderately severe discontinuation symptoms. Venlafaxine has been associated with clinically significant hypotension, electrocardiographic changes, arrhythmia, and acute ischemia (Johnson et al. 2006). The National Institute for Clinical Excellence in Great Britain has recommended that venlafaxine should not be given to older patients with preexisting heart disease and that patients taking higher doses should have their blood pressure and cardiac functions closely monitored (National Collaborating Centre for Mental Health 2004). In a study of older nursing home residents, Oslin et al. (2003) found that venlafaxine was less well tolerated and possibly less safe than sertraline and did not demonstrate increased efficacy.

Bupropion

Consensus guidelines support the use of bupropion in older depressed patients who cannot tolerate the side effects of or have not responded to an SSRI or SNRI (Alexopoulos et al. 2001). Bupropion is well tolerated and does not cause the gastrointestinal or sexual disturbances of SSRIs and SNRIs or the anticholinergic side effects of TCAs. The primary side effects are activation, sleep disturbance, and agitation. Bupropion has been associated with seizures, but they occurred primarily at higher dosages in younger patients with eating disorders. A 10-week study (Hewett et al. 2010) funded by the maker of extended-release bupropion demonstrated statistically significant improvements for bupropion, compared to placebo, in motivation and energy and in life satisfaction and contentment. Adverse events were mild to moderate. Bupropion has also been used to augment the effectiveness of other agents.

Psychostimulants

The principal role of psychostimulants in treating geriatric depression is to increase activity in patients who are apathetic and not participating in their rehabilitation after a stroke or hip fracture. They have also been used as an augmentation strategy with other first-line antidepressants. Lavretsky and Kumar (2001) used methylphenidate in an open trial to augment the effects of citalopram. They found that 8 of 10 elderly depressed patients showed clinically significant improvement by week 8, and no patient discontinued treatment.

Treatment of Depressed Older Patients With Dementia

Depression can coexist with dementia in an older patient. The evaluation of such a patient requires that the clinician consider whether the symptoms of "depression" are actually due to apathy and withdrawal because of the cognitive deficit rather than to a clinical depression. Even if clinical depression is present, alternatives to medication should be tried first, such as encouragement to participate in activities, more frequent family visits, or regular exercise. If a decision is made to try an antidepressant, the target symptoms should be clearly specified. The medication should be supervised or dispensed by a responsible caregiver, because the demented patient may be unable to remember to take the medication, may take more than is prescribed, or may stop taking it once the prescription runs out.

A number of investigators have tried antidepressants in depressed patients with dementia. An early study by Reifler et al. (1989) of Alzheimer's patients with and without depression found that imipramine, a TCA with strong anticholinergic properties, was no better (or worse) than placebo, although there was a high placebo response rate that might have affected the results. Raji and Brady (2001) studied mirtazapine for treatment of depression and comorbidities in three patients with Alzheimer's disease at an outpatient memory loss clinic. The patients had a prompt and sustained response, with complete remission of poor appetite, weight loss, sleep disturbance, and anxiety. Sad mood, anhedonia, and energy level also improved substantially. Lyketsos et al. (2003) studied sertraline in 44 outpatients with probable Alzheimer's disease and major depressive episodes. They concluded that sertraline was superior to placebo in these patients. They also found that with effective treatment of the depression, patients had lessened behavior disturbance and improved activities of daily living but not improved cognition. In a Cochrane review, Bains et al. (2002) looked at six studies with a total of 1,077 patients and concluded that the available evidence offered weak support to the contention that antidepressants are an effective treatment of patients with depression and dementia. They also noted the paucity of research and evidence in this area. Their conclusion was that clinicians should prescribe with caution given the potentially serious side effects of these medications in this population. Price and McAllister (1989) looked at ECT in elderly depressed patients with dementia. Overall, the patients achieved an 86% response rate, with only 21% experiencing a significant worsening of cognition. Most clinicians, however, reserve ECT as a last resort for these patients.

Treatment of Older Depressed Poststroke Patients

Depression is a common symptom in patients who have had a stroke. Although depression may an understandable response to the functional deficits and change in lifestyle that a stroke can cause, Robinson (2003) has shown that depression seems to be related to the brain changes caused by the stroke and occurs in approximately 20% of stroke patients. An early study by Lipsey et al. (1984) showed that nortriptyline produced a significantly greater improvement in depression than did placebo. Fruehwald et al. (2003) studied fluoxetine in 54 depressed patients ages 25–85 years following a stroke. They found that fluoxetine started within the first 2 weeks following a stroke showed no advantage in the first 3 months of treatment, but after 18 months of treatment, patients treated with fluoxetine were significantly less depressed than those treated with placebo. Starkstein et al. (2008) reviewed several controlled trials of treatment for poststroke depression and concluded that efficacy was demonstrated for sertraline, citalopram, and nortriptyline. Hackett et al. (2008) reviewed 16 RCTs comparing antidepressants with placebo or various forms of psychotherapy or ECT in 1,655 patients following a stroke. The analyses were complicated by the lack of standardized diagnostic and outcome criteria, as well as differing analytical methods. Some evidence suggested benefit for pharmacotherapy in terms of a complete remission of depression and a reduction (improvement) in scores on depression rating scales. However, not surprisingly, a significant increase in adverse events occurred.

Treatment of Depression in Patients With Parkinson's Disease

Parkinson's disease, the second most common neurodegenerative disorder after Alzheimer's disease, affects around 1 million persons in the United States (de Lau and Breteler 2006). Depression is quite common in patients with Parkinson's disease, occurring in up to 35% of the patients (Reijnders et al. 2008). Some of the depressive symptoms are associated with the physical symptoms, loss of functioning, and change in lifestyle caused by the Parkinson's disease. However, it is also hypothesized that the dopamine deficiency in the brain of patients with Parkinson's can lead directly to the symptoms of depression (Cummings 1992).

Weintraub et al. (2003) studied the recognition and treatment of depression in patients at a Parkinson's disease center. They found that one-third of subjects met criteria for a depressive disorder but that two-thirds of those were not currently receiving antidepressant treatment. One-quarter of the patients were taking an antidepressant, but almost half of them still met criteria for a depressive disorder. Their findings suggested that most depressed patients with Parkinson's disease are untreated and that their treatment is often inadequate or ineffective. Another study (Chen et al. 2007) looked at patients with Parkinson's disease treated through the Veterans Affairs health care system. They found that the presence of Parkinson's disease had little impact on the frequency and type of antidepressant treatment. They recommended that efforts to improve the care of depressed patients with Parkinson's disease should focus on improving recognition, ensuring adequacy of treatment, and evaluating the efficacy of existing antidepressants.

In a Cochrane review, Ghazi-Noori et al. (2003) looked at three randomized trials of oral antidepressants in 106 patients. They concluded that insufficient data were available on the effectiveness and safety of any antidepressant therapies in patients with Parkinson's disease and that RCTs were urgently required. They also noted that no trials of ECT were found. However, case reports (Faber 1997) have suggested that ECT can help not only symptoms of depression but also motor symptoms in patients with Parkinson's disease. Popeo and Kellner (2009) noted that ECT is hypothesized to act by enhancing dopamine neurotransmission, including increasing the sensitivity of dopamine receptors in patients with Parkinson's disease.

KEY CLINICAL CONCEPTS

- Symptoms of depression are common in older patients.
- Most older patients with depression present to their primary care doctor.
- A careful history and workup, if necessary, should rule out an underlying medical illness.
- No perfect antidepressant exists.
- Antidepressants differ more in their side effects than in their efficacy, and elderly patients can be more sensitive than younger patients to those side effects.
- Any antidepressant should be started at a low dosage and increased as needed and tolerated.
- As with younger patients, the first-choice agent is usually an SSRI or SNRI.
- Antidepressants can be effective in older patients with dementia, with Parkinson's disease, or following a stroke.
- ECT should be considered if the patient is refusing oral medications, is psychotic, or is not responding.

References

Alexopoulos GS, Katz IR, Reynolds CF 3rd, et al: Pharmacotherapy of depression in older patients: a summary of the expert consensus guidelines. J Psychiatr Pract 7:361–376, 2001

Alexopoulos GS, Kiosses DN, Heo M, et al: Executive dysfunction and the course of geriatric depression. Biol Psychiatry 58:204–210, 2005

Alexopoulos GS, Reynolds CF, Bruce ML, et al: Reducing suicidal ideation and depression in older primary care patients: 24-month outcomes of the PROSPECT study. Am J Psychiatry 166:882–890, 2009

Allard P, Gram L, Timdahl K, et al: Efficacy and tolerability of venlafaxine in geriatric outpatients with major depression: a double-blind, randomised 6-month comparative trial with citalopram. Int J Geriatr Psychiatry 19:1123–1130, 2004

American Psychiatric Association: Diagnostic and Statistical Manual of Mental Disorders, 4th Edition. Washington, DC, American Psychiatric Association, 1994

American Psychiatric Association: Practice Guideline for the Treatment of Patients With Major Depressive Disorder, 3rd Edition. Washington, DC, American Psychiatric Association, 2010. Available at: http://www.psychiatryonline.com/pracGuide/PracticePDFs/PG_Depression3rdEd.pdf. Accessed August 2011.

Areàn PA, Raue P, Mackin RS, et al: Problem-solving therapy and supportive therapy in older adults with major depression and executive dysfunction. Am J Psychiatry 167:1391–1398, 2010

Bains J, Birks JS, Dening TR: Antidepressants for treating depression in dementia. Cochrane Database of Systematic Reviews 2002, Issue 4. Art. No.: CD003944. DOI: 10.1002/14651858.CD003944.

Blumner KH, Marcus SC: Changing perceptions of depression: ten-year trends from the General Social Survey. Psychiatr Serv 60:306–312, 2009

Burrows AB, Salzman C, Satlin A, et al: A randomized, placebo-controlled trial of paroxetine in nursing home residents with non-major depression. Depress Anxiety 15:102–110, 2002

Chen P, Kales HC, Weintraub D, et al: Antidepressant treatment of veterans with Parkinson's disease and depression. J Geriatr Psychiatry Neurol 20:161–165, 2007

Chen SY, Hansen RA, Farley JF, et al: Follow-up visits by provider specialty for patients with major depressive disorder initiating antidepressant treatment. Psychiatr Serv 61:81–85, 2010

Conwell Y, Thompson C: Suicidal behavior in elders. Psychiatr Clin North Am 31:333–356, 2008

Cummings JL: Depression and Parkinson's disease: a review. Am J Psychiatry 149:443–454, 1992

de Lau LML, Breteler MMB: Epidemiology of Parkinson's disease. Lancet Neurol 5:525–535, 2006

Faber R: Electroconvulsive therapy in Parkinson's disease. Biol Psychiatry 42:262S, 1997

Fruehwald S, Gatterbauer E, Rehak P, et al: Early fluoxetine treatment of post-stroke depression: a three-month double-blind placebo-controlled study with an open-label long-term follow up. J Neurol 250:347–351, 2003

Gallo JJ, Lebowitz BD: The epidemiology of common late-life mental disorders in the community: themes for the new century. Psychiatr Serv 50:1158–1166, 1999

Gaynes BN, Warden D, Trivedi MH, et al: What did STAR*D teach us? Results from a large-scale, practical, clinical trial for patients with depression. Psychiatr Serv 60:1439–1445, 2009

Ghazi-Noori S, Chung TH, Deane K, et al: Therapies for depression in Parkinson's disease. Cochrane Database of Systematic Reviews 2003, Issue 2. Art. No.: CD003465. DOI: 10.1002/14651858.CD003465.

Hackett ML, Anderson CS, House A, et al: Interventions for treating depression after stroke. Cochrane Database of Systematic Reviews 2008, Issue 4. Art. No.: CD003437. DOI: 10.1002/14651858.CD003437.pub3.

Hanlon JT, Boudreau RM, Roumani YF, et al: Number and dosage of central nervous system medications on recurrent falls in community elders: the Health, Aging and Body Composition study. J Gerontol A Biol Sci Med Sci 64:492–498, 2009

Hewett K, Chrzanowski W, Jokinen R, et al: Double-blind, placebo-controlled evaluation of extended-release bupropion in elderly patients with major depressive disorder. J Psychopharmacol 24:521–529, 2010

Iosifescu DV, Bankier B, Fava M: Impact of medical comorbid disease on antidepressant treatment of major depressive disorder. Curr Psychiatry Rep 6:193–201, 2004

Johnson EM, Whyte E, Mulsant BH, et al: Cardiovascular changes associated with venlafaxine in the treatment of late-life depression. Am J Geriatr Psychiatry 14:796–802, 2006

Katz IR, Simpson GM, Curlik SM, et al: Pharmacologic treatment of major depression for elderly patients in residential care settings. J Clin Psychiatry 51(suppl):41–47, 1990

Lavretsky H, Kumar A: Methylphenidate augmentation of citalopram in elderly depressed patients. Am J Geriatr Psychiatry 9:298–303, 2001

Lenze EJ, Munin MC, Dew MA, et al: Apathy after hip fracture: a potential target for intervention to improve functional outcomes. J Neuropsychiatry Clin Neurosci 21:271–278, 2009

Lipsey JR, Robinson RG, Pearlson GD, et al: Nortriptyline treatment of post-stroke depression: a double-blind study. Lancet 1:297–300, 1984

Lyketsos CG, DelCampo L, Steinberg M, et al: Treating depression in Alzheimer disease: efficacy and safety of sertraline therapy, and the benefits of depression reduction: the DIADS. Arch Gen Psychiatry 60:737–746, 2003

Mottram PG, Wilson K, Strobl JJ: Antidepressants for depressed elderly. Cochrane Database of Systematic Reviews 2006, Issue 1. Art. No.: CD003491. DOI: 10.1002/14651858.CD003491.pub2.

Mulsant BH, Pollock BG: Psychopharmacology, in The American Psychiatric Publishing Textbook of Geriatric Psychiatry, 4th Edition. Edited by Blazer DG, Steffens DC. Washington, DC, American Psychiatric Publishing, 2010, pp 453–483

National Collaborating Centre for Mental Health: Management of Depression in Primary and Secondary Care (Clinical Guideline 23). London, UK, National Institute for Clinical Excellence, 2004

Nelson JC, Wohlreich MM, Mallincrodt CH, et al: Duloxetine for the treatment of major depressive disorder in older patients. Am J Geriatr Psychiatry 13:227–235, 2005

Nelson JC, Delucchi K, Schneider LS: Efficacy of second generation antidepressants in late-life depression: a meta-analysis of the evidence. Am J Geriatr Psychiatry 16:558–567, 2008

Oslin DW, Ten Have TR, Streim JE, et al: Probing the safety of medications in the frail elderly: evidence from a randomized clinical trial of sertraline and venlafaxine in depressed nursing home residents. J Clin Psychiatry 64:875–882, 2003

Popeo D, Kellner CH: ECT for Parkinson's disease. Med Hypotheses 73:468–469, 2009

Price TR, McAllister TW: Safety and efficacy of ECT in depressed patients with dementia: a review of clinical experience. Convuls Ther 5:61–74, 1989

Raji MA, Brady SR: Mirtazapine for treatment of depression and comorbidities in Alzheimer disease. Ann Pharmacother 35:1024–1027, 2001

Rapaport MH, Schneider LS, Dunner DL, et al: Efficacy of controlled-release paroxetine in the treatment of late-life depression. J Clin Psychiatry 64:1065–1074, 2003

Raskin J, Wiltse CG, Siegal A, et al: Efficacy of duloxetine on cognition, depression, and pain in elderly patients with major depressive syndrome: an 8-week, double-blind, placebo-controlled trial. Am J Psychiatry 164:900–909, 2007

Regier DA, Boyd JH, Burke JD Jr, et al: One-month prevalence of mental disorders in the United States: based on five Epidemiologic Catchment Area sites. Arch Gen Psychiatry 45:977–986, 1988

Reifler BV, Teri L, Raskind M, et al: Double-blind trial of imipramine in Alzheimer's disease patients with and without depression. Am J Psychiatry 146:45–49, 1989

Reijnders JS, Ehrt U, Weber WE, et al: A systematic review of prevalence studies of depression in Parkinson's disease. Mov Disord 23:183–189, 2008

Reynolds CF, Frank E, Perel JM, et al: Nortriptyline and interpersonal psychotherapy as maintenance therapies for recurrent major depression: a randomized controlled trial in patients older than 59 years. JAMA 281:39–45, 1999

Reynolds CF, Dew MA, Pollock BG, et al: Maintenance treatment of major depression in old age. N Engl J Med 354:1130–1138, 2006

Robinson RG: Poststroke depression: prevalence, diagnosis, treatment, and disease progression. Biol Psychiatry 54:376–387, 2003

Roose SP, Nelson JC, Salzman C, et al: Open-label study of mirtazapine orally disintegrating tablets in depressed patients in the nursing home. Curr Med Res Opin 19:737–746, 2003

Rosenberg C, Lauritzen L, Brix J, et al: Citalopram versus amitriptyline in elderly depressed patients with or without mild cognitive dysfunction: a Danish multicenter trial in general practice. Psychopharmacol Bull 40:63–73, 2007

Schatzberg AF, Kremer C, Rodrigues HE, et al: Double-blind, randomized comparison of mirtazapine and paroxetine in elderly depressed patients. Am J Geriatr Psychiatry 10:541–550, 2002

Starkstein SE, Mizrahi R, Power BD: Antidepressant therapy in post-stroke depression. Expert Opin Pharmacother 9:1291–1298, 2008

Steinmetz K, Coley K, Pollock BG: Assessment of the quantity and quality of geriatric information in the drug label for commonly prescribed drugs in the elderly. J Am Geriatr Soc 53:891–894, 2005

Unutzer J, Katon W, Callahan CM, et al: Collaborative care management of late-life depression in the primary care setting: a randomized controlled trial. JAMA 288:2836–2845, 2002

Weintraub D, Moberg PJ, Duda JE, et al: Recognition and treatment of depression in Parkinson's disease. J Geriatr Psychiatry Neurol 16:178–183, 2003

Wohlreich MM, Sullivan MD, Mallinckrodt CH, et al: Duloxetine for the treatment of major depressive disorder in elderly patients: treatment outcomes in patients with comorbid arthritis. Psychosomatics 50:402–412, 2009

Yesavage JA, Brink TL, Rose TL, et al: Development and validation of a geriatric depression screening scale: a preliminary report. J Psychiatr Res 17:37–49, 1982

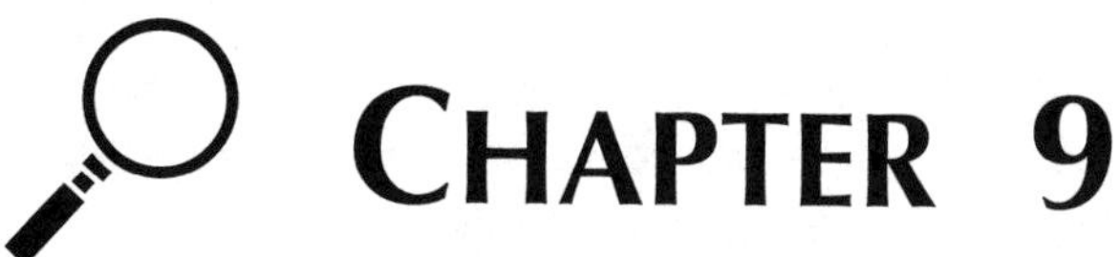

CHAPTER 9

Use of Antidepressants in Medically Ill Patients

Stacey B. Gramann, D.O., M.P.H.
Nancy Byatt, D.O., M.B.A.

MEDICALLY ILL PATIENTS commonly experience comorbid psychiatric illness, and chronic psychiatric illness is associated with an increase in comorbid medical conditions. Psychiatric symptoms are often precipitated by stressors that occur secondary to medical conditions; these stressors include loss of autonomy, health care–related financial stress, and decreased mobility or functioning. Untreated psychiatric illness leads to impairment in functioning and poor compliance with medications and medical care; such psychiatric barriers to medical care may lead to increased morbidity and mortality. Furthermore, depression itself may be an etiological factor in certain medical illnesses (Evans et al. 2005).

Over the past several decades, the U.S. Preventive Services Task Force has made efforts toward improved psychiatric screening, diagnosis, and treatment of comorbid psychiatric conditions in primary care settings (O'Connor et al. 2009). As psychiatric screening and diagnosis increase, antidepressants will likely be increasingly prescribed for the medically ill population. Given the rise of antidepressant use in individuals with comorbid medical and psychiatric illness, it is vital that practitioners use an evidence-based approach that takes into account the effect of antidepressant use on medical conditions, the impact that medical conditions have on psychiatric illness, and the complicated drug interactions that can occur in medically ill patients (Evans et al. 2005).

Medical Considerations

Drug-Drug Interactions

Medically ill patients are particularly susceptible to drug-drug interactions. Patients with chronic medical illnesses are often subject to polypharmacy, which increases the risk of drug-drug interactions. Further complicating matters, certain medications may induce or inhibit metabolism of other medications. Hepatic enzyme activity can be induced or inhibited, causing alterations in serum drug levels, which can then potentially affect the efficacy or toxicity of a drug. Medically ill patients may be more sensitive to such interactions and alterations in drug availability. Consequently, initiation and dosage adjustments of an antidepressant medication must be done conservatively, with consideration for potential interactions with other medications (Levenson 2005).

Pharmacokinetics

Pharmacokinetics refers to the processing of drugs through the body, beginning with absorption, followed by distribution and metabolism, and ending with excretion. In medically ill patients, diseases affecting the gastrointestinal tract, liver, kidneys, and heart can alter these processes. For instance, patients with liver cirrhosis, acute pancreatitis, bacterial pneumonia, and renal failure may have low serum protein levels, resulting in increased active drug availability and potential drug toxicity. Often, nutritional deficiencies and chronic illness lead to reduced protein binding, decreased metabolism, and reduced volume of distribution in medically ill patients. Consequently, availability of active antidepressant compounds may be increased, raising concern for potential toxicity and adverse effects (Levenson 2005).

Sexual Side Effects

Despite their efficacy for the treatment of depression, both selective serotonin reuptake inhibitors (SSRIs) and serotonin-norepinephrine reuptake inhibitors (SNRIs) can produce significant sexual side effects. Antidepressants with increased serotonergic activity carry the greatest risk, with sexual side effects being the most common adverse events experienced by individuals taking SSRIs (Delgado et al. 2005). Between 30% and 40% of patients taking antidepressant medications experience some form of sexual dysfunction during the course of treatment (Rothschild 2000). Three phases of the sexual arousal cycle can be affected for both genders: reduced interest in sex, decreased physiological arousal, and difficulty attaining orgasm. SSRI and SNRI medication effects on sexual arousal are thought to occur through increased serotonergic activity via 5-HT_2 and 5-HT_3 receptors, inhibiting orgasm and sexual desire. The noradrenergic effects of SNRIs do not appear to reduce the risk of developing sexual side effects (Clayton et al. 2006).

Sexual side effects can resolve spontaneously, but often treatment intervention is indicated. Several treatment approaches exist for patients experiencing treatment-induced sexual dysfunction (Table 9–1). Prior to attempting one of these treatment strategies, the practitioner must carefully consider the severity of a patient's psychiatric illness and the risk of worsening depressive symptoms or potential relapse with adjustment of antidepressant medication.

Akathisia

Akathisia, a side effect most commonly associated with antipsychotics, has also been noted to occur, although rarely, with the use of antidepressants. In case reports, akathisia has been associated with SSRIs, tricyclic antidepressants (TCAs), and venlafaxine. It is characterized by a sense of restlessness that can produce significant distress when severe. Akathisia is more likely to develop with the use of antidepressants in patients who have preexisting anxiety or panic disorders, who have a prior history of akathisia, who are receiving multiple akathisia-inducing medications, or who are female.

When akathisia is suspected, it should be addressed immediately. Treatment options include addition of a medication such as a β-blocker (e.g., propranolol 40–60 mg/day), a benzodiazepine, or an anticholinergic agent. If akathisia is distressing and continues to persist, other options are to switch to an alternative SSRI, switch to an alternative antidepressant class, or simply discontinue the akathisia-inducing antidepressant (Koliscak and Makela 2009).

Hyponatremia

Hyponatremia, which occurs more commonly with SSRIs than with other antidepressant classes, is a potentially serious adverse event that if untreated, can lead to delirium, seizures, and potentially death. The incidence of hyponatremia among patients taking an SSRI is reported to be 3–5 per 1,000 cases. Risk factors include female gender, older age, prior history of hyponatremia, and a current regimen including other medications that carry the risk of hyponatremia. Jacob and Spinler (2006) recommended careful clinical monitoring for symptoms including muscle cramps, fatigue, and confusion in individuals with such risk factors. Based on prior research, monitoring of serum sodium (Na^+) levels during the first 3–4 weeks of SSRI treatment may be beneficial in at-risk populations, because hyponatremia is most likely to develop during the initiation phase of treatment.

If hyponatremia is detected, based on a serum Na^+ level <130 mmol/L, treatment is then guided by three factors: underlying cause (e.g., malignancy, renal disease, surgery, medications), severity of onset (acute vs. chronic), and severity of presenting symptoms. In mild cases, treatment consists of fluid restriction, with monitoring of serum Na^+ levels and clinical symptoms. Aggressive treatment with hypertonic saline solution infusion may be indicated in more severe cases with neurological sequelae. Consequently, when an SSRI is suspected as the causal agent of hyponatremia, treatment is determined by the severity of the condition, and all underlying etiologies must be ruled out. In cases of SSRI-induced hyponatremia, discontinuation of the SSRI is often recommended, with the expectation that serum Na^+ levels should normalize within several days. A rechallenge with the same medication or an alternative SSRI frequently results in recurrence of hyponatremia (Jacob and Spinler 2006; Palmer et al. 2003).

Serotonin Syndrome

Serotonin syndrome, potentially the most adverse event associated with antidepressants, can occur with all four classes of antidepressants. It is caused by abnormally increased stimulation of 5-HT_{2A} and 5-HT_{1A} receptors in combination with elevated norepinephrine levels. Increased serotonergic and noradrenergic activity levels produce a syndrome of symptoms that begins with

TABLE 9–1. Treatment strategies for management of antidepressant-induced sexual dysfunction

Sexual side effect severity	Treatment strategies
Mild	1. Wait and monitor for symptoms to improve over time. 2. Decrease the dosage of the antidepressant medication. 3. Schedule sexual activity with dosing of antidepressant medication. • Target sexual activity when serum drug levels are lowest (between 1 hour before and 1 hour after daily administered medication). 4. Augment with another medication: • Bupropion • Buspirone • Amantadine
Severe	Switch to an alternative antidepressant medication with lower sexual side-effect profile: • Bupropion • Mirtazapine

Source. Data from Rothschild 2000.

milder symptoms, such as tachycardia, diaphoresis, mydriasis, and intermittent tremor. Without immediate treatment, symptoms can progress to hypertension, hyperthermia, tachycardia, and increased clonus and hyperreflexia. In severe cases, symptoms can progress to malignant hypertension, delirium, and potentially shock (Boyer and Shannon 2006).

Careful consideration is needed when prescribing antidepressants, because serotonin syndrome can develop after the first dose of an SSRI (Boyer and Shannon 2006). When a monoamine oxidase inhibitor (MAOI) is being prescribed, as frequently occurs in cases of treatment-refractory depression, serotonergic agents such as SSRIs, SNRIs, TCAs, and meperidine must be avoided. Before an MAOI can be initiated, the serotonergic agent must be adequately washed out. The practitioner also needs to consider the medication half-life when cross-tapering. For example, fluoxetine has the greatest half-life of the SSRIs, and its metabolite norfluoxetine remains active long after discontinuation of the medication. Therefore, the practitioner must consider the long half-life of fluoxetine when cross-tapering with other serotonergic agents to help prevent the patient from developing serotonin syndrome (Table 9–2) (Boyer and Shannon 2006).

Medically ill patients often take medications that carry a risk of serotonin syndrome. Linezolid, an antibiotic often prescribed for antibiotic-resistant bacterial infections, is structurally similar to toloxatone, an MAO-A inhibitor. As with MAOIs, linezolid taken in combination with SSRIs, SNRIs, or TCAs increases the risk of developing serotonin syndrome (Vinh and Rubinstein 2009).

General Considerations

Cardiovascular Disease

Approximately 20% of individuals with recent acute myocardial infarction have depression. Untreated depression in patients with a recent myocardial infarction can be a risk factor for recurrent myocardial infarction or cardiac-related mortality, regardless of cardiac disease severity (Taylor et al. 2005).

In the SADHART (Sertraline Antidepressant Heart Attack Randomized Trial), 369 subjects with major depressive disorder (MDD) and cardiac issues (myocardial infarction or unstable angina) received sliding dosages of sertraline (25–200 mg/day) over 24 weeks. Study results showed no evidence of any cardiac sequelae; however, sertraline was only slightly better than placebo in treating depression. These SADHART findings suggest that sertraline has a benign side-effect profile and is safe for treatment of depression in individuals with ischemic heart disease (Joynt and O'Connor 2005; Taylor et al. 2005). Furthermore, sertraline and other SSRIs may be cardioprotective, because SSRI-mediated serotonergic activity may have a positive anti-inflammatory effect on platelet function (Joynt and O'Connor 2005).

In recent years, general population trends show increased prescribing of SSRIs over TCAs in cardiac patients. This trend reflects a level of discretion by practitioners prescribing TCAs in cardiac patients, because TCAs can have a Type 1A antiarrythmic effect. Evidence varies regarding the cardiac effects of TCAs, with some studies suggesting that TCAs can lead to death in individuals with underlying ischemic heart disease (Benazon et al. 2005). Careful consideration is necessary when prescribing antidepressants to individuals with a history of cardiac arrythmias and ischemic heart disease, and antidepressant efficacy must be weighed against cardiac side-effect profiles. Of the antidepressants, the SSRIs, bupropion, and mirtazapine have the safest cardiac profiles. TCAs have the highest risk of adverse cardiac effects and therefore should be avoided in patients with a known history of ischemic heart disease or arrythmias (Summers et al. 2010).

TABLE 9–2. Signs and symptoms of serotonin syndrome

Syndrome severity	Common symptoms
Mild	Tachycardia, diaphoresis, mydriasis, intermittent tremor
Moderate	Hypertension, hyperthermia, tachycardia, increased clonus, hyperreflexia
Severe	Malignant hypertension, delirium, shock

Source. Data from Boyer and Shannon 2006.

Pulmonary Disease

Respiratory illness is often associated with psychiatric conditions, most commonly anxiety disorders. Panic disorder, generalized anxiety disorder, and specific phobia have been associated with asthma (Roy-Byrne et al. 2008). The prevalence rates of MDD are as high as 47% in asthma patients, compared with 20% in the general population. Untreated depression in individuals with asthma may lead to poor compliance with asthma treatment, which can then lead to increased risk of mortality secondary to asthma-related complications. This suggests that treatment of depression in asthma patients can improve treatment compliance and have a positive impact on both mental health and pulmonary disease (Brown et al. 2005).

Antidepressants have also been shown to have therapeutic effects on respiratory capacity and asthma symptoms via anti-inflammatory effects. In a study of panic disorder and lung function, subjects with panic disorder received a trial of an SSRI, followed by a washout period. During the SSRI treatment period, subjects had significantly higher forced expiratory lung volume and forced expiratory flow, suggesting that they had greater respiratory function with SSRI treatment (Nascimento et al. 2005). Fluoxetine and desipramine were shown to have anti-inflammatory effects in animal model studies, in which the medications prevented development of severe allergic asthma and septic shock by reducing tumor necrosis factor alpha production (Roumestan et al. 2007).

In a randomized controlled trial of 90 subjects with asthma receiving citalopram or placebo, citalopram treatment resulted in greater remission of depression. Furthermore, improvement in depressive symptoms was also shown to reduce asthma symptom severity (Brown et al. 2005). In a smaller pilot follow-up study, subjects who had not achieved remission of depression with citalopram were treated with bupropion. Bupropion was efficacious in treating anxiety and depression in asthma patients without exacerbating asthma symptoms (Brown et al. 2007). Animal model and clinical studies suggest that

SSRIs and TCAs are effective in treating depression in patients with comorbid asthma and have beneficial anti-inflammatory and respiratory effects and tolerable side-effect profiles. SSRIs and TCAs are often considered a first-line treatment option in individuals with anxiety and/or depression in addition to respiratory complications secondary to pulmonary disease (Levenson 2005).

Gastrointestinal Disease

Functional Gastrointestinal Disorders

Irritable bowel syndrome (IBS) is a very common functional gastrointestinal disorder that occurs in up to 20% of the North American population. The syndrome is characterized by altered bowel habits, associated with chronic, recurrent abdominal pain. Therapeutic modalities used for treatment include behavioral strategies, such as diet, psychotherapy, and stress reduction. In moderate to severe cases, antidepressants such as SSRIs and TCAs are often chosen. The serotonergic effects can modulate pain perception via the central nervous system and improve bowel transit and comorbid psychological distress associated with the syndrome (Rahimi et al. 2009).

Conflicting evidence exists regarding the efficacy of antidepressants in the treatment of functional gastrointestinal disorders. Clinical research has focused primarily on the effects of antidepressants on pain associated with gastrointestinal symptoms and overall quality of life and coping with such disorders. Studies have shown that treatment with SSRIs can slightly improve functional bowel pain and overall quality of life in patients with IBS. Studies have not found a significant improvement in other IBS-associated symptoms (Olden 2005). TCA treatment has been shown to significantly improve IBS-associated pain and symptoms and is therefore more commonly prescribed than other antidepressants in patients with IBS. Discretion must be used when prescribing TCAs, because anticholinergic side effects such as constipation may worsen IBS symptoms. Selective TCA prescribing, based on a patient's IBS symptoms and the TCA's side-effect profile, may decrease side-effect burden. For example, if a patient experiences chronic, recurrent diarrhea, tertiary amines such as imipramine or amitriptyline may be used, because they may slow bowel activity via anticholinergic effects. Based on the same methodology, secondary amines such as doxepin or desipramine may be prescribed in IBS patients with recurrent constipation, to avoid more anticholinergic side effects (Rahimi et al. 2009).

Hepatic Insufficiency

Individuals with a history of hepatic insufficiency or severe liver disease commonly develop shifts in fluid volume and disruptions in protein binding, leading to disrupted metabolism and excretion of medications. Medications with a lower risk of drug interactions and active metabolites should be used, given that patients with hepatic insufficiency are more vulnerable to drug interactions. Because they have a lower risk of drug interactions, SSRIs are the first-line treatment option for depression and anxiety in patients with hepatic insufficiency. Citalopram, escitalopram, and sertraline are most commonly recommended. Because of interactions with cytochrome P450 (CYP) isoenzymes, paroxetine and fluoxetine should be avoided in combination with other medications in individuals with hepatic insufficiency. When prescribing antidepressants, smaller loading and maintenance dosages of antidepressants should be prescribed, and patients should be monitored for clinical signs and symptoms of hepatotoxicity (Crone and Gabriel 2004).

Antidepressant-Induced Hepatotoxicity

Although drug-induced hepatotoxicity is rare, it can lead to fulminant liver failure and potentially death. Certain antidepressants can cause hepatotoxicity, even in healthy individuals with normal hepatic function. Acting as haptens on proteins, antidepressants may trigger an immune response on the hepatocyte cell membrane, which subsequently initiates immune-mediated cell death. For example, nefazodone has the most serious documented cases of hepatotoxicity and has a U.S. Food and Drug Administration (FDA) black box warning regarding risk of hepatic failure that can potentially lead to liver transplant or death (Desanty and Amabile 2007).

SSRIs are generally safe in individuals with hepatic insufficiency and have been shown to have no greater risk of hepatotoxicity than placebo. Several cases of paroxetine-induced hepatotoxicity have been reported, however. The SNRI duloxetine has been associated with mixed-type hepatic injury and hepatocellular injury. Individuals with a history of heavy alcohol consumption or chronic liver disease have an elevated risk of hepatotoxicity with duloxetine. Similarly, venlafaxine has been associated with elevated transaminase levels (>3 times the upper limit of normal). TCAs and MAOIs also have documented cases of drug-induced hepatotoxicity. In recent years, fewer cases have been reported, which may be due to decreased prescribing practices since the introduction of SSRIs (Desanty and Amabile 2007).

Antidepressants that carry the risk of hepatotoxicity should be avoided in patients with a known history of heavy alcohol use or liver disease. Routine laboratory testing of liver transaminases is not recommended, because this testing is unlikely to detect an acute hepatotoxic event. It is prudent, however, to educate patients on potential symptoms of hepatotoxicity, such as jaundice, anorexia, and gastrointestinal complaints, and to advise patients to immediately report such symptoms to their prescriber. Clinical discretion must be used when an antidepressant-induced hepatotoxic event is detected. The antidepressant should be discontinued when aspartate aminotransferase (AST) and alanine aminotransferase (ALT) levels are shown to be three times the upper limit of normal. When considering or planning discontinuation, the practitioner should weigh the risk of relapse and discontinuation syndrome against the risk of hepatotoxicity. Typically, a retrial of the antidepressant medication is not recommended (Desanty and Amabile 2007).

Renal Disease

Syndrome of Inappropriate Antidiuretic Hormone Secretion

The syndrome of inappropriate antidiuretic hormone secretion (SIADH) is a syndrome that causes hyponatremia. Hyponatremia is diagnosed by a serum Na^+ level <135 mmol/L and is classified into three subtypes: hypervolemic, isovolemic, and hypovolemic. SIADH is a hypovolemic hyponatremia and is marked by an abnormally elevated urine osmolality in comparison to serum osmolality. The most common causes of SIADH include malignant tumors, postoperative pain, protracted nausea, and pharmacological agents such as antidepressants. Symptoms of SIADH include generalized weakness, dizziness, nausea, lethargy, and headache. If SIADH is untreated, Na^+ levels can fall below 120 mmol/L, putting patients at severe risk of developing delirium, coma, and potentially death (Nirmalani et al. 2006).

SSRIs are the most common antidepressants associated with SIADH, with case reports having been published for each SSRI. Of the newer-generation SNRIs, venlafaxine has also been associated with SIADH in case reports. Development of SIADH with antidepressants most commonly occurs within the first 2–4 weeks of initiating the medication. SIADH may also develop later in the course of antidepressant treatment with dosage increases (Nirmalani et al. 2006).

Risk factors that increase the likelihood of SIADH with antidepressant treatment include older age, female gender, comorbid medical issues such as hypertension, and the use of antihypertensive agents and diuretics. Patients with comorbid medical issues such as hypertension may develop renal impairment with potential for fluid imbalances, thus exponentially increasing the risk of SIADH with concomitant antidepressant treatment. In addition, SSRIs such as fluoxetine, fluvoxamine, and paroxetine have inhibitory effects on CYP isoenzymes and should be avoided in such patients because of the potential of increasing serum diuretic levels and the risk of SIADH (Table 9–3) (Romero et al. 2007).

TABLE 9–3. Risk factors for syndrome of inappropriate antidiuretic hormone secretion (SIADH)

PATIENT RISK FACTORS	MEDICATIONS ASSOCIATED WITH SIADH
Older age	Antihypertensive agents
Female gender	Diuretics
Comorbid medical issues (hypertension)	SSRIs with inhibitory effects on cytochrome P450 isoenzymes • Fluoxetine • Fluvoxamine • Paroxetine

Source. Data from Romero et al. 2007.

Renal Insufficiency

Mental illness commonly occurs in individuals with renal disorders, with prevalence rates of mental illness in dialysis patients ranging from 20% to 83% (Baghdady et al. 2009). In patients with end-stage renal disease (ESRD), subsyndromal depression likely occurs in 25% and major depression in 5%–22%. Prevalence rates of comorbid renal disorders and psychiatric illness are likely to increase as the aging population expands. Practitioners need to understand the altered pharmacokinetics that occurs in renal disease patients and how this influences antidepressant prescribing practices (Cohen et al. 2004).

Absorption of medications can be impaired by excess gastric alkalinity in patients with ESRD. More severely ill renal patients may have lower volumes of distribution because of lower body mass and fluid volume. Patients with renal disease also have decreased protein binding. Such patients are at risk of having larger amounts of unbound, active drug metabolites circulating within the system, which increases the risk of side effects and toxicity. In addition to changes that occur in distribution volume and protein binding with worsening severity of renal disease, renal elimination and urinary excretion become significantly impaired (Cohen et al. 2004).

Given the changes in metabolism and excretion that occur in patients with ESRD, careful consideration must be taken when prescribing antidepressants. SSRIs are generally thought to be safe and effective in treating depression in such patients. Fluoxetine, sertraline, and citalopram are the most studied SSRIs in patients with ESRD. Despite the long half-life of fluoxetine, evidence suggests that changes in the serum levels of fluoxetine and its active metabolite norfluoxetine do not occur with impaired renal function. Sertraline has been shown to help prevent hemodialysis-related hypotension. Of the SSRIs, paroxetine raises the most concern, because levels can be elevated with renal impairment; therefore, an alternative SSRI should be considered. If using paroxetine in patients with renal impairment, a low starting dosage and conservative titration are recommended (Cohen et al. 2004).

The SNRI venlafaxine is excreted primarily in the urine, and therefore elimination is decreased in individuals with renal insufficiency and ESRD. Conservative loading and maintenance dosages should be used while the patient is monitored for the side effect of hypertension. Similarly, bupropion is excreted primarily through the urine; as a result, individuals receiving dialysis may have elevated levels of metabolites and a lower seizure threshold (Cohen et al. 2004).

TCAs are often prescribed to patients with ESRD, and dosage adjustments are not recommended. Patients should, however, be monitored for signs and symptoms of toxicity, because drug level tests may not detect toxicity if metabolism is affected. MAOIs are often avoided in patients with ESRD, due to a high risk of adverse events. In particular, patients receiving hemodialysis while taking MAOIs are at increased risk for hemodialysis-related hypotension. Treatment with MAOIs should be reserved for ESRD patients with treatment-resistant depression (Table 9–4) (Baghdady et al. 2009).

Endocrine Disease

Diabetes Mellitus

Diabetes mellitus patients have a 50%–100% increased risk of developing depression in comparison to the general population. Untreated depression in patients with diabetes has been associated with greater diabetic complications, increased health care costs, and increased mortality (Rubin et al. 2008). Conflicting evidence exists regarding the relationship between diabetes and comorbid depression . It is unclear whether depression affects the development of the diabetes and whether treatment of depression improves overall medical outcomes in patients with diabetes (Eaton 2002).

Patients with diabetes are frequently prescribed antidepressant medications because of the high comorbidity of depression and diabetes. Antidepressants are also often used for treatment of diabetic complications. For example, TCAs and duloxetine are prescribed for diabetic neuropathic pain. Despite the common use of antidepressants among diabetic patients, little is known about the direct effects of antidepressants on the development and progression of diabetes. In a multicenter study, 3,187 subjects at high risk of developing type 2 diabetes were followed to determine whether antidepressant exposure or depression itself accelerated development of diabetes (Rubin et al. 2008). The results indicated that antidepressant exposure increased the risk of developing type 2 diabetes. However, the study was limited because it did not include specific antidepressant classes and did not control for confounding variables such

TABLE 9–4. Management of antidepressant medications in patients with end-stage renal disease

Antidepressant class	Drug effects in ESRD	Treatment recommendations
SSRIs	Generally safe Special considerations: • *Paroxetine:* potential for elevated levels with renal impairment • *Sertraline:* shown to prevent hemodialysis-related hypotension	1. Consider these generally safe to prescribe. 2. Start at low dose and titrate conservatively.
Second-generation antidepressants	• *Venlafaxine:* decreased elimination in renal insufficiency and ESRD • *Bupropion:* potential for elevated levels of metabolites and lowered seizure threshold	1. Prescribe conservative loading and maintenance doses. 2. Monitor for side effect of hypertension with venlafaxine.
TCAs	Generally safe	Monitor for signs of toxicity.
MAOIs	High risk of hemodialysis-related hypotension	Reserve for ESRD patients with treatment-resistant depression.

Note. ESRD=end-stage renal disease; MAOI=monoamine oxidase inhibitor; SNRI=serotonin-norepinephrine reuptake inhibitor; SSRI=selective serotonin reuptake inhibitor; TCA=tricyclic antidepressant.
Source. Data from Cohen et al. 2004.

as depression. Despite limited research on direct effects of antidepressants on diabetes risk, side-effect profiles of antidepressants that may indirectly increase risk of diabetes should be considered. TCAs may indirectly cause diabetes through such side effects as weight gain and TCA-associated hyperglycemia. Such side effects should be considered before prescribing TCAs in patients with restricted physical activity, weight gain, and poor glycemic control. Alternatively, SSRIs have been shown to have an opposite effect, with previous studies suggesting that they may lower weight and improve insulin sensitivity in patients with type 2 diabetes (Rubin et al. 2008).

Thyroid

Major depression is commonly associated with thyroid disease. Forty percent of patients with hypothyroidism have depression, and 12%–50% of patients with depression have hypothyroidism (Carvalho et al. 2007). Triiodothyronine (T_3) augmentation (25–50 μg/day) is used for treatment-refractory depression (TRD), based on clinical observations that hypothyroidism often leads to depressed mood. Although T_3 is frequently used in clinical practice, studies are inconclusive and have not found evidence of a significant response to T_3 augmentation. The majority of studies investigated patients with TRD who had previously been treated with a TCA. In these studies, T_3 augmentation was shown to enhance response to TCAs in patients who were known to have a partial response to the medication. In the Sequenced Treatment Alternatives to Relieve Depression (STAR*D) study, T_3 augmentation was shown to have only modest benefit for treatment of TRD, and the effect was not significantly different from that with lithium augmentation (Nirenberg et al. 2006). Unlike T_3 augmentation, thyroxine (T_4) augmentation has not been shown to have an effect on depression (Carvalho et al. 2009).

Although important implications may exist for the treatment of depressed patients with comorbid thyroid disease, there is a dearth of information about how antidepressants such as SSRIs and TCAs interact with the hypothalamic-pituitary-thyroid axis and the central serotonergic system. TCA treatment may lead to a decrease in T_4 and free thyroxine (FT_4) but no changes in thyroid-stimulating hormone. With these changes, thyroid function remains in a euthyroid state. A study by Carvalho and colleagues sought to determine effects of SSRIs on T_3 function (Carvalho et al. 2009). However, research is currently in the early phases, and larger studies are needed to further explicate such neuroendocrine effects.

Cancer

Oncology patients often experience increased psychological distress, predisposing them to common psychiatric conditions such as mood and anxiety disorders. Prevalence rates range from 25% to 48% for posttraumatic stress disorder (PTSD) and from 5% to 42% for MDD among oncology patients. Antidepressant medication must be carefully considered, because cancer patients receiving combined antidepressant and anticancer drug therapy are at increased risk for drug interactions (Table 9–5) (Yap et al. 2011).

Several anticancer drug classes have been shown to have serious drug interactions with antidepressant medications. Selective estrogen receptor modulators, such as tamoxifen, have been shown to have significant interactions with SSRIs. Both fluoxetine and paroxetine have been shown to have strong inhibitory effects on CYP2D6 metabolism. When prescribed with fluoxetine or paroxetine, tamoxifen has significantly reduced metabolism through CYP2D6 to endoxifen, tamoxifen's more active metabolite. As a result, the combination of an SSRI and tamoxifen decreases efficacy of tamoxifen in the treatment of breast cancer, increases risk of relapse, and can potentially increase mortality (Henry et al. 2008). Other SSRIs and SNRIs, such as citalopram, escitalopram, fluvoxamine, venlafaxine, duloxetine, and mirtazapine, may also have mild to moderate inhibitory effects. The risks and benefits of antidepressant treatment should be weighed before antidepressants are prescribed in breast cancer patients receiving tamoxifen (Desmarais and Looper 2009).

TCAs prescribed in combination with tamoxifen may result in additive arrhythmogenic effects, increasing risk of QTc prolongation and torsades de pointes. Other classes of anticancer drugs that have a risk of drug interactions with antidepressants include topoisomerase inhibitors, tyrosine kinase inhibitors, and alkylating agents. Topoisomerase inhibitors such as irinotecan have been shown to decrease metabolism of SSRIs such as citalopram through the inhibition of CYP3A4 isoenzymes. The combination of irinotecan and citalopram has been associated with an increased risk of rhabdomyolysis due to elevated serum levels of citalopram. Therefore, patients receiving combination therapy with such medications should be closely monitored for the development of myopathy by clinical observation and monitoring of creatine phosphokinase levels (Yap et al. 2011).

Tyrosine kinase inhibitors such as imatinib may also reduce metabolism of certain SSRIs and TCAs through competitive inhibition of the CYP 3A4/5, 2C9, and 2D6 isoenzymes. The alkylating agent procarbazine may act as a mild MAO inhibitor, which can lead to serotonin syndrome if concomitantly prescribed with a TCA, SSRI, or SNRI. Consequently, recommendations for prescribing procarbazine are the same as for the MAOIs. Due to the risk of drug interactions, antidepressant treatment should be coordinated with the oncology treatment team. Patients should also be monitored closely for symptoms of drug toxicity (Yap et al. 2011).

Neurological Illness

Epilepsy

Epilepsy is a neurological disorder characterized by a chronic predisposition to developing seizures in conjunction with various co-occurring cognitive, psychological, neurobiological, and social effects as a result of the condition. Conflicting evidence exists regarding the effects of antidepressants on seizure activity (Jobe 2004). Previous research reveals an increased risk of seizures in patients taking TCAs, SSRIs, SNRIs, and MAOIs in therapeutic dosages and in overdose (Jobe and O'Connor 2005). Epidemiological studies have also shown that individuals taking antidepressants have a greater likelihood of developing seizures. A more recent suggestion is that the increased risk of seizures in patients taking antidepressants is due to preexisting noradrenergic and serotonergic deficits in such patients who require antidepressant therapy, and not due to the antidepressant itself. Alternatively, antidepressants may have anticonvulsant effects through serotonergic and noradrenergic activation (Jobe and Browning 2005).

TCAs and SSRIs may have antiepileptic treatment properties. Although studies supporting the efficacy of antidepressants in treating epilepsy are minimal, findings suggest that antidepressants may be protective against seizures. An exception is bupropion, an antidepressant known to reduce seizure threshold. Bupropion must therefore be avoided in patients with a known history of seizures or with a history of heavy alcohol use (Jobe and Browning 2005).

Multiple Sclerosis

Depression is more common in multiple sclerosis (MS) than in other chronic neurological conditions, with a 12-month prevalence of 15.7%. The lifetime risk of MDD in MS is 27%–54%. Evidence suggests that MDD has a negative impact on MS, resulting in elevated rates of subjective cognitive difficulties, poor performance on objective neuropsychological measures, lower quality of life, decreased functional status, disruption on social supports and family systems, and decreased adherence to treatment. It is therefore imperative that depression be diagnosed and treated adequately in persons with MS (Chwastiak and Ehde 2007).

Although antidepressant prescribing for patients with MS is similar to prescribing for the general population, there are some notable differences. Treatment of MDD in MS is complicated by MS treatments that cause psychiatric symptoms; these treatments include corticosteroids and interferon. Depressive symptoms can occur with initiation, long-term use, or discontinuation of corticosteroids. Antidepressants are often indicated for relief of psychiatric

TABLE 9–5. Drug-drug interactions: anticancer agents and antidepressants

Anticancer drug class	Potential drug interactions
Selective estrogen receptor modulators	
Tamoxifen	*SSRIs and SNRIs* Paroxetine and fluoxetine have severe inhibitory effects on tamoxifen. Citalopram, escitalopram, fluvoxamine, venlafaxine, duloxetine, and mirtazapine have mild to moderate inhibitory effects on tamoxifen. *TCAs* Combination of tamoxifen and TCAs leads to risk of arrythmogenic effects, QTc prolongation, and torsades de pointes.
Topoisomerase inhibitors	
Irinotecan	*SSRIs* Citalopram metabolism may be reduced via irinotecan inhibitory effects on CYP3A4. Elevated citalopram levels may lead to increased risk of rhabdomyolysis.
Tyrosine kinase inhibitors	
Imatinib	*SSRIs and TCAs* Imatinib may reduce metabolism of certain SSRIs and TCAs via inhibition of CYP 3A4/5, 2C9, and 2D6 isoenzymes.
Alkylating agents	
Procarbazine	*Procarbazine* may act as mild MAO inhibitor, and recommendation is to avoid prescribing TCAs, SSRIs, and SNRIs in combination with this agent.

Note. CYP=cytochrome P450; MAO=monoamine oxidase; SNRI=serotonin-norepinephrine reuptake inhibitor; SSRI=selective serotonin reuptake inhibitor; TCA=tricyclic antidepressant.
Source. Data from Desmais et al. 2009; Henry et al. 2008; Yap et al. 2011.

symptoms secondary to MS treatment, particularly if long-term treatment is indicated. Studies indicate that 90% of patients completely recover from depression once steroid treatment is discontinued; therefore, the indication for use of an antidepressant should be reevaluated upon discontinuation of steroid treatment (Sirois 2003). Given the clinical characteristics of MS, side effects of antidepressants may be particularly bothersome and lead to higher rates of nonadherence and premature treatment termination in clinical practice. Basing treatment options on side-effect profiles may decrease the side-effect burden (Chwastiak and Ehde 2007).

Traumatic Brain Injury

Traumatic brain injury (TBI) is a condition that can lead to serious cognitive, emotional, and behavioral consequences. In a minority of patients, such symptoms may persist for months to years after an injury (Silver et al. 2009). MDD may be the most common psychiatric disorder, occurring in 25% of patients with TBI. Research is limited on the efficacy of antidepressants in patients with TBI. Antidepressants may vary in efficacy and tolerability in patients with TBI due to postinjury alterations in neurochemistry. For example, because of alterations in brain chemistry, patients with TBI may be predisposed to develop increased seizure frequency when taking TCAs. Various studies have researched the effects of TCAs, MAOIs, SSRIs, and SNRIs in treating depression in patients with TBI. Because of small sample sizes and various limitations associated with studying TBI, no particular class of antidepressant has been shown to be superior in patients with TBI and comorbid depression. Considering that a significant proportion of patients with TBI have depression and that antidepressants are commonly prescribed, further research is required on the efficacy and side-effect profile of antidepressants in such patients (Fann et al. 2009).

Delirium

Delirium is an acute medical disorder, characterized by impairment of attention and global cognitive functioning. When prescribing antidepressants, the practitioner should consider the relationship between delirium and MDD. First, it is difficult to diagnose MDD in the context of delirium because symptoms overlap, particularly in patients with hypoactive delirium. Initiation of antidepressant treatment must be approached cautiously in such cases, and often should be avoided (Leonard et al. 2009). Second, patients with a history of delirium are at increased risk of developing anxiety and depressive symptoms up to 2 years following the episode of delirium (Davydow et al. 2008). Lastly, depression is identified as an established risk factor for delirium and may increase morbidity and mortality in elderly patients who develop delirium (Givens et al. 2009). Consequently, the role of antidepressants must be carefully considered when prescribed to patients with or at risk for delirium. At-risk patients include those with comorbid medical illnesses or dementia, older patients, and those receiving multiple medications consistent with polypharmacy (Cancelli et al. 2009).

Several antidepressants have been associated with an increased risk of developing delirium. For example, antidepressants with anticholinergic side effects, such as TCAs, may lead to delirium in patients at risk for delirium. Although the underlying mechanism is unknown, it is proposed to be an imbalance in neurotransmission of various neurotransmitters, including serotonin, noradrenaline, dopamine, γ-aminobutyric acid (GABA), and cholinergic activity (Cancelli et al. 2009). Electrolyte abnormalities caused by antidepressants have also been suggested to cause delirium in patients taking antidepressants. SSRIs, venlafaxine, and mirtazapine at therapeutic dosages have been noted to cause delirium by inducing hyponatremia (Cancelli et al. 2009; Thomas and Oster 2009).

Migraines

Migraines are commonly associated with comorbid psychiatric conditions, including MDD, bipolar disorder, and anxiety disorders. A migraine is characterized by the classic symptom of moderate to severe headache, lasting 4–72 hours. Additional symptoms may include photophobia, phonophobia, osmophobia, nausea, and vomiting. Approximately 15% of patients who have migraines may experience symptoms of aura, which may affect vision, sensation, and language (Silverstein 2009).

Pharmacological treatment of migraines includes both acute and prophylactic approaches and often a combination of both. Antidepressants can be used as preventive therapy to reduce the frequency, severity, and duration of migraine episodes. TCAs are the most common antidepressant class used for prophylactic treatment of migraines. They have been shown to be an effective treatment, with evidence of direct analgesic effect, not secondary to antidepressant effect as suggested in previous studies. The mechanism of analgesic effect is unknown. Both tertiary and secondary amines have been recommended. Of the tertiary amines, both amitriptyline and doxepin can be used. The recommended dosage range is 10–300 mg/day, with 10 mg at bedtime as the starting dose. The secondary amines nortriptyline and protriptyline have also been shown to be effective for treatment of migraines. Treatment options may be made based on side-effect profiles. SSRIs have also been used for prophylactic treatment of migraines, although limited evidence supports treatment efficacy. Most commonly, SSRIs have been limited to treatment of individuals sensitive to TCA side-effect profiles or in combination treatment of TRD (Silverstein 2009).

Chronic Pain

Research has shown an association between chronic pain disorders and depression. Ninety-two percent of depressed patients experience clinical pain symptoms. Eighty percent of depressed patients presenting to a primary care practice present initially with a chief complaint of physical pain symptoms (Bär et al. 2005). As in the treatment of migraines, TCAs are the most commonly prescribed antidepressant class for treatment of chronic pain syndromes. Amitriptyline is often prescribed for pain syndromes such as neuropathic pain. Recommended dosages range from 25 to 100 mg/day of amitriptyline or an equivalent dosage of an alternative TCA. Therapeutic dosages for treatment of pain are often lower than recommended dosages for depression. Although the use of TCAs for chronic pain is well established, TCAs have a side-effect profile that must be considered (Kroenke et al. 2009).

Newer antidepressant agents such as duloxetine and venlafaxine have been more recently studied as treatment options for chronic pain. Duloxetine has been shown to have significant analgesic effect in comparison to placebo for treatment of diabetic pain neuropathy in several randomized controlled trials. Although previous theories suggested that antidepressants treat pain through antidepressant effects, duloxetine may have a direct analgesic effect. Duloxetine has FDA approval for treatment of both fibromyalgia and neuropathic pain. Venlafaxine may also be used for pain treatment but currently does not have FDA approval (Kroenke et al. 2009). Venlafaxine, like TCAs, has been shown to have moderate efficacy for treatment of neuropathic pain, with a number needed to treat of 3, suggesting that it has significant analgesic properties and that for every three patients prescribed the medication, at least one patient will have significant analgesic effect (Saarto and Wiffen 2007).

Human Immunodeficiency Virus

According to the National HIV Cost and Services Utilization Study, approximately 48% of individuals with HIV experience psychiatric illness. Untreated psychiatric illness such as MDD in HIV-infected individuals can lead to poor adherence with medications and medical care, resulting in worsening disease progression (Repetto and Petitto 2008). Research has shown that treating depression in HIV-infected individuals can improve antiretroviral therapy adherence and potentially reduce morbidity (Dalessandro et al. 2007).

Various antidepressant classes, including TCAs, SSRIs, and newer-generation antidepressants such as duloxetine, mirtazapine, and bupropion, have been studied in HIV-infected individuals. SSRIs are commonly prescribed for treatment of MDD and anxiety in individuals with HIV. Studies have shown SSRIs to be as effective as TCAs in treating depression, with the benefit of having a more tolerable side-effect profile. Fluoxetine, paroxetine, sertraline, and citalopram have been shown to be effective in treating depression and potentially reducing somatic symptoms, without proven effects on CD4 cell counts (Repetto and Petitto 2008).

SSRIs have the potential for drug interactions with certain highly active antiretroviral therapy medications. Consequently, careful consideration is necessary when prescribing SSRIs to individuals receiving antiretrovirals such as ritonavir, efavirenz, or saquinavir. Both protease inhibitors and non-nucleoside reverse transcriptase inhibitors can interact with the CYP isoenzyme system, affecting metabolism of SSRIs and increasing the risk of serotonin syndrome. Similarly, SSRIs such as fluoxetine can interact with the CYP2D6 isoenzyme, potentially increasing ritonavir levels. Acknowledging the potential risk of drug interactions is important when prescribing SSRIs in HIV-infected individuals. When prescribing SSRIs in combination with antiretrovirals, the practitioner should start with low loading doses and titrate slowly and conservatively while monitoring for any clinical signs of serotonin toxicity (Repetto and Petitto 2008).

TCAs have also been shown to be effective in treating major depression in HIV-infected individuals. Although imipramine was found to be superior to placebo in treatment efficacy for MDD, without having an effect on CD4 cell counts, high discontinuation rates occurred because of the side-effect profile. TCAs such as imipramine can be prescribed for treatment of depression in HIV-infected individuals, but in view of the side-effect profile, they are best reserved for treatment-refractory cases (Repetto and Petitto 2008).

More recently, newer-generation antidepressants, including the SNRIs venlafaxine and duloxetine, have been studied in HIV-infected patients. In addition to having proven efficacy for treating depression, both medications may also be effective in treating HIV-associated pain syndromes. When prescribing duloxetine in individuals with HIV, one should closely monitor for signs and symptoms of hepatotoxicity. Other newer-generation antidepressants, including bupropion, nefazodone, and mirtazapine, have also been studied. Mirtazapine has been shown to be effective in treating depression and, like the SNRIs, may have additional therapeutic benefits, including treating HIV-associated nausea and weight loss (Repetto and Petitto 2008).

Steroid-Induced Psychiatric Symptoms

Synthetic glucocorticosteroids have been shown to produce psychiatric symptoms consistent with various psychiatric conditions, including psychotic disorders, manic or depressive episodes, and delirium. Prevalence rates of psychiatric symptoms with steroid treatment vary widely, between 1.3% and 62%. In the most severe cases, steroid-induced psychiatric conditions can lead to suicide. Mania is the most common psychiatric condition induced by steroids, but risk of depression substantially increases with long-term steroid treatment (Fietta et al. 2009).

Steroid-induced psychiatric symptoms commonly occur within the first weeks of treatment but may occur at any time during the course of treatment, including during the period of steroid withdrawal. Research has shown an increased risk of psychiatric symptoms at prednisone dosages ≥20 mg/day, with greatest risk occurring at dosages ≥40 mg/day. Treatment of steroid-induced psychiatric symptoms typically involves reduction and discontinuation of the steroid medication, with resolution of psychiatric symptoms occurring within approximately 2 weeks. However, adjunctive psychopharmacological management may be indicated if psychiatric symptoms are severe. Antidepressants including SSRIs and the SNRI venlafaxine have been shown to be effective in treating steroid-induced psychiatric symptoms. Alternatively, study results of TCAs have been equivocal (Fietta et al. 2009).

Burns and Hospital-Based Trauma

Prevalence rates of PTSD are approximately 22% in patients hospitalized in the intensive care unit (ICU). Patients may develop symptoms of PTSD as a result of traumatic experiences with critical care procedures such as endotracheal intubation and physical restraints. Predictors of post-ICU PTSD include prior psychiatric illness, ICU administration of benzodiazepines, and memories consistent with delirium or an associated psychotic episode (Davydow et al. 2008). PTSD frequently occurs in acute hospital care settings, particularly the ICU, where there are several risk factors for PTSD. Risk factors include increased use of centrally acting medications that alter sensorium, such as benzodiazepines, opiates, and corticosteroids; multiple critical care procedures; and delirium (Davydow et al. 2008).

Little information is available regarding selection of antidepressant medications for treatment of PTSD in the hospital setting. However, both SSRIs and SNRIs are first-line treatments for PTSD in the general population. Of the SSRIs, both sertraline and paroxetine have received FDA approval for this indication. Randomized, double-blind, placebo-controlled studies have demonstrated efficacy of fluoxetine, paroxetine, and sertraline in treating PTSD. Studies have shown that these SSRIs can improve quality of life and functional impairment but may have limited efficacy in treating sleep disturbances and nightmares. The newer-generation antidepressant mirtazapine has also been shown to be superior to placebo in treating PTSD, and it may have additional benefits in treating sleep disturbances. Based on the research, after 12 weeks of treatment with an SSRI, 20%–40% of patients may fail to respond, and approximately 30% of patients will achieve remission. Thus, in patients diagnosed with PTSD, long-term therapy with an SSRI or SNRI medication is recommended to increase remission rates and prevent relapse (Davidson 2006). Further research is needed to explicate the implications of prescribing such antidepressants to critical care patients who are at risk of developing acute stress disorder and PTSD.

Conclusion

With increased efforts to improve screening and diagnosis of depression in medically ill patients, a growing number of psychiatrists and general practitioners will be treating depression in this patient population with unique needs and often complicated medical issues. In response, practitioners must strengthen their knowledge about prescribing antidepressant medications in this special population. Prescribing in this population can be met with serious challenges, because medically ill patients are more likely to have alterations in pharmacokinetics, which increase the potential for drug toxicity. The practitioner will often encounter iatrogenic challenges in addition to the physiological challenges of prescribing. Often, medically ill patients are taking multiple medications, a situation that raises the potential for dangerous drug-drug interactions and adverse events such as serotonin syndrome or SIADH. Furthermore, such patients have an increased likelihood of being hospitalized in critical care settings and of undergoing hospital procedures, either of which can lead to other psychiatric issues such as delirium, further complicating treatment. An evidence-based approach to prescribing antidepressants in medically ill patients can be achieved by understanding the pharmacokinetic alterations, potential for adverse events and drug-drug interactions, and special needs of patients with specific medical conditions, as reviewed in this chapter.

KEY CLINICAL CONCEPTS

- Initiation of antidepressant medication must be done cautiously in medically ill patients, with consideration of drug-drug interactions and alterations in drug metabolism and availability.
- Medically ill patients have a greater risk of developing adverse effects and toxicity from antidepressant medications.
- Polypharmacy is common among medically ill patients and can increase the risk of drug-drug interactions, as well as adverse effects such as hyponatremia and serotonin syndrome.
- SADHART and other studies suggest that SSRIs are safe and may be cardioprotective in patients with a history of ischemic heart disease.
- Antidepressants have been shown to be beneficial in patients with pulmonary disease and to have positive effects on respiratory capacity and asthma symptoms.

- SSRIs are the first-line treatment option for anxiety and depression in patients with hepatic insufficiency.
- As diabetes mellitus increases, prescribers should carefully consider the metabolic profiles of antidepressants that may indirectly increase risk of diagnoses or worsen illness.
- Serious drug interactions can occur in cancer patients receiving antidepressants and anticancer medications. Selective estrogen receptor modulators such as tamoxifen may have reduced efficacy when prescribed in combination with SSRIs such as fluoxetine and paroxetine.
- Both FDA- and non–FDA-approved antidepressants, such as TCAs, duloxetine, and venlafaxine, have been shown to be effective in treating various forms of chronic pain.
- Acknowledging the potential risk of drug interactions is important when prescribing SSRIs in HIV-infected individuals. When prescribing SSRIs in combination with antiretrovirals, the practitioner needs to prescribe cautiously, monitoring for any clinical signs of serotonin toxicity.

References

Baghdady NT, Banik S, Swartz SA, et al: Psychotropic drugs and renal failure: translating the evidence for clinical practice. Adv Ther 26:404–424, 2009

Bär KJ, Brehm S, Boettger MK, et al: Pain perception in major depression depends on pain modality. Pain 117:97–103, 2005

Benazon NR, Mamdani MM, Coyne JC: Trends in prescribing antidepressants following myocardial infarction, 1993–2002. Psychosom Med 67:916–920, 2005

Boyer EW, Shannon M: The serotonin syndrome. N Engl J Med 352:1112–1120, 2006

Brown ES, Vigil L, Khan DA, et al: A randomized trial of citalopram versus placebo in outpatients with asthma and major depressive disorder: a proof of concept study. Biol Psychiatry 58:865–870, 2005

Brown ES, Vornik LA, Khan DA, et al: Bupropion in the treatment of outpatients with asthma and major depressive disorder. Int J Psychiatry Med 37:23–28, 2007

Cancelli I, Beltrame M, Gigli GL, et al: Drugs with anticholinergic properties: cognitive neuropsychiatric side-effects in elderly patients. Neurol Sci 30:87–92, 2009

Carvalho AF, Cavalcante JL, Castelo MS, et al: Augmentation strategies for treatment-resistant depression: a literature review. J Clin Pharm Ther 32:415–428, 2007

Carvalho AG, Bahls SC, Boeving A, et al: Effects of selective serotonin reuptake inhibitors on thyroid function in depressed patients with primary hypothyroidism or normal thyroid function. Thyroid 19:691–697, 2009

Chwastiak LA, Ehde DM: Psychiatric issues in multiple sclerosis. Psychiatr Clin North Am 30:803–817, 2007

Clayton A, Keller A, McGarvey EL: Burden of phase-specific sexual dysfunction with SSRIs. J Affect Disord 91:27–32, 2006

Cohen LM, Tessier EG, Germain MJ, et al: Update on psychotropic medication use in renal disease. Psychosomatics 45:34–48, 2004

Crone CC, Gabriel GM: Treatment of anxiety and depression in transplant patients. Clin Pharmacokinet 43:361–394, 2004

Dalessandro M, Conti CM, Gambi F, et al: Antidepressant therapy can improve adherence to antiretroviral regimens among HIV-infected and depressed patients. J Clin Psychopharmacol 27:58–61, 2007

Davidson JT: Pharmacologic treatment of acute and chronic stress following trauma: 2006. J Clin Psychiatry 67 (suppl 2):34–39, 2006

Davydow DS, Gifford JM, Desai SV, et al: Posttraumatic stress disorder in general intensive care unit survivors: a systematic review. Gen Hosp Psychiatry 30:421–434, 2008

Delgado PL, Brannan SK, Mallinckrodt CH, et al: Sexual functioning assessed in 4 double-blind placebo- and paroxetine-controlled trials of duloxetine for major depressive disorder. J Clin Psychiatry 66:686–696, 2005

Desanty KP, Amabile CM: Antidepressant-induced liver injury. Ann Pharmacother 41:1201–1211, 2007

Desmarais JE, Looper KJ: Interactions between tamoxifen and antidepressants via cytochrome P450 2D6. J Clin Psychiatry 70:1688–1697, 2009

Eaton WW: Epidemiologic evidence on the comorbidity of depression and diabetes. J Psychosom Res 53:903–906, 2002

Evans DL, Charney DS, Lewis L, et al: Mood disorders in the medically ill: scientific review and recommendations. Biol Psychiatry 58:175–189, 2005

Fann JR, Hart T, Schomer KG: Treatment of depression after traumatic brain injury: a systematic review. J Neurotrauma 26:2383–2402, 2009

Fietta P, Fietta P, Delsante G: Central nervous system effects of natural and synthetic glucocorticoids. Psychiatry Clin Neurosci 63:613–622, 2009

Givens JL, Jones RN, Inouye SK: The overlap of depression and delirium in older hospitalized patients. J Am Geriatr Soc 57:1347–1353, 2009

Henry NL, Stearns V, Flockhart DA, et al: Drug interactions and pharmacogenomics in the treatment of breast cancer and depression. Am J Psychiatry 165:1251–1255, 2008

Jacob S, Spinler SA: Hyponatremia associated with selective serotonin reuptake inhibitors in older adults. Ann Pharmacother 40:1618–1622, 2006

Jobe PC: Affective disorder and epilepsy comorbidity: implications for development of treatment and diagnostic procedures. Clin EEG Neurosci 35:53–68, 2004

Jobe PC, Browning RA: The serotonergic and noradrenergic effects of antidepressant drugs are anticonvulsant, not proconvulsant. Epilepsy Behav 7:602–619, 2005

Joynt KE, O'Connor CM: Lessons from SADHART, ENRICHD, and other trials. Psychosom Med 67 (suppl 1):S63–S66, 2005

Koliscak LP, Makela EH: Selective serotonin reuptake inhibitor–induced akathisia. J Am Pharm Assoc 49:E28–E38, 2009

Kroenke K, Krebs EE, Bair MJ: Pharmacotherapy of chronic pain: a synthesis of recommendations from systematic reviews. Gen Hosp Psychiatry 31:206–219, 2009

Leonard M, Spiller J, Keen J, et al: Symptoms of depression and delirium assessed serially in palliative-care inpatients. Psychosomatics 50:506–514, 2009

Levenson JL (ed): The American Psychiatric Publishing Textbook of Psychosomatic Medicine. Washington, DC, American Psychiatric Publishing, 2005

Nascimento I, Nardi AE, Valença AM, et al: Effect of antipanic drugs on pulmonary function in patients with panic disorder, in 2005 New Research Program and Abstracts, American Psychiatric Association 158th Annual Meeting, Atlanta, GA, May 21–26, 2005. Arlington, VA, American Psychiatric Association, 2005

Nirenberg AA, Fava M, Trivedi MH, et al: A comparison of lithium and T3 augmentation following two failed medication treatments for depression: a STAR*D report. Am J Psychiatry 163:1519–1530, 2006

Nirmalani A, Stock SL, Catalano GC: Syndrome of inappropriate antidiuretic hormone associated with escitalopram therapy. CNS Spectr 11:429–432, 2006

O'Connor EA, Whitlock EP, Bell TL, et al: Screening for depression in adult primary care settings: a systematic evidence review. Ann Intern Med 151:793–803, 2009

Olden KW: The use of antidepressants in functional gastrointestinal disorders: new uses for old drugs. CNS Spectr 10:891–897, 2005

Palmer BF, Gates JR, Lader M: Causes and management of hyponatremia. Ann Pharmacother 37:1694–1702, 2003

Rahimi R, Nikfar S, Rezaie A, et al: Efficacy of tricyclic antidepressants in irritable bowel syndrome: a meta-analysis. World J Gastroenterol 15:1548–1553, 2009

Repetto MJ, Petitto JM: Psychopharmacology in HIV-infected patients. Psychosom Med 70:585–592, 2008

Romero S, Pintor L, Serra M, et al: Syndrome of inappropriate secretion of antidiuretic hormone due to citalopram and venlafaxine. Gen Hosp Psychiatry 29:81–84, 2007

Rothschild AJ: Sexual side effects of antidepressants. J Clin Psychiatry 61 (supp 11):28–36, 2000

Roumestan C, Michel A, Bichon F, et al: Anti-inflammatory properties of desipramine and fluoxetine. Respir Res 8:35, 2007

Roy-Byrne PP, Davidson KW, Kessler RC, et al: Anxiety disorders and comorbid medical illness. Gen Hosp Psychiatry 30:208–225, 2008

Rubin RR, Ma Y, Marrero DG, et al: Elevated depression symptoms, antidepressant medicine use, and risk of developing diabetes during the diabetes prevention program. Diabetes Care 31:420–426, 2008

Saarto T, Wiffen PJ: Antidepressants for neuropathic pain. Cochrane Database of Systematic Reviews 2007, Issue 4. Art. No.: CD005454. DOI: 10.1002/14651858.CD005454.pub2.

Silver JM, McAllister TW, Arciniegas DB: Depression and cognitive complaints following traumatic brain injury. Am J Psychiatry 166:653–661, 2009

Silverstein SD: Preventative migraine. Neurol Clin 27:429–443, 2009

Sirois F: Steroid psychosis: a review. Gen Hosp Psychiatry 25:27–33, 2003

Summers KM, Martin KE, Watson K: Impact and clinical management of depression in patients with coronary artery disease. Pharmacotherapy 30:304–322, 2010

Taylor CB, Marston EY, Catellier D, et al: Effects of antidepressant medication on morbidity and mortality in depressed patients after myocardial infarction. Gen Hosp Psychiatry 62:792–798, 2005

Thomas C, Oster P: Depression-delirium overlap. J Am Geriatr Soc 57:2357–2358, 2009

Vinh DC, Rubinstein E: Linezolid: a review of safety and tolerability. J Infect 59:S59–S74, 2009

Yap KY, Tay WL, Chui WK, et al: Clinically relevant drug interactions between anticancer drugs and psychotropic agents. Eur J Cancer Care (Engl) 20:6–32, 2011

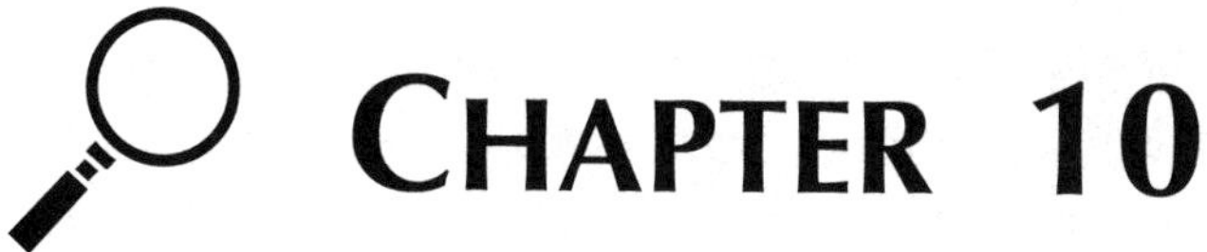

CHAPTER 10

Use of Antidepressants During Pregnancy and Lactation

Kristina M. Deligiannidis, M.D.

Antidepressant Use During Pregnancy

Depressive and anxiety disorders are prevalent in women during pregnancy and the postnatal (i.e., postpartum) period. Up to 18.4% of women experience depression during pregnancy (i.e., antenatal depression), with 12.7% of those women suffering from major depression; an estimated 19.2% of mothers within the first several weeks after delivery experience a major or minor depressive disorder (Gavin et al. 2005). Similarly, the prevalence rate of anxiety disorders is estimated to be 21.7% during the third trimester of pregnancy and 11.1% over the first 3 postnatal months (Borri et al. 2008; Reck et al. 2008).

Both psychological and pharmacological therapies for depressive and anxiety disorders are effective during pregnancy and in the postnatal period. Guidelines on the management of depression during pregnancy have been published (Yonkers et al. 2009), but no treatment guidelines are available for anxiety disorders during pregnancy. Psychotherapy alone may be an appropriate treatment for some women, whereas antidepressant therapy may be indicated in others. The aim of effective treatment is to minimize maternal and fetal exposure to psychiatric illness by optimally treating it with the minimum effective dosage regimen (Deligiannidis 2010).

Patterns of Antidepressant Use During Pregnancy

Of the 4,265,555 births registered in the United States in 2006, almost two-thirds of the infants were exposed to one or more medications prenatally. In utero exposure to antidepressants increased from 2.0% in 1996 to 7.6% in 2004 and 2005 (Andrade et al. 2008). Because the majority of women who take antidepressants during pregnancy do so for the treatment of depression rather than for anxiety disorders (Chambers et al. 1996), this chapter focuses on antidepressant treatment of perinatal depressive disorders.

Almost half of women prescribed an antidepressant early in pregnancy stopped their medication by the end of the first trimester (Oberlander et al. 2006). Similarly, in an observational study of over 29,000 women, almost 60% discontinued their antidepressant in the first trimester and 11% stopped thereafter (Ververs et al. 2006). Women who discontinue successful antidepressant treatment to avoid further exposure to the fetus risk higher rates (68%) of depression recurrence than do women who maintain their antidepressant therapy during pregnancy (25.6%) (Cohen et al. 2006).

Potential Risks of Undertreated or Untreated Perinatal Depressive and Anxiety Disorders

A comprehensive discussion that includes the potential risks of untreated mental illness for the mother and fetus/infant and the potential risks, benefits, and alternatives to antidepressant treatment is essential to well-informed, quality patient care. Antenatal depression is associated with increased risk of underutilization of prenatal care; maternal substance use, preeclampsia, inadequate weight gain, and preterm birth; increased risk for delivery of an infant who is of low birth weight or who is small for gestational age; elective termination of the pregnancy; and postpartum depression and anxiety. Children exposed to untreated perinatal depression are at a higher risk of developmental delay, impaired language development, and lower IQ scores (Deave et al. 2008; Paulson et al. 2009). Emotional and functional disability that is due to postpartum depression adversely impacts infant socioemotional and cognitive development. Furthermore, maternal depression negatively impacts other children in the family, because one-third of school-age children suffer from depressive, anxiety, or disruptive disorders while their mother is depressed (Pilowsky et al. 2006).

Untreated antenatal anxiety has been associated with elevated maternal corticotropin-releasing hormone and infant cortisol (Brennan et al. 2008); maternal cigarette smoking, caffeine consumption, and unhealthy eating (Lobel et al. 2008); preterm labor, preterm birth, and low birth weight (Grote et al. 2010); reductions in gray matter density in young children (Buss et al. 2010); and changes in infant behavior and child temperament (Beydoun and Saftlas 2008).

Potential Risks Associated With Antidepressant Treatment During Pregnancy

Observational study designs, including single-case reports, case series, registries, prospective cohorts, and meta-analyses, have been used to investigate various reproductive outcomes (e.g., miscarriage, birth defects) from fetal exposure to antidepressants. Unfortunately, few studies have differentiated reproductive outcomes associated with maternal depression from those associated with antidepressant exposure; this remains a critical area for further research.

Clinicians must translate the results of an expanding evidence base when discussing treatment options with pregnant women or women of childbearing age. To help women make an informed treatment decision, the clinician should discuss the U.S. Food and Drug Administration (FDA) antidepressant risk category and provide an overview of the current research literature findings. Before prescribing for patients of childbearing age, I inquire about contraception and discuss the potential risks of first-trimester medication exposure, because more than half of pregnancies are unplanned and most women learn of their pregnancy at a time when significant neurodevelopment has already occurred.

Current FDA regulations require that drug labeling include a "Pregnancy" subsection within the "Use in Specific Populations" section. The drug's teratogenic and other effects on pregnancy are described in that section, and each drug is classified under one of five pregnancy categories (A, B, C, D, or X) on the basis of the risks described. The five FDA teratogenic risk classifications are described in Table 10–1, and the teratogenic risk classification of selective serotonin reuptake inhibitors (SSRIs) and serotonin-norepinephrine reuptake inhibitors (SNRIs), tricyclic antidepressants (TCAs) and tetracyclic antidepressants, and monoamine oxidase inhibitors (MAOIs) and other antidepressants are listed in Tables 10–2, 10–3, and 10–4, respectively. All SSRIs and SNRIs currently approved by the FDA are classified as risk category C, except paroxetine, which is category D. No psychotropic medications have been classified as category A, indicating that they are safe for use during pregnancy.

One shortcoming of the current classification system is that the risk categories do not specify the dosage and/or duration of gestational exposure that is associated with teratogenic risk. In an effort to give clinicians more complete information about drug effects during pregnancy and lactation, the FDA recently proposed eliminating the current pregnancy categories (A, B, C, D, and X) and replacing them with a pregnancy and lactation subsection on drug labels. The proposed pregnancy subsection would include the following: fetal risk summary, clinical considerations, and risks associated with inadvertent exposure. The proposed lactation subsection would include an infant risk summary and clinical considerations, with respective supporting data (Shuren 2008). For those interested in viewing the full FDA proposal with a fictitious example of the projected pregnancy and lactation subsections, it may be viewed at the FDA Web site: www.fda.gov/Drugs/DevelopmentApprovalProcess/DevelopmentResources/Labeling/ucm093307. htm.

Four main categories of potential risks of medications used during pregnancy—spontaneous abortion (miscarriage) and adverse birth outcome measures, neonatal teratogenesis (major and minor malformations), neonatal toxicity or neonatal behavioral symptoms, and long-term neurodevelopmental sequelae—are discussed in the following subsections. Additionally, other perinatal adverse events are discussed.

Spontaneous Abortion (Miscarriage) and Adverse Birth Outcome Measures

The overall spontaneous abortion rate in the United States is 15%–20%, which means that 15%–20% of recognized pregnancies result in miscarriage. As maternal age increases, the frequency of spontaneous abortion increases further. The incidence of miscarriage for women younger than 35 years is 15%; ages 35–39 years, 20%–25%; ages 40–44 years, approximately 51%; and ages 45 and older, greater than 75% (Nybo Andersen et al. 2000).

The evidence base regarding the risks and safety of antidepressants during pregnancy is complex. Study results are mixed and often conflict because of the use of different study designs, which may be underpowered, may eval-

TABLE 10–1. FDA teratogenic risk classification for drugs

A	Studies in pregnant women have not shown an increased risk of fetal abnormalities, and the possibility of fetal harm appears remote.
B	Either animal-reproduction studies have demonstrated a fetal risk and studies in pregnant women have not shown that the drug increases the risk of fetal abnormalities or animal-reproduction studies have not demonstrated a fetal risk but there are no controlled studies in pregnant women. The drug should be used only when clearly needed.
C	Either animal studies have demonstrated teratogenic, embryocidal, or other effects and there are no controlled studies in women or studies in women and animals are not available. The drug should be used only if the potential benefit outweighs the potential risk to the fetus.
D	Positive evidence of human fetal risk exists based on adverse reaction data from investigational or marketing experience or studies in humans. The potential benefits from the use of the drug in pregnant women may be acceptable despite its potential risk.
X	Animal-reproduction and/or human studies have demonstrated fetal abnormalities or there is evidence of fetal risk based on human experience or both, and the risk of the use of the drug during pregnancy outweighs any potential benefit. The drug is contraindicated for use in pregnant women or women who may become pregnant.

Note. FDA=U.S. Food and Drug Administration.
Source. Adapted from Shuren J: "Content and Format of Labeling for Human Prescription Drug and Biological Products: Requirements for Pregnancy and Lactation Labeling." Federal Register, May 29, 2008. Available at: www.federalregister.gov/articles/2008/05/29/E8-11806/content-and-format-of-labeling-for-human-prescription-drug-and-biological-products-requirements-for. Accessed May 17, 2011.

uate drug exposure during different trimesters and at varying dosages and durations, may evaluate different outcome measures, and may or may not control for the presence or severity of maternal depressive illness.

Several studies have investigated the potential association between antidepressant use during pregnancy and spontaneous abortion rate. Two meta-analyses reported an increased risk of spontaneous abortion associated with antidepressant use (Hemels et al. 2005; Rahimi et al. 2006). Hemels et al. (2005) found an increased risk of spontaneous abortion in 1,534 women exposed to antidepressants compared with 2,033 women not exposed (12.4% and 8.7%, respectively). The number needed to harm (NNH) was 26. Nonsignificant differences in risk ratios were found between antidepressant classes,

TABLE 10–2. FDA teratogenic risk classification[a] of selective serotonin reuptake inhibitor (SSRI) and serotonin-norepinephrine reuptake inhibitor (SNRI) antidepressants

SSRIs	
Citalopram	C
Escitalopram	C
Fluoxetine	C
Fluoxetine weekly	C
Fluvoxamine	C
Fluvoxamine CR	C
Paroxetine	D
Paroxetine CR	D
Sertraline	C
SNRIs	
Desvenlafaxine	C
Duloxetine	C
Venlafaxine	C
Venlafaxine ER	C
Venlafaxine XR	C

Note. CR=controlled release; ER=extended release; FDA=U.S. Food and Drug Administration; XR=extended release.
[a]See drug classification descriptions in Table 10–1.

including SSRIs, TCAs, and dual-action agents (i.e., trazodone, venlafaxine, and nefazodone).

In two recent Canadian studies with different study designs, an increased risk of spontaneous abortion was identified in association with antidepressant use. Einarson et al. (2009b) identified a miscarriage rate of 13% in a group of women exposed to antidepressants in early pregnancy versus 8% in the nonexposed group. Nakhai-Pour et al. (2010) reported a differential risk among antidepressant classes; the lowest risk was associated with SSRIs (odds ratio [OR]=1.61), a greater risk was associated with SNRIs (OR=2.11), and the greatest risk was associated with combined use of different classes of antidepressants (OR=3.51).

In a small study with bupropion, Chun-Fai-Chan et al. (2005) also reported an increased risk of spontaneous abortion in exposed versus nonexposed groups (14.7% vs. 4.5%). In a small study of mirtazapine use during the first trimester, Djulus et al. (2006) did not find a significant difference in spontaneous abortion

TABLE 10–3. FDA teratogenic risk classification[a] of tricyclic and tetracyclic antidepressants

Tricyclic antidepressants	
Amitriptyline	C
Amoxapine	C
Clomipramine	C
Desipramine	—[b]
Doxepin	C
Imipramine	D
Nortriptyline	D
Protriptyline	—[b]
Trimipramine	C
Tetracyclic antidepressants	
Maprotiline	B

Note. FDA=U.S. Food and Drug Administration.
[a]See drug classification descriptions in Table 10–1.
[b]Not classified by the FDA.

rates between mirtazapine-exposed, other antidepressant–exposed, or nonexposed groups; however, Yaris et al. (2004) reported one spontaneous abortion in a woman taking mirtazapine in combination with other psychotropics.

Other individual studies have been done with fluoxetine (Chambers et al. 1996); fluvoxamine, sertraline, and paroxetine (Kulin et al. 1998); citalopram (Sivojelezova et al. 2005); and venlafaxine (Einarson et al. 2001; Yaris et al. 2004). Either the medications did not result in an increased risk of miscarriage, or no miscarriages were reported in the small case series evaluated.

In summary, several studies have demonstrated an increased rate of spontaneous abortion in depressed women exposed to antidepressants. However, the majority of studies could not determine if the increased rate of spontaneous abortion was associated with maternal depression or antidepressant exposure, because the studies did not control for maternal depression. Also, the overall range of rates of spontaneous abortion in women treated with antidepressants did not exceed the overall national rate of 15%–20%.

Regarding other birth outcomes, SSRI, SNRI, and TCA use in pregnancy is associated with an almost twofold increased risk of low birth weight (LBW) (i.e., <2,500 g) (Källén 2004; Reis and Källén 2010). LBW deliveries are considered small for gestational age (SGA) when the weight is below the 10th percentile for gestational age; these infants are at higher risk of perinatal mortality and morbidity. Although most studies have found an association be-

TABLE 10–4. FDA teratogenic risk classification[a] of MAOIs and other antidepressants

MAOIs	
Isocarboxazid	C
Phenelzine	C
Selegiline	C
Tranylcypromine	C
Other	
Bupropion hydrobromide	C
Bupropion hydrochloride	C
Bupropion hydrochloride SR	C
Bupropion hydrochloride XR	C
Mirtazapine	C
Nefazodone	C
Trazodone	C
Vilazodone	C

Note. FDA=U.S. Food and Drug Administration; MAOI=monoamine oxidase inhibitor; SR=sustained release; XR=extended release.
[a]See drug classification descriptions in Table 10–1.

tween antidepressant use during pregnancy and LBW, not all studies have found an increased risk of SGA deliveries (Chambers et al. 1996; Källén 2004; Oberlander et al. 2006; Reis and Källén 2010; Wisner et al. 2009).

Preterm birth, which refers to a birth that occurs prior to 37 completed weeks of gestation, is the leading cause of infant mortality in the United States. In 2006 in the United States, 12.8% of live births were preterm. Most studies have found an association between SSRI, SNRI, or TCA use during pregnancy and reduced gestational age or preterm birth (Källén 2004; Lund et al. 2009; Reis and Källén 2010; Simon et al. 2002; Suri et al. 2007), but not all studies have confirmed that finding (Oberlander et al. 2006; Pastuszak et al. 1993). An early study demonstrated a threefold increased rate of preterm birth when fluoxetine was used during late pregnancy (14.3%) compared with when the antidepressant was discontinued earlier in pregnancy (4.1%) or not used at all (5.9%) (Chambers et al. 1996); however, this study lacked a comparison group of women with untreated maternal depression.

Studies that have controlled for the effects of maternal depression either by inclusion of depressed women who chose not to take an antidepressant or by the use of propensity score matching have not found an increased risk of preterm birth in antidepressant-exposed women (Oberlander et al. 2006). Wisner et al. (2009) found an increased risk of preterm birth for depressed women with or without SSRI treatment (23% and 21%, respectively) compared with women without depression or SSRI exposure (6%).

Neonatal Teratogenesis (Major and Minor Malformations)

In the United States, 1 of every 28 infants is born with a birth defect that results in physical or mental disability or death. Major birth defects or malformations are structural or functional abnormalities that usually require medical or surgical intervention. Antidepressants that affect serotonergic tone could theoretically have teratogenic effects because serotonin is important in several aspects of early embryonic development, including cell cleavage, neural tube development, cell migration and differentiation of the neural crest and branchial arch, and cardiac development.

Minor birth defects are estimated to be 10–20 times more common than major birth defects. Twenty percent of infants with one or more minor birth defects have a major birth defect, and the occurrence of three or more minor birth defects is associated with major structural malformations and neurodevelopmental abnormalities. Minor birth defects generally do not require medical or surgical treatment.

Most studies have not found an association between structural malformations (major or minor) and use of TCAs or SSRIs during pregnancy (Chambers et al. 1996; Davis et al. 2007; Einarson et al. 2001, 2008, 2009a; Ericson et al. 1999; Kulin et al. 1998; Pastuszak et al. 1993; Simon et al. 2002; Wichman et al. 2009). However, the use of certain individual SSRIs during pregnancy has been associated with a small increased absolute risk of rare defects, such as anencephaly, craniosynostosis, omphalocele, cystic kidney, and right ventricular outflow tract obstruction defects (Alwan et al. 2007; Källén and Otterblad Olausson 2007; Louik et al. 2007).

A large population-based cohort study in Denmark demonstrated an increased prevalence of septal heart defects among children born to mothers who were prescribed more than one type of SSRI (2.1%) than in children born to mothers prescribed any one SSRI (0.9%) or not taking an SSRI (0.5%). As the percentages indicate, prescription of a single SSRI taken during the first trimester slightly increased the prevalence of infant septal heart defects; the NNH was large (246). By comparison, prescription of more than one type of SSRI was associated with an NNH of 48, a clinically meaningful increased risk of harm. The use of more than one type of SSRI could represent either a cross-taper from one SSRI to another or the use of two SSRIs concurrently, but this study could not, by design, distinguish between these two possibilities. When the results were analyzed by specific antidepressant, a slightly increased prevalence of septal heart defects was found for children of women who used sertraline (1.5%) or citalopram (1.1%) but not fluoxetine (0.6%) or paroxetine (0.3%). No specific SSRI was significantly associated with overall major malformations or noncardiac malformations. The authors suggested that SSRIs as a class may be associated with a small increased risk of cardiac malformations (Pedersen et al. 2009).

Some studies have shown that compared with use of other antidepressants, use of paroxetine during early pregnancy is associated with an increased risk of overall major malformations and major cardiac malformations, especially atrial and ventricular septal defects (Alwan et al. 2007; Bakker et al. 2010; Bérard et al. 2007; Cole et al. 2007a; Källén et al. 2007; Wurst et al. 2010), but not all studies agree (Diav-Citrin et al. 2008; Einarson et al. 2008; Kornum et al. 2010; Pedersen et al. 2009; Ramos et al. 2008; Wisner et al. 2009). In the September 2009 joint publication of the American Psychiatric Association and the American College of Obstetricians and Gynecologists, it was noted that the link between paroxetine use during the first trimester and cardiac abnormalities was not strong (Yonkers et al. 2009). A case-control analysis of major malformations in the National Birth Defects Prevention Study also showed a statistically significant association between paroxetine and anencephaly, omphalocele, and gastroschisis, but the overall number of exposed cases was small, which limited the strength of these findings (Alwan et al. 2007). In contrast, Louik and colleagues (2007) were not able to replicate the finding of an association between paroxetine and omphalocele. Paroxetine, in its immediate- and extended-release forms, is the only SSRI that is classified in the FDA's teratogenic risk category D.

Other studies have found an increased risk of omphalocele and cardiac septal defects with use of sertraline during early pregnancy and increased risk of congenital heart defects with use of fluoxetine (Diav-Citrin et al. 2008; Louik et al. 2007; Oberlander et al. 2008b). Oberlander et al. (2008b) reported that the risk of congenital heart disease was greater when SSRIs are used concomitantly with benzodiazepines than when either an SSRI or a benzodiazepine is used alone during pregnancy; perhaps the combination causes competitive inhibition of hepatic metabolism, leading to increased drug levels and increased neonatal risk. Reis and Källén (2010) reported a higher risk of cardiovascular defects after clomipramine exposure than after SSRI or SNRI exposure.

Fewer data exist regarding use of bupropion, venlafaxine, duloxetine, trazodone, nefazodone, and mirtazapine during pregnancy, and further research is needed to assess potential fetal risk. Limited studies thus far have not shown an association between the drugs and an increased risk of congenital malformations (Chun-Fai-Chan et al. 2005; Cole et al. 2007b; Djulus et al. 2006; Einarson et al. 2001, 2003; Lennestal and Källén 2007), with the exception of an increased risk of left outflow tract heart defects associated with bupropion use (Alwan et al. 2010).

Five meta-analyses have investigated the risk for major malformations in association with antidepressant use during pregnancy. Four of these studies found no statistically significant increased risk of major malformations when mothers took antidepressants during the first trimester (Addis and Koren 2000; Einarson and Einarson 2005; O'Brien et al. 2008; Rahimi et al. 2006). The fifth meta-analysis found an increased risk of cardiac malformations in infants exposed to paroxetine in the first trimester, although the apparently higher incidence of cardiac defects in neonates whose mothers used paroxetine may be an artifact of the more frequent use of paroxetine by anxious mothers (Bar-Oz et al. 2007; Ramos et al. 2008).

Limited data are available on the risk of minor malformations associated with antidepressant exposure during pregnancy (Casper et al. 2003; Chambers et al. 1996). The current evidence base is mixed and requires further investigation.

In summary, the SSRIs and possibly the TCAs may confer increased risks for some specific major malformations; however, based on the current evidence, these malformations are rare and the absolute risks appear small. Unfortunately, the use of MAOIs during pregnancy has not been systematically studied. SNRIs, bupropion, mirtazapine, nefazodone, and trazodone need further investigation before the risks associated with their use may be fully understood.

Future studies will require larger sample sizes to better identify particular patterns of teratogenesis; if individual antidepressants or classes of antidepressants are teratogenic, specific birth defects will be isolated consistently and with reproducibility across studies. Larger sample sizes will correct a current shortcoming of the evidence base, which is that some of the malformation types have been grouped together to have enough power to detect a difference in risk. For example, some studies have grouped together all septal defects or, even more broadly, all congenital heart disease, although these categories encompass a variety of birth defects and a range of severity. Studies may not indicate whether the reported increased risk for cardiac defects is for minor, moderate, or severe forms, which carry varying medical risks to the infant.

Neonatal Toxicity or Neonatal Behavioral Symptoms

Late in utero exposure to SSRIs and SNRIs is associated with several behavioral and neurological signs and symptoms in the neonate, including tremor, shivering, hypertonia, feeding difficulties, irritability, respiratory disturbances, hyperreflexia, excess crying, and sleep disturbance. The syndrome, which has been termed the *neonatal behavioral syndrome* or *poor neonatal adaptation syndrome,* can develop within hours to days; is usually mild, transient, and self-limited; and resolves within days to weeks. Premature neonates, who have lung and central nervous system (CNS) immaturity, may be more susceptible to the risk of respiratory symptoms, seizure, and irritability due to in utero antidepressant exposure (Ferreira et al. 2007). For term and preterm neonates, the behavioral syndrome can be severe and include seizure, dehydration, and respiratory distress requiring intubation. Most infants receive supportive medical care in the special care nursery or in the neonatal intensive care unit during this time.

Compared with SSRIs and SNRIs, TCAs have been associated with increased perinatal complications, which include respiratory distress, neonatal convulsions, and hypoglycemia (Källén 2004). Neonatal adaptation syndrome has been associated with the use of many of the SSRIs and SNRIs and has most often been reported with late exposure to paroxetine, fluoxetine, and venlafaxine, although not all studies are in agreement (Maschi et al. 2008; Wisner et al. 2009). In one study, nearly 22% of neonates exposed to paroxetine in the third trimester had complications that necessitated intensive treatment and prolonged hospitalization. The most prevalent symptoms, which resolved within 1–2 weeks, were respiratory distress, hypoglycemia, and jaundice. In the comparison group of neonates born to women not using paroxetine during the third trimester, only 5.5% experienced complications requiring treatment and hospitalization (Costei et al. 2002). A prospective case-control study that compared rates of neonatal behavioral symptoms in neonates with late pregnancy antidepressant exposure with those of matched controls without antidepressant exposure reported an increased risk of neonatal behavioral symptoms associated with late pregnancy exposure (Galbally et al. 2009). Similarly, compared with early exposure to fluoxetine during pregnancy, late exposure was associated with a higher incidence of neonatal adaptation syndrome (8.9% vs. 31.5%) (Chambers et al. 1996).

Compared with neonates of untreated mothers, neonates exposed during the third trimester to SSRIs or venlafaxine had a higher rate of CNS and respiratory symptoms. CNS effects, reported in 63.2% of exposed infants, included tremors, agitation, spasms, hypotonia, irritability, sleep disturbances, apnea/bradycardia, and tachypnea. Respiratory effects, including indrawing, apnea/bradycardia, and tachypnea, were noted in 43.2% of exposed neonates (Ferreira et al. 2007). Similarly, maternal use of SSRIs, SNRIs, or mirtazapine was associated with an increased risk for respiratory problems, low 5-minute Apgar score, and hypoglycemia; this risk was higher if the exposure was later rather than earlier in pregnancy (Lennestal et al. 2007).

The above-mentioned studies and others (Boucher et al. 2008; Davis et al. 2007; Oberlander et al. 2004) that have found an association between the in utero use of antidepressants and neonatal behavioral symptoms have not investigated the potential impact of maternal psychiatric illness on the occurrence of the neonatal syndrome. However, a large population-based study compared outcomes of infants of depressed mothers treated with SSRIs with those of infants of depressed mothers not treated with medication and nonexposed controls, thus controlling for potential confounders such as disease severity, maternal psychotropic medication use, and concurrent illness (Oberlander et al. 2006). The incidence of symptoms or behavioral syndrome in infants born to depressed mothers who had not been exposed to SSRIs was similar to that in infants born to depressed mothers who had been exposed to SSRIs, with the exception of respiratory distress. Thus, as Tuccori and colleagues (2009) have pointed out, previous studies had not controlled for the severity of depression, and the use of SSRIs during pregnancy may not be associated with an increased risk for neonatal behavioral syndrome.

Not all infants exposed to antidepressants in pregnancy develop the syndrome. The infant serotonin transporter (SLC6A4) promoter genotype moderates specific adverse outcomes, such as reduced Apgar score, birth weight, and respiratory problems in neonates with prenatal SSRI exposure (Oberlander et al. 2008a), and may be one factor that influences why some infants develop the syndrome whereas others do not.

Other Perinatal Adverse Events

Persistent pulmonary hypertension of the newborn (PPHN) is a rare but potentially fatal disorder characterized by suprasystemic pulmonary vascular resistance causing right-to-left shunting at the level of the ductus arteriosus and the foramen ovale, which leads to a cycle of hypoxemia, acidosis, and further pulmonary vasoconstriction. PPHN occurs in 1–2 per 1,000 live births and can be fatal in 4%–33% of cases. PPHN may be primary or secondary to a variety of disorders, including congenital heart disease, intrapartum hypoxia, infection, pulmonary hypoplasia, and drug exposure. Infants with PPHN present within 12 hours of birth with cyanosis and mild respiratory distress but can develop severe respiratory failure requiring intubation and mechanical ventilation. Goals of treatment include reducing the right-to-left shunt by improving the systemic blood pressure and administering pulmonary vasodilators to prevent neurological damage from severe hypoxemia, irreversible hypoxia, or myocardial failure (Greenough and Khetriwal 2005; Walsh-Sukys et al. 2000).

In utero drug exposure can cause varying degrees of neonatal respiratory distress; even mild respiratory distress may represent the presence of PPHN and not poor neonatal adaptation syndrome per se (Boucher et al. 2009; Koren and Boucher 2009). The accumulation of SSRIs in the lungs may result in high circulating levels of serotonin which, through its vasoconstrictive effects, increases pulmonary vascular resistance and may cause proliferation of smooth muscle cells in the fetal lung. In utero fluoxetine exposure in rodents induces pulmonary hypertension as a result of a developmentally regulated increase in pulmonary vascular smooth muscle proliferation (Fornaro et al. 2007); this finding is in contrast to the current understanding that fluoxetine protects against pulmonary hypertension in adult rodents through its effects on the serotonin transporter (Zhu et al. 2009).

Chambers et al. (1996) first reported that late in utero exposure to fluoxetine was associated with an increased risk of PPHN when compared with first-trimester exposure (2.7% vs. 0%), especially when compared with the prevalence found in the general population (0.1%–0.2%). A subsequent case-control study also found that in utero use of SSRIs (i.e., citalopram, fluoxetine, paroxetine, and sertraline) after the 20th week of pregnancy was significantly associated with PPHN (adjusted OR=6.1) but that in utero use of SSRIs or other antidepressants (i.e., TCAs, bupropion, venlafaxine, and trazodone) used prior to 20 weeks' gestation was not (Chambers et al. 2006). Furthermore, the risk for PPHN in infants was increased when infants had been exposed to SSRIs in both early and late gestation (Källén and Olausson 2008; Reis and Källén 2010) instead of early or late gestation alone. Exposure to non-SSRIs was not associated with PPHN.

In a 2009 retrospective cohort study of U.S. hospital registry data, the prevalence of PPHN was no different among infants whose mothers had been exposed to antidepressants in the third trimester of pregnancy (2.14 per 1,000) than among infants whose mothers had not been exposed (2.72 per 1,000) (Andrade et al. 2009). Other studies have reported no association between maternal antidepressant use and PPHN, and some indicate that mode of delivery (i.e., vaginal delivery vs. cesarean section) is associated with PPHN rather than maternal antidepressant use (Wichman et al. 2009; Wilson et al. 2011).

Other perinatal adverse events that may be associated with in utero antidepressant use include QTc interval prolongation, seizures, and bleeding complications. SSRIs affect cardiac repolarization and have been associated with reversible QTc prolongation in children and adults. In a recent prospective cohort study, 10% of neonates exposed to SSRIs in the immediate antepartum period had QTc prolongation (i.e., 12%–44% prolongation) compared with later electrocardiogram (ECG) tracings, which had normalized. This was a clinically significant finding, because prolongation of the QTc interval by more than 30% of baseline in adults predisposes to torsades de pointes (Dubnov-Raz et al. 2008); because the ECG was performed soon after delivery, the drug effect likely reflected a condition that was present in utero. The authors noted that none of the infants had serious adverse effects but suggested that ECG monitoring be considered in infants exposed to SSRIs during pregnancy.

Two cases of seizures were reported in neonates born to mothers taking venlafaxine during pregnancy. Seizures occurred within 24 hours of birth, were self-limited, and, because no other cause for seizure was found, were attributed to maternal use of venlafaxine (Pakalapati et al. 2006). Larger studies that have reported on the incidence of convulsions or seizure disorder in neonates with prenatal exposure to TCAs or SSRIs have not found such an association (Oberlander et al. 2006; Simon et al. 2002).

A few case reports have described neonatal subarachnoid and/or intraventricular hemorrhage after late gestational use of paroxetine or fluoxetine, but the relationship between antidepressant use and hemorrhagic effects is understudied and uncertain. A population-based nested case-control study did not find an association between postpartum hemorrhage and SSRI use during pregnancy (Salkeld et al. 2008), and a large birth registry study did not find an increased risk of neonatal intracerebral hemorrhage or peripartum bleeding in women who used antidepressants during pregnancy (Reis and Källén 2010).

Long-Term Neurodevelopmental Sequelae

Few studies have investigated the potential risk of long-term neurobehavioral, cognitive, and motor development sequelae from prenatal exposure to antidepressants, but initial findings are reassuring. A recent systematic review that examined longer-term neurodevelopmental teratogenic effects in children exposed to antidepressants prenatally found no evidence of adverse effects on neurocognition or emotional development (Gentile and Galbally 2011). However, two studies have found impaired psychomotor development following in utero exposure to antidepressants (Casper et al. 2003; Mortensen et al. 2003). Another study demonstrated that exposure to bupropion during pregnancy, especially in the second trimester, was associated with an increased risk of attention-deficit/hyperactivity disorder, whereas exposure to SSRIs was not (Figueroa 2010). Most recently, prenatal exposure to antidepressants, especially during the first trimester, was associated with an increased risk of autism spectrum disorders in exposed children, though the absolute risk appears small (Croen et al. 2011). Limitations of the study included a reliance on medical records so that the investigators did not validate actual use of antidepressants by the mothers or conduct evaluations of the children.

Summary

In summary, the use of antidepressants during pregnancy involves complex clinical decisions based on the risks and benefits and alternatives to pharmacological treatment. Risks are inherent from either the use of antidepressants during pregnancy or untreated depression. Careful, individualized discussions with the patient regarding the growing evidence base regarding risks and safety in the context of her treatment preferences are vital to delivering the best clinical care to the patient and her developing child.

Clinical Management Approaches to Depression During Pregnancy and the Postpartum Period

Guidelines for the management of depression during pregnancy have been published by representatives from the American Psychiatric Association and the American College of Obstetricians and Gynecologists (Yonkers et al. 2009). Depending on the clinical situation, women might be initiating, continuing, or tapering an antidepressant during pregnancy. For patients with mild to moderate depression during pregnancy, individual and group psychotherapy, including cognitive-behavioral therapy or interpersonal therapy, sometimes as monotherapy, has been shown to be effective. For patients with moderate symptoms of depression, antidepressant medication is often recommended in combination with psychotherapy. The choice of an antidepressant will depend on the stage of gestation; history of successful or failed antidepressant trials, which may guide antidepressant selection; risk versus safety profile of the antidepressant; and the patient's symptoms and treatment preference. For patients with severe depression, active suicidal ideation, or psychosis, a multimodal treatment approach may include pharmacotherapy, psychotherapy, and psychiatric hospitalization.

Women who have a history of severe, recurrent depression are at high risk of relapse if they stop treatment. For women who prefer to taper antidepressant therapy, are euthymic, and do not have a history of severe, recurrent depression, a trial of medication taper may be suitable, with close monitoring for reemergence of symptoms. Some women may choose to taper and discontinue antidepressant treatment and utilize psychotherapy during the pregnancy to maintain euthymia (Yonkers et al. 2009).

Women who require antidepressant treatment should receive the minimal *effective* dose to maximally treat depression and minimize maternal and fetal exposure to antidepressants and the effects of undertreated depression. Treatment often needs to be adjusted throughout pregnancy. Two-thirds of pregnant women undergoing antidepressant monotherapy may require dosage increases, especially after 20 weeks' gestation (Hostetter et al. 2000), to treat depressive symptoms or maintain euthymia. One contributing factor may be the more rapid metabolism of the medication; in particular, changes in

CYP metabolic activity appear to lower SSRI plasma levels and may impact treatment response during pregnancy (Sit et al. 2008). CYP3A4 is induced during pregnancy (Tracy et al. 2005), and CYP2D6 has been reported to be induced (Anderson 2005; Tracy et al. 2005; Wadelius et al. 1997). Lower trough levels of fluoxetine and citalopram in pregnancy than in the postpartum period may be due to pregnancy-associated demethylation by CYP2D6 (Heikkinen et al. 2002, 2003) and may contribute to the emergence or worsening of depressive symptoms during pregnancy.

In addition to changes in antidepressant metabolism, other physiological or psychosocial changes frequently experienced during pregnancy likely contribute to the need for dosage adjustments during this period. I have the patient continue taking the dose that was effective early in pregnancy (or prepregnancy) as she progresses through pregnancy, while monitoring for depressive symptoms at least monthly, and base dosage adjustments on clinical presentation (Deligiannidis 2010).

In 2004, the FDA instructed antidepressant manufacturers to issue warnings about perinatal complications associated with antidepressant use. Antidepressant drug labels recommend considering discontinuation of antidepressants in the third trimester to reduce the risk of neonatal behavioral syndrome and/or PPHN. However, tapering antidepressants in the third trimester may precipitate relapse or postpartum-onset depression, especially in high-risk individuals (Moses-Kolko et al. 2005). In a study that compared neonates of mothers who did taper in the third trimester with those who did not, there was no difference in neonatal symptoms among the two groups (Warburton et al. 2010). Discontinuing clinically necessary antidepressant treatment in women near term is not supported by scientific evidence at this time, does not appear to reduce the risk of neonatal symptoms, and places women at risk of complications from untreated depression or from relapse. I recommend women to continue antidepressant treatment in late pregnancy into the postpartum period if they have depressive symptoms in late pregnancy or are at elevated risk for depression relapse.

The return to the prepregnancy metabolic state in the immediate postpartum period may result in increased antidepressant blood levels and manifest as antidepressant side effects, especially when an increased dosage that was used during pregnancy is continued postpartum. Some authors have suggested that to help prevent postpartum mood exacerbations, a woman should continue the SSRI dose used in pregnancy, in the absence of adverse effects, to at least 6 weeks postpartum (Hostetter et al. 2000). My practice is to have the patient continue the dose used in pregnancy into the postpartum and to monitor her for the emergence of side effects or depression by telephone communication during the first postpartum week, and then every 2–4 weeks via office visits as clinically indicated. Dosage adjustments should be based on clinical presentation, and I use standardized assessments of depression (e.g., the Edinburgh Postnatal Depression Scale, Quick Inventory of Depressive Symptomatology—Self Report) throughout pregnancy and the postpartum period to inform treatment decisions (Deligiannidis 2010).

Antidepressant Use During Lactation

Benefits of Breast-Feeding

Human breast milk contains the optimal balance of fats, carbohydrates, protein, micronutrients, immunoglobulin, digestive enzymes, and hormones needed for infant growth and development. The World Health Organization recommends that children should be breast-fed for their first 2 years of life. The American Academy of Pediatrics, the American Academy of Family Physicians, and the American Dietetic Association (James et al. 2009) recommend exclusive breast-feeding for the first 6 months of life and breast-feeding with complementary food from 6 months until at least 12 months of age and as long thereafter as desired. In the United States, only 32% of infants are breast-fed exclusively through 3 months of age, and only 12% of infants are breast-fed through 6 months of age (Stuebe and Schwarz 2010).

Breast-feeding is associated with numerous health benefits for both mother and child. For the child, breast-feeding is associated with a reduced risk of otitis media, gastroenteritis, lower respiratory tract infection, sudden infant death syndrome, necrotizing enterocolitis, asthma, obesity, and postneonatal mortality. Breast-feeding is also associated with improved maternal outcomes, including a reduced risk of postpartum bleeding, ovarian and premenopausal breast cancer, type 2 diabetes, metabolic syndrome, and postpartum depression (Stuebe and Schwarz 2010).

Potential Risks Associated With Antidepressant Use During Lactation

Several factors that affect antidepressant drug concentration in breast milk include pH (most psychotropic drugs including antidepressants are alkaline), protein content, and lipid content (most psychotropic drugs including antidepressants are lipophilic). Each of these factors varies throughout the postpartum period and at different times during a feeding. For example, hind milk has higher lipid content than fore milk and thus may have higher drug concentrations. Several factors affect infant drug exposure risk, such as drug absorption rate into maternal circulation, diffusion rate from maternal circulation to breast milk, and infant drug absorption via milk consumption. Nursing mothers produce about 600–1,000 mL of milk daily.

These physiological factors are important in understanding how drug exposure risk in lactation is evaluated and reported in the literature. The milk-to-plasma drug ratio is often used as a measure of translactal passage and, due to the above factors, varies for the same drug depending on whether the milk aliquot consisted of hind or fore milk and how much drug was absorbed into the maternal circulation and diffused into the breast milk at the time of sampling. The relative infant dose (RID), another measure commonly reported, is a measure of the daily dose of drug received by an infant through breast milk, expressed as a percentage of the weight-adjusted maternal daily dosage. A low RID does not necessarily mean that an infant will be unaffected.

All antidepressants have translactal passage from maternal plasma to breast milk and then are metabolized by the infant. Neonatal CYP activity is about one-half that found in adults, and each liver enzyme system matures at a different rate in the infant. Isoenzymes important for antidepressant metabolism include CYP2D6, which gains activity during the third trimester or just after birth. CYP3A4 and CYP2C19 also gain functional activity after birth, and CYP1A2 appears 3–4 months after birth (Oesterheld 1998). Premature infants have premature livers and thus premature hepatic enzymes. Infants who are poor metabolizers of CYP isoenzymes may be at increased risk of developing side effects due to impaired hepatic metabolism. However, findings from initial studies of serum concentrations of paroxetine and citalopram in infants who are poor metabolizers of CYP2D6 or CYP2C19 have been reassuring (Berle et al. 2004).

In the postpartum period, women may request consultation on the continuation of an antidepressant that was used during pregnancy or, if a new depressive episode develops, on the initiation of antidepressant therapy during lactation. For many reasons, they may also be considering the option of continuing breast-feeding or changing to formula feeding of their infant. Clinically, I find that most women who take an antidepressant during pregnancy will continue to use it in the postpartum period regardless of whether or not they choose to breast-feed.

In 2001, the American Academy of Pediatrics (AAP) Committee on Drugs published its position on the use of medications during lactation. The AAP recently retired their policy statement on medications during lactation. At the time of this writing, no new policy statement had been released. In 2001, the committee reported that for the TCAs, most of the SSRIs and SNRIs, and trazodone, the "effects on a nursing infant are unknown" and "may be of concern." A few antidepressants, including maprotiline, citalopram, escitalopram, duloxetine, venlafaxine, and mirtazapine, were not listed as having a category from the AAP. The committee did not issue a caution against prescribing antidepressants to nursing mothers, but noted that because these medications "affect neurotransmitter function in the developing central nervous system, it may not be possible to predict long-term neurodevelopmental effects" (American Academy of Pediatrics Committee on Drugs 2001, pp. 776–777). Few studies have investigated the potential long-term neurodevelopmental effects secondary to antidepressant exposure through breast milk. However, few long-term effects have been reported in infants who had been exposed to these agents in utero. In utero SSRI exposure is associated with maternal serum concentrations that are at least 5–10 times greater than exposure through breast milk (Berle et al. 2004). Platelet serotonin uptake is not decreased in breast-fed infants who were exposed to sertraline or fluoxetine through breast milk, so it is unlikely that there is significant serotonin blockade in the infant brain because it shares the same serotonin transporter present in platelets (Epperson et al. 2001, 2003). Table 10–5 lists the maternal dosage range, RID, and reported adverse effects for several of the most commonly prescribed TCAs, SSRIs, SNRIs, and other antidepressants.

Published milk-to-plasma ratios and infant serum levels of the TCAs vary widely, but there are no reports of adverse effects in breast-fed infants of mothers treated with the TCAs amitriptyline, nortriptyline, imipramine, desipramine, or clomipramine (Fortinguerra et al. 2009). Nortriptyline and imipramine have the most evidence of safety in lactation. I would not recommend the use of doxepin because there have been case reports of respiratory depression, sedation, hypotonia, and poor suckling/swallowing and weight loss (Frey et al. 1999).

Among newer antidepressants, sertraline, paroxetine, and fluvoxamine are considered safer alternatives for the treatment of depression in lactation because they have the lowest degree of translactal passage and fewest reported adverse effects compared to other antidepressants. Citalopram, escitalopram, and fluoxetine are not recommended as first-line treatment of depression during lactation because of their longer half-life or reported adverse effects in infants (Fortinguerra et al. 2009).

Data are limited (or absent) for bupropion, venlafaxine, desvenlafaxine, duloxetine, trazodone, and the MAOIs. The rate of venlafaxine/desvenlafaxine excretion into human breast milk was reported to be higher than that for other antidepressants. Desvenlafaxine is excreted into breast milk at a much higher rate than venlafaxine and contributes disproportionately to the RID and thus is the largest contributor to infant exposure (Newport et al. 2009).

In lactating women with mild to moderate postpartum depression, nonpharmacological therapies such as interpersonal therapy or cognitive-behavioral therapy are considered first-line therapies. Antidepressant therapy with or without psychotherapy is recommended for lactating women with moder-

TABLE 10–5. Antidepressant excretion into human breast milk and compatibility with breast feeding

Drug	Maternal dosage (mg/day)	Relative infant dose (%)	Reported adverse effects
TCAs			
Amitriptyline	75–175	0.2–1.9	None located
Clomipramine	75–150	0.4–4.0	None located
Desipramine	300	2.0	None located
Doxepin	150–200	2.5	Respiratory depression, sedation, paleness, poor suckling and swallowing, hypotonia, vomiting and weight loss
Imipramine	75–200	0.1–7.5	None located
Nortriptyline	125	0.6–3.0	None located
Tetracyclic antidepressants			
Maprotiline	100–150	<0.1–1.6	None located
SSRIs			
Citalopram	18–60	1.0–10.9	Drowsiness, weight loss, uneasy sleep
Escitalopram	5–20	2.9–8.3	Necrotizing enterocolitis
Fluoxetine	10–80	0.8–16.3	Colic, fussiness, drowsiness, decreased weight gain, decreased rooting behavior, decreased nursing, difficult to arouse, moaning, drowsiness
Fluvoxamine	42–200	0.1–1.6	None located
Paroxetine	10–50	0.1–5.5	Irritability, alertness, constipation, sleepiness
Sertraline	25–200	<0.1–3.6	Discontinuation symptoms after nursing cessation
SNRIs			
Duloxetine	80	0.1	None located
Venlafaxine	75–400	3.5–9.22	None located
Desvenlafaxine	50–100	5.7–7.4	None located

TABLE 10–5. Antidepressant excretion into human breast milk and compatibility with breast feeding *(continued)*

DRUG	MATERNAL DOSAGE (MG/DAY)	RELATIVE INFANT DOSE (%)	REPORTED ADVERSE EFFECTS
Other antidepressants			
Bupropion	150–300	5.7	Seizure
Mirtazapine	3–120	0.5–4.4	Weight gain, sedation
Trazodone	50	0.4	

Note. SNRI=serotonin-norepinephrine reuptake inhibitor; SSRI=selective serotonin reuptake inhibitor; TCA=tricyclic antidepressant.
Source. Davis et al. 2009; Fortinguerra et al. 2009; U.S. National Library of Medicine 2011.

ate to severe postpartum depression. If a woman has had an effective trial of an antidepressant in the past, then that antidepressant may be reinitiated at one-half the usual starting dose to prevent side effects (Lanza di Scalea and Wisner 2009). For women who have not had a trial of antidepressant therapy in the past, paroxetine and sertraline are recommended first-line agents. A comprehensive personalized risk-benefit discussion should include the risks of undertreated or untreated depression for the mother and infant; the benefits of treated depression for both mother and infant; the benefits of breast-feeding for mother and child and the risks to the mother's or child's health associated with discontinuing breast-feeding; the risks of translactal antidepressant exposure to the infant; and nonpharmacological interventions if clinically appropriate.

Additionally, in my practice, I speak with the infant's pediatrician to discuss the possible adverse effects from antidepressant exposure so the infant can be monitored. Before maternal treatment is initiated, a pediatric evaluation of the child's baseline behavior, sleep, feeding, and alertness should be completed.

In summary, exposure to antidepressants during lactation is associated with less risk for the infant than that associated with their use in pregnancy. Based on the available evidence, breast-feeding should not generally be discouraged in women using some of the antidepressants discussed above as long as the infant is monitored by his or her pediatric provider for possible adverse effects.

KEY CLINICAL CONCEPTS

- Up to 18.4% of women suffer from depression during pregnancy, and 19.2% of mothers within the first several weeks after delivery experience postpartum depression.
- Untreated antenatal depression is associated with increased risk of underutilization of prenatal care, maternal inadequate weight gain, substance use, preeclampsia, and preterm birth; increased risk for delivery of an infant who is of low birth weight or who is small for gestational age; elective termination of the pregnancy; and postpartum depression and anxiety.
- Pregnant women who require antidepressant treatment should receive the minimal *effective* dose to maximally treat depression and minimize maternal and fetal exposure to antidepressants and the effects of undertreated depression.
- The SSRIs and possibly the TCAs may confer increased risks for some specific major malformations, but based on the current evidence, these malformations are rare and the absolute risks appear small.
- Late in utero exposure to SSRIs and SNRIs may be associated with several behavioral and neurological signs and symptoms in the neonate, such as tremor, shivering, hypertonia, feeding difficulties, irritability, respiratory disturbances, hyperreflexia, excess crying, and sleep disturbance.
- Data suggest that the use of antidepressants in pregnancy is associated with an increased risk of persistent pulmonary hypertension of the newborn.
- Two-thirds of pregnant women undergoing antidepressant monotherapy may require dose increases, especially after 20 weeks' gestation, to treat depressive symptoms or maintain euthymia.
- Women who discontinue successful antidepressant treatment to avoid further exposure to the fetus risk higher rates of depression recurrence than do women who maintain their antidepressant therapy during pregnancy.
- There are no reports of adverse effects in breast-fed infants of mothers treated with the TCAs amitriptyline, nortriptyline, imipramine, desipramine, and clomipramine.

- Among newer antidepressants, sertraline, paroxetine, and fluvoxamine are considered safer alternatives for the treatment of depression in lactation because they have the lowest degree of translactal passage and fewest reported adverse effects compared to other antidepressants.

References

Addis A, Koren G: Safety of fluoxetine during the first trimester of pregnancy: a meta-analytical review of epidemiological studies. Psychol Med 30:89–94, 2000

Alwan S, Reefhuis J, Rasmussen SA, et al: Use of selective serotonin-reuptake inhibitors in pregnancy and the risk of birth defects. N Engl J Med 356:2684–2692, 2007

Alwan S, Reefhuis J, Botto LD, et al: Maternal use of bupropion and risk for congenital heart defects. Am J Obstet Gynecol 203:52.e1–e6, 2010

American Academy of Pediatrics Committee on Drugs: Transfer of drugs and other chemicals into human milk. Pediatrics 108:776–789, 2001

Anderson GD: Pregnancy-induced changes in pharmacokinetics: a mechanistic-based approach. Clin Pharmacokinet 44:989–1008, 2005

Andrade SE, Raebel MA, Brown J, et al: Use of antidepressant medications during pregnancy: a multisite study. Am J Obstet Gynecol 198:194.e1–e5, 2008

Andrade SE, McPhillips H, Loren D, et al: Antidepressant medication use and risk of persistent pulmonary hypertension of the newborn. Pharmacoepidemiol Drug Saf 18:246–252, 2009

Bakker MK, Kerstjens-Frederikse WS, Buys CH, et al: First-trimester use of paroxetine and congenital heart defects: a population-based case-control study. Birth Defects Res A Clin Mol Teratol 88:94–100, 2010

Bar-Oz B, Einarson T, Einarson A, et al: Paroxetine and congenital malformations: meta-analysis and consideration of potential confounding factors. Clin Ther 29:918–926, 2007

Bérard A, Ramos E, Rey E, et al: First trimester exposure to paroxetine and risk of cardiac malformations in infants: the importance of dosage. Birth Defects Res B Dev Reprod Toxicol 80:18–27, 2007

Berle JO, Steen VM, Aamo TO, et al: Breastfeeding during maternal antidepressant treatment with serotonin reuptake inhibitors: infant exposure, clinical symptoms, and cytochrome P450 genotypes. J Clin Psychiatry 65:1228–1234, 2004

Beydoun H, Saftlas AF: Physical and mental health outcomes of prenatal maternal stress in human and animal studies: a review of recent evidence. Paediatr Perinat Epidemiol 22:438–466, 2008

Borri C, Mauri M, Oppo A, et al: Axis I psychopathology and functional impairment at the third month of pregnancy: results from the Perinatal Depression-Research and Screening Unit (PND-ReScU) study. J Clin Psychiatry 69:1617–1624, 2008

Boucher N, Bairam A, Beaulac-Baillargeon L: A new look at the neonate's clinical presentation after in utero exposure to antidepressants in late pregnancy. J Clin Psychopharmacol 28:334–339, 2008

Boucher N, Koren G, Beaulac-Baillargeon L: Maternal use of venlafaxine near term: correlation between neonatal effects and plasma concentrations. Ther Drug Monit 31:404–409, 2009

Brennan PA, Pargas R, Walker EF, et al: Maternal depression and infant cortisol: influences of timing, comorbidity and treatment. J Child Psychol Psychiatry 49:1099–1107, 2008

Buss C, Davis EP, Muftuler LT, et al: High pregnancy anxiety during mid-gestation is associated with decreased gray matter density in 6–9-year-old children. Psychoneuroendocrinology 35:141–153, 2010

Casper RC, Fleisher BE, Lee-Ancajas JC, et al: Follow-up of children of depressed mothers exposed or not exposed to antidepressant drugs during pregnancy. J Pediatr 142:402–408, 2003

Chambers CD, Johnson KA, Dick LM, et al: Birth outcomes in pregnant women taking fluoxetine. N Engl J Med 335:1010–1015, 1996

Chambers CD, Hernandez-Diaz S, Van Marter LJ, et al: Selective serotonin-reuptake inhibitors and risk of persistent pulmonary hypertension of the newborn. N Engl J Med 354:579–587, 2006

Chun-Fai-Chan B, Koren G, Fayez I, et al: Pregnancy outcome of women exposed to bupropion during pregnancy: a prospective comparative study. Am J Obstet Gynecol 192:932–936, 2005

Cohen LS, Altshuler LL, Harlow BL, et al: Relapse of major depression during pregnancy in women who maintain or discontinue antidepressant treatment. JAMA 295:499–507, 2006

Cole JA, Ephross SA, Cosmatos IS, et al: Paroxetine in the first trimester and the prevalence of congenital malformations. Pharmacoepidemiol Drug Saf 16:1075–1085, 2007a

Cole JA, Modell JG, Haight BR, et al: Bupropion in pregnancy and the prevalence of congenital malformations. Pharmacoepidemiol Drug Saf 16:474–484, 2007b

Costei AM, Kozer E, Ho T, et al: Perinatal outcome following third trimester exposure to paroxetine. Arch Pediatr Adolesc Med 156:1129–1132, 2002

Croen LA, Grether JK, Yoshida CK, et al: Antidepressant use during pregnancy and childhood autism spectrum disorders. Arch Gen Psychiatry July 4, 2011 (Epub)

Davis MF, Miller HS, Nolan PE Jr : Bupropion levels in breast milk for 4 mother-infant pairs: more answers to lingering questions. J Clin Psychiatry 70:297–298, 2009

Davis RL, Rubanowice D, McPhillips H, et al: Risks of congenital malformations and perinatal events among infants exposed to antidepressant medications during pregnancy. Pharmacoepidemiol Drug Saf 16:1086–1094, 2007

Deave T, Heron J, Evans J, et al: The impact of maternal depression in pregnancy on early child development. BJOG 115:1043–1051, 2008

Deligiannidis KM: Therapeutic drug monitoring in pregnant and postpartum women: recommendations for SSRIs, lamotrigine, and lithium. J Clin Psychiatry 71:649–650, 2010

Diav-Citrin O, Shechtman S, Weinbaum D, et al: Paroxetine and fluoxetine in pregnancy: a prospective, multicentre, controlled, observational study. Br J Clin Pharmacol 66:695–705, 2008

Djulus J, Koren G, Einarson TR, et al: Exposure to mirtazapine during pregnancy: a prospective, comparative study of birth outcomes. J Clin Psychiatry 67:1280–1284, 2006

Dubnov-Raz G, Juurlink DN, Fogelman R, et al: Antenatal use of selective serotonin-reuptake inhibitors and QT interval prolongation in newborns. Pediatrics 122:e710–e715, 2008

Einarson TR, Einarson A: Newer antidepressants in pregnancy and rates of major malformations: a meta-analysis of prospective comparative studies. Pharmacoepidemiol Drug Saf 14:823–827, 2005

Einarson A, Fatoye B, Sarkar M, et al: Pregnancy outcome following gestational exposure to venlafaxine: a multicenter prospective controlled study. Am J Psychiatry 158:1728–1730, 2001

Einarson A, Bonari L, Voyer-Lavigne S, et al: A multicentre prospective controlled study to determine the safety of trazodone and nefazodone during pregnancy. Can J Psychiatry 48:106–110, 2003

Einarson A, Pistelli A, DeSantis M, et al: Evaluation of the risk of congenital cardiovascular defects associated with use of paroxetine during pregnancy. Am J Psychiatry 165:749–752, 2008

Einarson A, Choi J, Einarson TR, et al: Incidence of major malformations in infants following antidepressant exposure in pregnancy: results of a large prospective cohort study. Can J Psychiatry 54:242–246, 2009a

Einarson A, Choi J, Einarson TR, et al: Rates of spontaneous and therapeutic abortions following use of antidepressants in pregnancy: results from a large prospective database. J Obstet Gynaecol Can 31:452–456, 2009b

Epperson [C]N, Czarkowski KA, Ward-O'Brien D, et al: Maternal sertraline treatment and serotonin transport in breast-feeding mother-infant pairs. Am J Psychiatry 158:1631–1637, 2001

Epperson CN, Jatlow PI, Czarkowski K, et al: Maternal fluoxetine treatment in the postpartum period: effects on platelet serotonin and plasma drug levels in breastfeeding mother-infant pairs. Pediatrics 112:e425, 2003

Ericson A, Kallen B, Wiholm B: Delivery outcome after the use of antidepressants in early pregnancy. Eur J Clin Pharmacol 55:503–508, 1999

Ferreira E, Carceller AM, Agogue C, et al: Effects of selective serotonin reuptake inhibitors and venlafaxine during pregnancy in term and preterm neonates. Pediatrics 119:52–59, 2007

Figueroa R: Use of antidepressants during pregnancy and risk of attention-deficit/hyperactivity disorder in the offspring. J Dev Behav Pediatr 31:641–648, 2010

Fornaro E, Li D, Pan J, et al: Prenatal exposure to fluoxetine induces fetal pulmonary hypertension in the rat. Am J Respir Crit Care Med 176:1035–1040, 2007

Fortinguerra F, Clavenna A, Bonati M: Psychotropic drug use during breastfeeding: a review of the evidence. Pediatrics 124:e547–e556, 2009

Frey OR, Scheidt P, von Brenndorff AI: Adverse effects in a newborn infant breast-fed by a mother treated with doxepin. Ann Pharmacother 33:690–693, 1999

Galbally M, Lewis AJ, Lum J, et al: Serotonin discontinuation syndrome following in utero exposure to antidepressant medication: prospective controlled study. Aust N Z J Psychiatry 43:846–854, 2009

Gavin NI, Gaynes BN, Lohr KN, et al: Perinatal depression: a systematic review of prevalence and incidence. Obstet Gynecol 106:1071–1083, 2005

Gentile S, Galbally M: Prenatal exposure to antidepressant medications and neurodevelopmental outcomes: a systematic review. J Affect Disord 128:1–9, 2011

Greenough A, Khetriwal B: Pulmonary hypertension in the newborn. Paediatr Respir Rev 6:111–116, 2005

Grote NK, Bridge JA, Gavin AR, et al: A meta-analysis of depression during pregnancy and the risk of preterm birth, low birth weight, and intrauterine growth restriction. Arch Gen Psychiatry 67:1012–1024, 2010

Heikkinen T, Ekblad U, Kero P, et al: Citalopram in pregnancy and lactation. Clin Pharmacol Ther 72:184–191, 2002

Heikkinen T, Ekblad U, Palo P, et al: Pharmacokinetics of fluoxetine and norfluoxetine in pregnancy and lactation. Clin Pharmacol Ther 73:330–337, 2003

Hemels ME, Einarson A, Koren G, et al: Antidepressant use during pregnancy and the rates of spontaneous abortions: a meta-analysis. Ann Pharmacother 39:803–809, 2005

Hostetter A, Stowe ZN, Strader JR Jr, et al: Dose of selective serotonin uptake inhibitors across pregnancy: clinical implications. Depress Anxiety 11:51–57, 2000

James DC, Lessen R, American Dietetic Association: Position of the American Dietetic Association: promoting and supporting breastfeeding. J Am Diet Assoc 109:1926–1942, 2009

Källén B: Neonate characteristics after maternal use of antidepressants in late pregnancy. Arch Pediatr Adolesc Med 158:312–316, 2004

Källén B, Olausson PO: Maternal use of selective serotonin re-uptake inhibitors and persistent pulmonary hypertension of the newborn. Pharmacoepidemiol Drug Saf 17:801–806, 2008

Källén BA, Otterblad Olausson P: Maternal use of selective serotonin re-uptake inhibitors in early pregnancy and infant congenital malformations. Birth Defects Res A Clin Mol Teratol 79:301–308, 2007

Koren G, Boucher N: Adverse effects in neonates exposed to SSRIs and SNRI in late gestation—Motherisk Update 2008. Can J Clin Pharmacol 16:e66–67, 2009

Kornum JB, Nielsen RB, Pedersen L, et al: Use of selective serotonin-reuptake inhibitors during early pregnancy and risk of congenital malformations: updated analysis. Clin Epidemiol 2:29–36, 2010

Kulin NA, Pastuszak A, Sage SR, et al: Pregnancy outcome following maternal use of the new selective serotonin reuptake inhibitors: a prospective controlled multicenter study. JAMA 279:609–610, 1998

Lanza di Scalea T, Wisner KL: Antidepressant medication use during breastfeeding. Clin Obstet Gynecol 52:483–497, 2009

Lennestal R, Källén B: Delivery outcome in relation to maternal use of some recently introduced antidepressants. J Clin Psychopharmacol 27:607–613, 2007

Lobel M, Cannella DL, Graham JE, et al: Pregnancy-specific stress, prenatal health behaviors, and birth outcomes. Health Psychol 27:604–615, 2008

Louik C, Lin AE, Werler MM, et al: First-trimester use of selective serotonin-reuptake inhibitors and the risk of birth defects. N Engl J Med 356:2675–2683, 2007

Lund N, Pedersen LH, Henriksen TB: Selective serotonin reuptake inhibitor exposure in utero and pregnancy outcomes. Arch Pediatr Adolesc Med 163:949–954, 2009

Maschi S, Clavenna A, Campi R, et al: Neonatal outcome following pregnancy exposure to antidepressants: a prospective controlled cohort study. BJOG 115:283–289, 2008

Mortensen JT, Olsen J, Larsen H, et al: Psychomotor development in children exposed in utero to benzodiazepines, antidepressants, neuroleptics, and anti-epileptics. Eur J Epidemiol 18:769–771, 2003

Moses-Kolko EL, Bogen D, Perel J, et al: Neonatal signs after late in utero exposure to serotonin reuptake inhibitors: literature review and implications for clinical applications. JAMA 293:2372–2383, 2005

Nakhai-Pour HR, Broy P, Bérard A: Use of antidepressants during pregnancy and the risk of spontaneous abortion. CMAJ 182:1031–1037, 2010

Newport DJ, Ritchie JC, Knight BT, et al: Venlafaxine in human breast milk and nursing infant plasma: determination of exposure. J Clin Psychiatry 70:1304–1310, 2009

Nybo Andersen AM, Wohlfahrt J, Christens P, et al: Maternal age and fetal loss: population based register linkage study. BMJ 320(7251):1708–1712, 2000

Oberlander TF, Misri S, Fitzgerald CE, et al: Pharmacologic factors associated with transient neonatal symptoms following prenatal psychotropic medication exposure. J Clin Psychiatry 65:230–237, 2004

Oberlander TF, Warburton W, Misri S, et al: Neonatal outcomes after prenatal exposure to selective serotonin reuptake inhibitor antidepressants and maternal depression using population-based linked health data. Arch Gen Psychiatry 63:898–906, 2006

Oberlander TF, Bonaguro RJ, Misri S, et al: Infant serotonin transporter (SLC6A4) promoter genotype is associated with adverse neonatal outcomes after prenatal exposure to serotonin reuptake inhibitor medications. Mol Psychiatry 13:65–73, 2008a

Oberlander TF, Warburton W, Misri S, et al: Major congenital malformations following prenatal exposure to serotonin reuptake inhibitors and benzodiazepines using population-based health data. Birth Defects Res B Dev Reprod Toxicol 83:68–76, 2008b

O'Brien L, Einarson TR, Sarkar M, et al: Does paroxetine cause cardiac malformations? J Obstet Gynaecol Can 30:696–701, 2008

Oesterheld JR: A review of developmental aspects of cytochrome P450. J Child Adolesc Psychopharmacol 8:161–174, 1998

Pakalapati RK, Bolisetty S, Austin MP, et al: Neonatal seizures from in utero venlafaxine exposure. J Paediatr Child Health 42:737–738, 2006

Pastuszak A, Schick-Boschetto B, Zuber C, et al: Pregnancy outcome following first-trimester exposure to fluoxetine (Prozac). JAMA 269:2246–2248, 1993

Paulson JF, Keefe HA, Leiferman JA: Early parental depression and child language development. J Child Psychol Psychiatry 50:254–262, 2009

Pedersen LH, Henriksen TB, Vestergaard M, et al: Selective serotonin reuptake inhibitors in pregnancy and congenital malformations: population based cohort study. BMJ 339:B3569, 2009

Pilowsky DJ, Wickramaratne PJ, Rush AJ, et al: Children of currently depressed mothers: a STAR*D ancillary study. J Clin Psychiatry 67:126–136, 2006

Rahimi R, Nikfar S, Abdollahi M: Pregnancy outcomes following exposure to serotonin reuptake inhibitors: a meta-analysis of clinical trials. Reprod Toxicol 22:571–575, 2006

Ramos E, St-André M, Rey E, et al: Duration of antidepressant use during pregnancy and risk of major congenital malformations. Br J Psychiatry 192:344–350, 2008

Reck C, Struben K, Backenstrass M, et al: Prevalence, onset and comorbidity of postpartum anxiety and depressive disorders. Acta Psychiatr Scand 118:459–468, 2008

Reis M, Källén B: Delivery outcome after maternal use of antidepressant drugs in pregnancy: an update using Swedish data. Psychol Med 40:1723–1733, 2010

Salkeld E, Ferris LE, Juurlink DN: The risk of postpartum hemorrhage with selective serotonin reuptake inhibitors and other antidepressants. J Clin Psychopharmacol 28:230–234, 2008

Shuren J: Content and format of labeling for human prescription drug and biological products: requirements for pregnancy and lactation labeling. Federal Register, May 29, 2008. Available at: www.federalregister.gov/articles/2008/05/29/E8-11806/content-and-format-of-labeling-for-human-prescription-drug-and-biological-products-requirements-for. Accessed May 17, 2011.

Simon GE, Cunningham ML, Davis RL: Outcomes of prenatal antidepressant exposure. Am J Psychiatry 159:2055–2061, 2002

Sit DK, Perel JM, Helsel JC, et al: Changes in antidepressant metabolism and dosing across pregnancy and early postpartum. J Clin Psychiatry 69:652–658, 2008

Sivojelezova A, Shuhaiber S, Sarkissian L, et al: Citalopram use in pregnancy: prospective comparative evaluation of pregnancy and fetal outcome. Am J Obstet Gynecol 193:2004–2009, 2005

Stuebe AM, Schwarz EB: The risks and benefits of infant feeding practices for women and their children. J Perinatol 30:155–162, 2010

Suri R, Altshuler L, Hellemann G, et al: Effects of antenatal depression and antidepressant treatment on gestational age at birth and risk of preterm birth. Am J Psychiatry 164:1206–1213, 2007

Tracy TS, Venkataramanan R, Glover DD, et al: Temporal changes in drug metabolism (CYP1A2, CYP2D6 and CYP3A activity) during pregnancy. Am J Obstet Gynecol 192:633–639, 2005

Tuccori M, Testi A, Antonioli L, et al: Safety concerns associated with the use of serotonin reuptake inhibitors and other serotonergic/noradrenergic antidepressants during pregnancy: a review. Clin Ther 31:1426–1453, 2009

U.S. National Library of Medicine: TOXNET: Toxicology data network. Drugs and lactation database (LactMed). Available at: http://toxnet.nlm.nih.gov/cgi-bin/sis/htmlgen?LACT. Accessed May 17, 2011.

Ververs T, Kaasenbrood H, Visser G, et al: Prevalence and patterns of antidepressant drug use during pregnancy. Eur J Clin Pharmacol 62:863–870, 2006

Wadelius M, Darj E, Frenne G, et al: Induction of CYP2D6 in pregnancy. Clin Pharmacol Ther 62:400–407, 1997

Walsh-Sukys MC, Tyson JE, Wright LL, et al: Persistent pulmonary hypertension of the newborn in the era before nitric oxide: practice variation and outcomes. Pediatrics 105:14–20, 2000

Warburton W, Hertzman C, Oberlander TF: A register study of the impact of stopping third trimester selective serotonin reuptake inhibitor exposure on neonatal health. Acta Psychiatr Scand 121:471–479, 2010

Wichman CL, Moore KM, Lang TR, et al: Congenital heart disease associated with selective serotonin reuptake inhibitor use during pregnancy. Mayo Clin Proc 84:23–27, 2009

Wilson KL, Zelig CM, Harvey JP, et al: Persistent pulmonary hypertension of the newborn is associated with mode of delivery and not with maternal use of selective serotonin reuptake inhibitors. Am J Perinatol 28:19–24, 2011

Wisner KL, Sit DK, Hanusa BH, et al: Major depression and antidepressant treatment: impact on pregnancy and neonatal outcomes. Am J Psychiatry 166:557–566, 2009

Wurst KE, Poole C, Ephross SA, et al: First trimester paroxetine use and the prevalence of congenital, specifically cardiac, defects: a meta-analysis of epidemiological studies. Birth Defects Res A Clin Mol Teratol 88:159–170, 2010

Yaris F, Kadioglu M, Kesim M, et al: Newer antidepressants in pregnancy: prospective outcome of a case series. Reprod Toxicol 19:235–238, 2004

Yonkers KA, Wisner KL, Stewart DE, et al: The management of depression during pregnancy: a report from the American Psychiatric Association and the American College of Obstetricians and Gynecologists. Gen Hosp Psychiatry 31:403–413, 2009

Zhu SP, Mao ZF, Huang J, et al: Continuous fluoxetine administration prevents recurrence of pulmonary arterial hypertension and prolongs survival in rats. Clin Exp Pharmacol Physiol 36:E1–E5, 2009

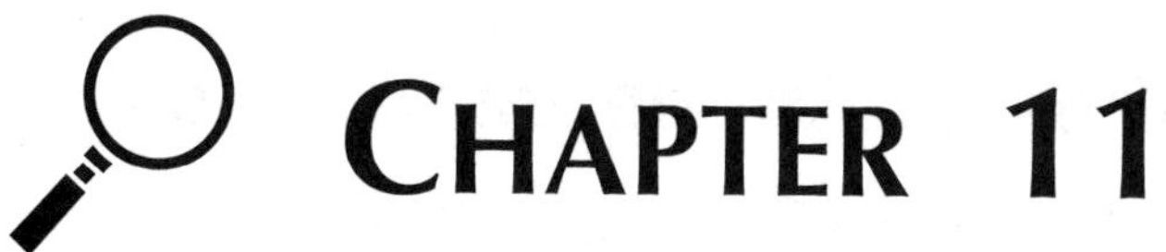

CHAPTER 11

Use of Antidepressants in Patients Receiving Nursing Care

Judith Shindul-Rothschild, Ph.D., R.N.P.C.

PATIENTS PRESCRIBED antidepressants are provided nursing care in a wide range of practice settings and specialties. Most antidepressants are prescribed by physicians and advanced practice nurses (APNs) in specialties other than psychiatry. For nurse practitioners (NPs) in primary care, pediatric offices, rural health, and long-term-care facilities, evidence-based guidelines are key to optimizing treatment outcomes for patients. In this chapter, I describe best practices for APNs who prescribe antidepressants, with a focus on providing evidence-based, patient-focused care across the life span. I also identify empirically based nursing interventions to assess serious adverse effects and enhance treatment adherence for culturally diverse populations prescribed antidepressants.

Prescription of Antidepressants by Advanced Practice Nurses

APNs, a group that includes NPs and advanced practice psychiatric nurses (APPNs), are legally authorized to independently prescribe medications in 14 states and to prescribe with some physician collaboration in all states and the District of Columbia (American College of Physicians 2009). Consistent with the legal scope of prescriptive authority, a national survey of NPs found that 13.7% do not consult with a physician for any patient encounters (Scudder 2006). Antidepressants are among the most commonly prescribed class of medication by NPs (Cipher et al. 2006; Scudder 2006) and the most commonly prescribed class by APPNs (Glod and Manchester 2000).

In a survey of prescribing practices among APPNs for major depression, almost all (97.3%) of the APPNs stated that their usual first choice of medication would be a selective serotonin reuptake inhibitor (SSRI) (Wolfe et al. 2008). If the patient was nonresponsive to an SSRI, 61.6% of APPNs stated that their next step would be to increase the dosage, 17% would switch to another SSRI, 10% would switch to a non-SSRI agent, and 6.2% would choose an augmentation strategy (Wolfe et al. 2008). Antidepressant prescribing practices self-reported by APPNs are consistent with practice guidelines for the treatment of major depression published by the American Psychiatric Association (APA; American Psychiatric Association 2010) and the American College of Physicians (Qaseem et al. 2008).

Prescribing patterns of APPNs and psychiatrists, including selection of antidepressant, dosing, duration of treatment, and documentation of treatment, are comparable (Feldman et al. 2003). When patients are in integrated treatment for psychopharmacology and psychotherapy, prescriptions of SSRIs are very similar between psychiatrists and APPNs (Jacobs 2005). In split treatment, psychiatrists are more likely to prescribe other classes of antidepressant medication (55%) than are APPNs (32%), which may reflect the complexity of cases referred to psychiatrists (Jacobs 2005).

Data from the 1996–2006 National Ambulatory Medical Care Survey indicated that prescriptions to adults for two or more antidepressants and antidepressant-antipsychotic combinations significantly increased during the decade (Mojtabai and Olfson 2010). Despite the lack of research on the safety and efficacy of polypharmacy in children, from 1996 to 2007, polypharmacy in children who were diagnosed with a major mental illness rose significantly to 32.2% of all pediatric visits (Comer et al. 2010). The most common polypharmacy practice in pediatrics is the simultaneous prescription of an antidepressant with a psychostimulant or an antipsychotic medication (Comer et al. 2010).

Studies that compare the polypharmacy and augmentation strategies used by psychiatrists versus APPNs suggest that APPNs are more conservative in their prescribing practices. From 2004 to 2007, psychotropic medications from different classes were concomitantly prescribed to pediatric patients by 15.8% of APNs versus 78.2% of psychiatrists (Comer et al. 2010). Jacobs (2005) reported that in an adult population, almost half (48%) of APPNs used monotherapy compared with 10% of psychiatrists. Similarly, a retrospective study of psychotropic claims data found that psychiatrists were significantly more likely than APPNs to augment and switch antidepressant medication, whereas APPNs were significantly less likely than psychiatrists to prescribe two or more antidepressants concomitantly (Feldman et al. 2003).

A study of prescribing clinicians in Nebraska suggests that the antidepressant prescribing practices of APNs are closely aligned with those of physicians in the same specialty (Bhatia et al. 2008). Prior to the issuance of a black box warning by the U.S. Food and Drug Administration (FDA) on the risk of suicidality among adolescents prescribed SSRIs, family NPs and family medicine physicians were the most likely to prescribe antidepressants to children and adolescents (79.8%), compared with APPNs and psychiatrists (71.3%) and pediatric NPs and pediatricians (69.1%). However, after the black box warning, psychiatric clinicians (71.3%) were the most likely to prescribe antidepressants, followed by family medicine clinicians (68.3%) and pediatric clinicians (65.5%). APPNs and psychiatrists were also more likely than family or pediatric clinicians to initially prescribe medication approved by the FDA for use with pediatric patients. Only a fraction (7.5%) of all clinicians followed guidelines by the FDA to have weekly follow-up visits with pediatric patients started on an antidepressant (Bhatia et al. 2008).

In general, prescribing practices for the use of antidepressants are similar for APPNs and psychiatrists, and both follow the APA treatment guideline for major depression (American Psychiatric Association 2010). One notable difference is that APPNs are more likely than psychiatrists to avoid polypharmacy in both pediatric and adult populations. APPNs are also less likely to prescribe antidepressants "off label" to youth than are NPs in other clinical specialties. Despite efforts through use of evidence-based protocols and quality initiatives to minimize polypharmacy and "off-label" prescribing in youth, these practices have increased significantly over the past decade (Comer et al. 2010). In light of these trends, an important observation is that studies indicate that APPNs do adhere to evidence-based practice and therefore can be a valuable resource to APNs in other specialties and physicians in primary care.

Promoting Evidence-Based Use of Antidepressants Through Collaborative Practice Models

In the majority of states, laws governing the prescriptive authority of APNs mandate collaboration with physicians. The principles of collaboration defined by the American College of Physicians (2009) include communicating in face-to-face contact, through electronic medical records (EMR), and via email. Effective communication between physicians and APNs is foundational to promoting evidence-based practice, especially among nonpsychiatric specialties.

Nurses and physicians express confidence in the ability of each profession to assess and treat depression; however, both nurses and physicians agree that communicating clinical symptoms of depression and interdisciplinary collaboration are problematic (Brown et al. 2006). Kerber et al. (2008) found that when nurses use the Geriatric Depression Scale or Minimum Data Set to properly identify nursing home residents exhibiting symptoms of depression, older adults remain undertreated by primary care providers (PCPs).

An example of a best-practice model to improve PCP and nurse collaboration is the TRaining In the Assessment of Depression (TRIAD) intervention (Brown et al. 2010). The aim of TRIAD is to improve depression recognition and communication between nurses and physicians working with long-term-care patients, using the Outcome and Assessment Information Set (OASIS) as a screening instrument. Home care nurses who received training to assess depression and use OASIS were significantly more likely to identify at-risk patients and to initiate referrals to physicians, which improved clinical outcomes for depressed older adults (Brown et al. 2010). A best-practice model to improve collaboration between PCPs and psychiatric clinicians is a patient-centered medical home in which teams of multidisciplinary providers collectively care for a patient population.

In a collaborative care model for homebound, depressed older adults, an APPN conducted an initial assessment using the Hamilton Depression Rating Scale (Ham-D) and the Geriatric Depression Scale (GDS). Following the initial screening and assessment, the APPN and PCP were in frequent contact to reevaluate medication that could be contributing to depressive symptoms and the efficacy of antidepressant treatment. When the APPN-PCP collaborative model was initiated, 39% of homebound study participants were prescribed inadequate dosages of antidepressant medication and were receiving an average of 10 medications to treat medical and psychiatric conditions. Enhanced collaboration in the APPN-PCP model promoted timely assessment of the risks and benefits of pharmacological treatment and dosage adjustments to improve antidepressant efficacy. Knight and Houseman (2008) reported that homebound older adults who received the APPN-PCP collaborative model intervention had significantly greater improvement in depression scores than did homebound elders who did not receive the APPN-PCP model of care. The Centers for Disease Control Task Force on Community Preventive Services (2009) has concluded that strong evidence exists to recommend collaborative models of care for the treatment of homebound older adults suffering from major depression.

The Massachusetts Consortium on Depression in Primary Care (MCDPC) sought to improve the treatment of depression in primary care using a collaborative care model that included PCPs, mental health clinicians, and case managers (Upshur and Weinreb 2008). Intake assessment and screening in the MCDPC study was conducted by PCPs with the nine-item Patient Health Questionnaire (PHQ-9). Although there was initial resistance by PCPs to use the PHQ-9, the MCDPC study found that use of the PHQ-9 improved communication among the PCPs, mental health providers, and case managers because it allowed them to quickly identify depressive symptoms. Collaboration between PCPs, mental health providers, and case managers was facilitated by regular phone consultation and face-to-face contacts. PCPs reported that caring for depressed patients was less burdensome using a collaborative care model because a case manager was available to assist with patient management (see Table 11–1 for another example of collaborative care).

A collaborative care model similar to the one described in the MCDPC has been studied in a population of depressed adolescents (Richardson et al. 2009). PCPs identified at-risk youth who were screened with the PHQ-9 and referred to a nurse case manager with expertise in depression for mental health evaluation. Nurse case managers were supervised by a child psychiatrist or psychologist by phone or in person. Interdisciplinary team meetings involving psychiatric and primary care clinicians were conducted weekly for new patients or patients with treatment-resistant depression. All clinicians documented treatment and consultation using an electronic medical record. The authors concluded that the collaborative care model is feasible to implement in primary care and significantly improved treatment outcomes for depressed adolescents.

Studies suggest that collaborative care models can be effective in promoting evidence-based treatment for depressed individuals across the life span (Gilbody et al. 2006). The Centers for Disease Control Task Force on Community Preventive Services (2009) recommends a collaborative care model for treatment of adults with depression in primary care because of the clear benefit of the model in promoting evidence-based practice and improving patient outcomes. Key components of collaborative care include screening with easy-to-administer standardized instruments, on-site case management by a mental

TABLE 11–1. National Registry of Evidence-based Programs and Practices: Partners in Care

Partners in Care (PIC) is based on collaborative care models, in which there is increased collaboration among primary care clinicians, mental health specialists, nurses, and patients. PIC is suitable for use with teenagers through older adults.

PIC educates primary care providers on evidence-based treatment of depression and provides access to mental health specialists. Mental health specialists include a depression nurse specialist who provides case management and acts as a nurse expert leader to provide education, supervision, and clinical support in case of emergencies. The depression nurse specialist is involved administratively and clinically in the PIC model. Psychiatrists provide consultation and are available to take referrals of complex cases.

Health care organizations participating in PIC receive the following:

- The Clinician Guide to Depression Assessment and Management in Primary Care, which gives primary care providers information regarding assessment and treatment, and references on education, medications, and psychotherapy
- Pocket-sized Quick Reference Cards, which summarize key points from the clinician guide and include information on antidepressants, including dosages, side effects, and typical costs
- Individual and group cognitive-behavioral therapy manuals
- Guidelines and Resources for the Depression Nurse Specialist, containing instructions, forms, and materials needed to carry out case management
- Patient education brochures, suitable for use with patients with major depression, as well as patients who feel sad but do not have the full-blown illness

Source. Adapted from SAMHSA's National Registry of Evidence-based Programs and Practices: "Partners in Care." November 2009. Available at: www.nrepp.samhsa.gov/ViewIntervention.aspx?id=126. Accessed August 15, 2010; and RAND Partners in Care: "Planning to Implement the PIC Approach." August 17, 2010. Available at: www.rand.org/health/projects/pic/approach.html. Accessed August 4, 2011.

health specialist, regular supervision and/or consultation by mental health clinicians, and timely communication among all members of the treatment team. In primary care settings, organizational barriers and clinician behavior have been identified as factors that hinder the implementation of evidence-based guidelines for the treatment of depression (Henke et al. 2008). One significant organizational barrier to effective communication among clinicians involves

TABLE 11–2. Description of Telemedicine-Based Collaborative Care from the National Registry of Evidence-based Practices

Telemedicine-Based Collaborative Care is designed to improve depression treatment outcomes in rural primary care practices that lack on-site mental health specialists. The intervention uses telecommunication technologies to facilitate collaboration between primary care providers and a depression care team that consists of nurses, pharmacists, APPNs, and psychiatrists. Nurse practitioners and primary care physicians screen patients for depression, make diagnoses, and prescribe antidepressants. Patients in treatment for depression have biweekly contacts with a registered nurse (RN) case manager. RN interviews are guided by a Web-based decision support system (NetDSS) that includes evidence-based instruments and scripts. RN case managers provide patient education, assessment, and evaluation of treatment adherence. Psychiatrists and APPNs provide clinical supervision for RNs and consultation to primary care providers through teleconferencing. Interactive video is used by APPNs and psychiatrists to conduct patient interviews and to provide evidence-based psychotherapy.

Note. APPN=advanced practice psychiatric nurses; RN=registered nurse.
Source. Adapted from SAMHSA's National Registry of Evidence-based Programs and Practices: "Telemedicine-Based Collaborative Care." January 2010. Available at: www.nrepp.samhsa.gov/ViewIntervention.aspx?id=127. Accessed August 15, 2010.

time constraints. The American College of Physicians (2009) recommends that physicians and nurses use a variety of information technologies to facilitate timely communication among all members of the treatment team (e.g., a description of telemedicine-based collaborative care is provided in Table 11–2).

Evidence-Based Guidelines: Implications for Nursing Practice

Depression Screening and Treatment

Children and Adolescents

The U.S. Preventive Services Task Force (USPSTF), a division of the Agency for Healthcare Research and Quality, issued separate depression screening guidelines for adolescents ages 12–18 years and children ages 7–11 years (U.S. Preventive Services Task Force 2009b; see Table 11–3). The USPSTF clinical guidelines for adolescents support routine depression screening only when "systems" are in place for proper diagnosis, treatment, and evaluation of major depressive disorders (U.S. Preventive Services Task Force 2009b, p. 1223). The challenge for NPs is to properly identify those adolescents who can be effectively managed in a primary care setting versus those whose treatment should be managed by child and family psychiatric nurse specialists (Raphel 2009). Risk factors that PCPs should consider in making a referral to mental health specialists include a history of suicide, parental depression, comorbid mental disorders (e.g., substance abuse), chronic medical conditions, and having experienced a major loss or stressful life event (U.S. Preventive Services Task Force 2009b).

The Patient Health Questionnaire for Adolescents (PHQ-A) and the Beck Depression Inventory—Primary Care (BDI-PC) were both found to have good sensitivity and specificity in adolescent populations and are recommended by the USPSTF (2009b) for routine screening. The USPSTF does not recommend routine depression screening for children, because currently insufficient evidence exists on the accuracy of depression screening instruments for use in children. Treatment guidelines endorse the use of medications alone or in combination with cognitive-behavioral and interpersonal therapies for adolescents with major depression. The USPSTF guidelines for adolescents stress that because of the potential risk of increased suicidality associated with SSRIs, these antidepressants should be prescribed only if clinical monitoring is available. Clinical monitoring by APNs should be once a week for the first month after starting an SSRI and once a month when symptoms have stabilized (Hamrin and Magorno 2010). The USPSTF states that insufficient scientific evidence exists on the risks and benefits of psychotherapy and medication for children under age 11 who meet the criteria for major depression.

The USPSTF (2009b) acknowledges a need for further research on the efficacy of collaborative care models to improve outcomes for depressed children and adolescents when compared with usual care by PCPs. The Academy of Pediatrics Task Force on Mental Health (Foy et al. 2010) recommends that mental health specialists assume treatment responsibility for children with major depressive disorder in a "shared care model" that includes a communication protocol to facilitate progress monitoring among PCPs, care providers in schools, and mental health specialists. A key feature of collaborative care models in pediatric primary care is that child or family psychiatric NPs assume responsibility for medication management and mental health treatment when children exhibit unsafe behaviors; have a family history of suicide or abuse; have treatment-resistant or recurrent depression; or have severe psychosocial stress, comorbid substance abuse, hypomania, or psychotic symptoms (Hamrin and Magorno 2010).

Although few studies have investigated the efficacy of collaborative care models, randomized controlled trials have reported that when close collaboration

TABLE 11–3. Screening and treatment for major depressive disorder in children and adolescents: clinical summary of U.S. Preventive Services Task Force Recommendation

POPULATION	ADOLESCENTS (12–18 YEARS)	CHILDREN (7–11 YEARS)
Recommendation	Screen (when systems for diagnosis, treatment, and follow-up are in place) Grade: B	No recommendation. Grade: I (insufficient evidence).
Risk assessment	Risk factors for major depressive disorder (MDD) include parental depression, having comorbid mental health or chronic medical conditions, and having experienced a major negative life event.	
Screening tests	The following screening tests have been shown to do well in teens in primary care settings: • Patient Health Questionnaire for Adolescents (PHQ-A) • Beck Depression Inventory—Primary Care Version (BDI-PC)	Screening instruments perform less well in younger children.
Treatments	Among pharmacotherapies fluoxetine, a selective serotonin reuptake inhibitor (SSRI), has been found efficacious. However, because of risk of suicidality, SSRIs should be considered only if clinical monitoring is possible. Various modes of psychotherapy, and pharmacotherapy combined with psychotherapy, have been found efficacious.	Evidence on the balance of benefits and harms of treatment of younger children is insufficient for a recommendation.

Source. Reprinted from U.S. Preventive Services Task Force: "Screening and Treatment for Major Depressive Disorder in Children and Adolescents: Clinical Summary of U.S. Preventive Services Task Force Recommendation." AHRQ Publication No. 09–05130-EF-3, March 2009. Available at: www.uspreventiveservicestaskforce.org/uspstf09/depression/chdeprsum.htm. Accessed August 21, 2010.

exists between PCPs and mental health specialists, the treatment outcomes for depressed adolescents improve, primarily because adolescents receive more psychotherapy than when they receive usual care (Williams et al. 2009). Pediatric NPs have an important role in ruling out medical or pharmacological etiologies for behavioral symptoms and in referring children or adolescents to mental health specialists early in the course of depression (Hamrin and Magorno 2010). Competencies for pediatric PCPs proposed by the American Academy of Pediatrics (2009) include applying evidence-based interventions for depressed children and adolescents, with a caveat that pediatric providers must refer psychiatric emergencies or children who exhibit severe and complex behaviors to mental health specialists.

In the primary care setting, nurses certified as child and adolescent psychiatric NPs, family psychiatric NPs, and psychiatric clinical nurse specialists offer expertise in psychiatric evaluation, the prescription of antidepressants, and psychotherapy for children and their families (Raphel 2009). The colocation of APPNs in pediatric offices, school-based clinics, and other primary care settings facilitates consultation with PCPs, especially in communities where shortages in child mental health specialists can lead to delays in referrals for treatment. Surveys of mental health administrators have identified multiple benefits of medication management by APPNs in pediatric practices; benefits include cost-effectiveness, improved family satisfaction, and easier access to specialized psychiatric treatment (Kaye et al. 2009). To promote colocation of APPNs or other mental health specialists in primary care practices, the American Academy of Child and Adolescent Psychiatry (2010; see "Web Resources" later in this chapter) proposes several reforms to insurance payment policies for mental health services. As these new models of health care delivery become more widely adopted, nurses must be prepared to practice in an environment that requires greater collaborative skills, innovative use of information technology, and a thorough knowledge of evidence-based practice (Delaney 2010).

Adults

The mandate of the USPSTF is to analyze the scientific evidence on the efficacy of clinical preventive services, including depression screening, counseling, and medication treatment (U.S. Preventive Services Task Force 2010). On the basis of this analysis, national experts convened by the USPSTF use standardized grading criteria to formulate recommendations that are considered the "gold standard" for clinical preventive services (Table 11–4; see also Table 11–5). The USPSTF recommendations are the basis of clinical guidelines endorsed by the American Academy of Nurse Practitioners, the National As-

TABLE 11–4. Screening for depression in adults: clinical summary of U.S. Preventive Services Task Force Recommendation

POPULATION	NONPREGNANT ADULTS 18 YEARS OR OLDER	
Recommendation	Screen when "staff-assisted depression care supports"* are in place to assure accurate diagnosis, effective treatment, and follow-up. Grade: B	Do not routinely screen when "staff-assisted depression care supports"* are not in place. Grade: C
Risk assessment	Persons at increased risk for depression are considered at risk throughout their lifetime. Groups at increased risk include persons with other psychiatric disorders, including substance misuse; persons with a family history of depression; persons with chronic medical diseases; and persons who are unemployed or of lower socioeconomic status. Also, women are at increased risk compared with men. However, the presence of risk factors alone cannot distinguish depressed patients from nondepressed patients.	
Screening tests	Simple screening questions may perform as well as more complex instruments. Any positive screening test result should trigger a full diagnostic interview using standard diagnostic criteria.	
Timing of screening	The optimal interval for screening is unknown. In older adults, significant depressive symptoms are associated with common life events, including medical illness, cognitive decline, bereavement, and institutional placement in residential or inpatient settings.	

TABLE 11–4. Screening for depression in adults: clinical summary of U.S. Preventive Services Task Force Recommendation *(continued)*

POPULATION	NONPREGNANT ADULTS 18 YEARS OR OLDER
Balance of harms and benefits	Limited evidence suggests that screening for depression in the absence of staff-assisted depression care does not improve depression outcomes.

*"Staff-assisted depression care supports" refers to clinical staff that assists the primary care clinician by providing some direct depression care and/or coordination, case management, or mental health treatment.

Source. Reprinted from U.S. Preventive Services Task Force: "Screening for Depression in Adults: Clinical Summary of U.S. Preventive Services Task Force Recommendation." AHRQ Publication No. 10–05143-EF-3, December 2009. Available at: www.uspreventiveservicestaskforce.org/uspstf09/adultdepression/addeprsum.htm. Accessed August 31, 2009.

TABLE 11–5. USPSTF recommendation grades and suggestions

Grade	Grade definition	Suggestions for practice
A	The USPSTF recommends the service. There is high certainty that the net benefit is substantial.	Offer or provide this service.
B	The USPSTF recommends the service. There is high certainty that the net benefit is moderate or there is moderate certainty that the net benefit is moderate to substantial.	Offer or provide this service.
C	The USPSTF recommends against routinely providing the service. There may be considerations that support providing the service in an individual patient. There is at least moderate certainty that the net benefit is small.	Offer or provide this service only if other considerations support offering or providing the service in an individual patient.
D	The USPSTF recommends against the service. There is moderate or high certainty that the service has no net benefit or that the harms outweigh the benefits.	Discourage the use of this service.
I statement	The USPSTF concludes that the current evidence is insufficient to assess the balance of benefits and harms of the service. Evidence is lacking, of poor quality, or conflicting, and the balance of benefits and harms cannot be determined.	Read the clinical considerations section of USPSTF Recommendation Statement. If the service is offered, patients should understand the uncertainty about the balance of benefits and harms.

Note. USPSTF=U.S. Preventive Services Task Force.

Source. Reprinted from Trinite T, Loveland-Cherry C, Marion L: "U.S. Preventive Services Task Force: An Evidence-Based Prevention Resource for Nurse Practitioners." AHRQ Publication No. 09–05138-EF, July 2009. Originally published in *Journal of the American Academy of Nurse Practitioners* 21:301–306, 2009. Available at: www.uspreventiveservicestaskforce.org/uspstf09/epbnursep/epbnursep.htm. Accessed August 31, 2010.

sociation of Pediatric Nurse Practitioners, and medical associations representing medical specialties in primary care.

In 2009, the USPSTF examined the scientific evidence for the benefits and harms of screening and treating adults with depression in primary care. The USPSTF concluded that there is a "moderate" benefit to screening non-pregnant adults for depression in primary care settings when "staff-assisted depression supports" are in place. The USPSTF further noted that when "staff-assisted depression supports" were absent, the impact on patient outcomes was "small" (U.S. Preventive Services Task Force 2009a, p. 791). The superiority of collaborative care models in improving treatment outcomes was the basis for the USPSTF to recommend routine screening of adults for depression in primary care only "when staff-assisted depression care supports are in place to assure accurate diagnosis, effective treatment and follow-up" (U.S. Preventive Services Task Force 2009a, p. 791). The USPSTF clinical guidelines for the treatment of adult depression in primary care (see Table 11–4) are endorsed both by the Centers for Disease Control Task Force on Community Preventive Services (2009) and by the American College of Preventive Medicine (2009), which has issued a position statement in which all primary care practices are urged to incorporate collaborative care with mental health clinicians to ensure proper diagnosis and treatment of patients with major depression.

The USPSTF (2009a) describes the lowest level of "staff-assisted depression care support" as a nurse who conducts depression screening and advises PCPs about referral resources for mental health treatment (p. 785). The highest level of "staff-assisted depression care" support includes visits with a cognitive-behavioral therapist in combination with regular evaluations by an APPN or psychiatrist for ensuring medication efficacy and treatment adherence. The USPSTF (2009a) does not specify the frequency of screening, psychotherapy, or medication evaluation, but does recommend that screening be repeated in patients with a history of depression, comorbid substance abuse, somatization, and chronic pain. Barriers to implementation of the USPSTF recommendations in primary care include time constraints, inadequate reimbursement for counseling services, and timely access to mental health specialists (Trinite et al. 2009).

Older Adults

Under the sponsorship of the Hartford Institute for Geriatric Nursing (HIGN) and the New York University College of Nursing, nurse experts have developed a series of educational and evidence-based materials for care of the older adult with depression (see depression section of "Evidence-Based Geriatric Nursing Protocol for Best Practice," developed by the HIGN 2008, listed in Web Resources below). The HIGN protocol emphasizes that for all levels of depression, nursing interventions include evaluating the efficacy of medication and documenting the patient's response by readministering a depression screening tool (Kurlowicz and Harvath 2008). A nurse's role includes educating patients and families about the goals of pharmacological treatment and monitoring medication side effects to promote treatment adherence (Kurlowicz and Harvath 2008). The protocol stresses the value of interdisciplinary collaboration and lists social workers, geropsychiatric APNs, geriatric psychiatrists, and psychologists as potential mental health resources (Kurlowicz and Harvath 2008).

The HIGN protocol specifically recommends the Geriatric Depression Scale—Short Form (GDS-SF) because of its validity, wide availability, and ease of administration (Kurlowicz and Harvath 2008). The protocol states that an older adult who has a GDS-SF score of 11 or greater, as well as any older adult who expresses suicidal ideation, psychosis, or substance abuse, should be referred for a comprehensive psychiatric evaluation. Evidence-based interventions that are recommended include treatment with antidepressants; cognitive-behavioral, interpersonal, and brief psychodynamic psychotherapies; and group and family therapies. The protocol notes that hospitalization or electroconvulsive therapy may be warranted for older adults with severe depression. An older adult with a GDS-SF score between 6 and 10 is less severely depressed, and the protocol directs the nurse to refer the older adult to a mental health clinician for psychotherapy and to an APPN or psychiatrist for an evaluation to determine whether medication treatment is indicated (Kurlowicz and Harvath 2008).

The HIGN has identified the Beers Criteria I and II for Potentially Inappropriate Medication Use in Older Adults as a best-practice screening tool for nurses in all settings to reduce the incidence of drug-related adverse events among older adults (Molony 2009). The Centers for Medicare and Medicaid Services uses the Beers Criteria in federal oversight of long-term-care facilities to evaluate compliance with medication-related quality outcomes. Antidepressants in the 2002 Beers Criteria I of 66 potentially inappropriate drugs for older adults include amitriptyline (Elavil), chlordiazepoxide-amitriptyline (Limbitrol), perphenazine-amitriptyline (Triavil), and daily doses of fluoxetine (Prozac) (Fick et al. 2003). Tricyclic antidepressants (TCAs) are not recommended for use in the older adult because of their high anticholinergic properties, whereas the SSRI fluoxetine is not recommended because of its long half-life and risk of central nervous system (CNS) stimulation and increased agitation (Molony 2009).

Beers Criteria II lists medications to be avoided when an older adult is diagnosed with a specific medical or health condition. Bupropion is contraindicated in older adults with a history of seizure disorders because it can lower the seizure threshold. The high anticholinergic and sedative properties of imipramine, doxepin, and amitriptyline have been associated with an increased risk of falls in older adults (Woolcott et al. 2009), and these medications are contraindicated in older adults with a history of syncope episodes, ataxia, or impaired mobility. TCAs are also contraindicated in older adults with a history of arrhythmias because of the potential to cause QT interval changes and proarrhythmic side effects (Molony 2008).

Despite the wide dissemination of the Beers Criteria I and II over the past decade, a study of 39 potentially inappropriate medications used among 17,971 community-dwelling older adults found that amitriptyline ranked ninth among the most frequently prescribed inappropriate medications (Fick et al. 2008). The use of medications listed in the Beers Criteria was significantly (P<0.01) associated with drug-related problems among older adults, including acute depression (odds ratio [OR]=7.77; 95% CI=2.26–26.69), falls (OR=4.05; 95% CI=1.89–8.69), syncope (OR=3.01; 95% CI=2.41–3.74), and bradycardia (OR=2.92; 95% CI=1.81–4.72) (Fick et al. 2008). Use of the Beers Criteria should be standard nursing practice, especially for psychiatric nurses, because many of drugs included in Beers Criteria I are in the CNS class and are used to treat behavioral symptoms. Nurses have a professional responsibility to monitor the efficacy and adverse effects of medications and thereby have a central role of interceding to minimize the use of potentially inappropriate medications, especially among older adults (Table 11–6).

Adverse Effects Associated With Antidepressants

Falls

Falling in older adults is a serious adverse event associated with the use of antidepressants (Kerse et al. 2008). Side effects of antidepressants that contribute to increasing the risk for falls include sedation, confusion, blurred vision, orthostatic hypotension, cardiac rhythm changes, and changes in gait (Howland 2009). In community-residing older adults, antidepressants were the most prescribed (6.2%) class of CNS medication; over 5 years, almost a quarter of older adults (24.1%) took two or more CNS agents, and an additional 18.9% of older adults were prescribed such agents at high dosages (Hanlon et al. 2009). Community-dwelling older adults taking an SSRI were 61.6% more likely to report falling, and the risk of injury from a fall was 4.96 (95% CI, 2.13–7.36) (Kerse et al. 2008, p. 3).

Almost half of nursing home residents (46.3%) are prescribed multiple antidepressants, placing antidepressants second behind laxatives as the class of medications most likely to show evidence of polypharmacy (Dwyer 2009). In nursing home residents, the odds of falling increased 3.4-fold (95% CI, 1.2–

TABLE 11–6. Nursing best practices to promote use of Beers Criteria I and II

- Include the following in nursing assessment: a comprehensive medication evaluation of prescription and nonprescription medications and of complementary treatments. Repeat medication evaluation at each transition of care and end of life.
- Avoid polypharmacy to minimize drug-drug interactions and adverse events.
- Post the Beers Criteria I and II where medications are ordered or dispensed.
- Incorporate the Beers Criteria I and II into electronic medication ordering systems.
- Evaluate falls, agitation, and injury to assess if the patient has been taking a medication contained in the Beers Criteria I and II.
- Reevaluate medications on Beers Criteria I and II and consider safer alternatives.
- Promote the use of nonpharmacological alternatives to manage behavioral symptoms.
- Educate patient and family about importance of adhering to prescribed treatment and about drug interactions with over-the-counter medications and alternative treatments.
- Evaluate and monitor laboratory data. Use the following Cockcroft-Gault formula to determine whether creatinine clearance is low and whether medication should be prescribed at a reduced dosage. For women, multiply answer by 0.85.

$$\frac{(140-\text{age in years}) \times \text{lean body weight in kg}}{\text{serum creatinine in mg/dL} \times 72}$$

Source. Molony 2009; Razzi 2009.

9.5) within 1–3 days of an antidepressant medication change or start (Sorock et al. 2009).

In hospital settings, falling ranked sixth among 20 sentinel events tracked by the Joint Commission (2010). A study of psychiatric inpatients found no statistical difference in the use of SSRIs between patients who fell and those who did not; however, men prescribed SSRIs were significantly more likely to fall than men not prescribed SSRIs (P<0.011) (Estrin et al. 2009). Other risk factors significantly associated with falls in psychiatric inpatients included use of four or more medications (P<0.001); use of antihypertensive medication (P<0.003); use of clonazepam (P<0.001); and physical complaints on the day of the fall, such as urinary frequency or incontinence (P<0.005), generalized weakness ($P<0.009$), mental status impairment ($P<0.017$), and dizziness ($P<0.017$) (Estrin et al. 2009). Risk of falls was also significantly associated with older age ($P<0.008$), bipolar disorder ($P<0.001$), history of syncope ($P<0.028$), and impaired mobility ($P<0.037$) (Estrin et al. 2009).

The Hendrich II Fall Risk Model has been identified as a best-practice approach for use in the older adult by HIGN and the American Geriatrics Society (Hendrich 2007). An evaluation of three fall-risk assessment tools used in acute care hospitals—the Morse Fall Scale, St. Thomas Risk Assessment Tool, and Hendrich II—found that only the Hendrich II had strong sensitivity (70%) and an acceptable level of specificity (61.5%) (Kim et al. 2007). The Hendrich II incorporates some, but not all, of the risk factors associated with falls among psychiatric inpatients.

The Hendrich II consists of eight weighted factors that are summed to provide a measure of risk. Patients are considered at high risk for falls if they receive a score on the Hendrich II of 5 or greater. The risk factor with the greatest weight (a score of 4) is "confusion, disorientation, and impulsivity," which includes inappropriate behavior, agitation, poor concentration, and changes in level of consciousness (Hendrich 2007, p. 56). The risk factor "symptomatic depression" does not refer to a history or diagnosis of major depression, but rather to current evidence of mood symptoms, such as tearfulness, withdrawal, or feeling overwhelmed; patients receive a score of 2 on this risk factor (Hendrich 2007, p. 56). The risk factors "any administered antiepileptics" and "any administered benzodiazepines" are given a score of 2 and 1, respectively. Physiological alterations such as "dizziness/vertigo" and "altered elimination" each receive a score of 1. Balance on the Hendrich II is evaluated with the "Get Up and Go Test," which is measured on a scale from 1 to 4, based on the patient's ability to rise from a sitting to a standing position, walk approximately 10 feet, turn and walk back to the original position, and sit down (Hendrich 2007, p. 56). Finally, on the Hendrich II, male gender is considered an independent risk factor and is given a score of 1.

In a psychiatric hospital that implemented a fall prevention program and included use of the Morse Fall Scale, the number of falls remained high. Subsequently, Knight and Coakley (2010) modified the fall prevention program to include a nursing assessment for fall risk that incorporated risk factors sensitive to a psychiatric population. The fall risk assessment that they devised included screening for two or more mood stabilizers and antipsychotics, an acute loading mood stabilizer, beta-blockers, and polypharmacy defined as greater than 10 medications. In addition to a review of the medication regimen, the nursing assessment included risk factors such as confusion, vertigo, or dizziness included in the Hendrich II, as well as tachycardia (>100 in past 24 hours) and postural hypotension (>20 mmHg) (Knight and Coakley 2010).

Psychiatric inpatients identified with the nursing fall assessment tool as being at risk were reviewed by the multidisciplinary team. The senior psychiatrist reviewed all cases deemed to be at risk due to polypharmacy and consulted with prescribing clinicians about reevaluating the medication treatment regimen. The fall risk assessment tool that triggered consultation with senior psychiatrists to minimize polypharmacy decreased the fall rate from 4.83 per 1,000 patient days to 0.46 the following quarter (Knight and Coakley 2010). Hendrich (2007) cautioned that polypharmacy cannot always predict falling. However, studies of falls among psychiatric patients suggest that polypharmacy may be a risk factor for this population (Estrin et al. 2009; Knight and Coakley 2010). Although the Hendrich II contains many of the risk factors associated with falls in psychiatric patients, additional nursing research is needed to validate the Hendrich II, as well as other screening tools, with samples of psychiatric patients.

In "Prevention of Falls and Fall Injury in the Older Adult," a nursing best-practice guideline, the Registered Nurses Association of Ontario (2005) recommends that nurses conduct periodic medication reviews and classify clients at high risk who are prescribed TCAs, SSRIs, trazodone, or more than five medications (see "Web Resources" later in this chapter). A clinical practice algorithm to reduce fall risk in the elderly states that SSRIs are the preferred class of antidepressants to minimize fall risk and if the older adult is nonresponsive to treatment with SSRIs, then nortriptyline should be considered because of its low anticholinergic effects (Bulat 2008).

Starting dosages of SSRIs in the older adult should be as much as 50% lower than in younger adults, and slowly titrated to minimize side effects that can increase fall risk (Darowski et al. 2009). Additional evidence-based nursing interventions to minimize fall risk include remedying environmental factors (e.g., obstructed or slippery walking areas, poor lighting, loose footwear) and balance training using Tai Chi, free weights, or resistance bands (Van Leuven 2010).

Antidepressant Poisoning

Antidepressants are among the most common prescription medications taken intentionally or unintentionally in overdose (Nelson et al. 2007). In 2008, antidepressants ranked third of the top 25 substances associated with fatalities (Bronstein et al. 2009). Amitriptyline and bupropion accounted for the most antidepressant fatalities (5 each), followed by lithium (4), doxepin and nortriptyline (3 each), and SSRIs (2) (Bronstein et al. 2009). TCAs are highly toxic in overdose, and a 2-week supply of TCAs can be lethal. A study of TCA overdose found that 71% of patients died before emergency medical services arrived, and an additional 13% were dead on arrival to the hospital (Callaham and Kassel 1985). It is critical that nurses appropriately refer patients suspected of

TCA poisoning to emergency medical services because the toxic effects can result in grand mal seizures, coma, cardiac arrhythmias, and death (Wolfe et al. 2008).

Although SSRIs accounted for the fewest fatalities, this class of antidepressants accounted for the vast majority of single-poison exposures (20,011 cases) reported to U.S. Poison Control Centers (Bronstein et al. 2009). Treatment in a health care facility was required for 9,739 cases of SSRI poisoning, and in approximately 1,263 of these cases patients experienced moderate sequelae (e.g., vital sign abnormalities, agitation, lethargy) or major sequelae (e.g., significant cardiovascular abnormalities, delirium, coma, seizures) (Bronstein et al. 2009). Unlike poisoning with medications from other classes of antidepressants, SSRI poisonings were more likely in children than adults, with 31% reported for children younger than age 6 years and 27% for children and adolescents ages 6–19 years, compared with 42% for adults over age 19 (Bronstein et al. 2009).

Guidelines for TCA and SSRI poisoning were developed by the American Association of Poison Control Centers in consultation with nurse experts representing the Emergency Nurses Association and the National Association of School Nurses, as well as the Centers for Disease Control, the FDA, and 17 medical specialty organizations (Nelson et al. 2007; Wolfe et al. 2008). The objective of the guidelines is to assist poison control clinicians, many of whom are registered nurses, in providing immediate recommendations and triage for TCA or SSRI poisoning victims and their families (see Web Resources at end of this chapter).

Serotonin Syndrome

Serotonin syndrome is a potentially life-threatening drug interaction that may occur after one dose of a serotonergic medication in a treatment-naive patient but that generally arises when two or more serotonergic drugs are ingested simultaneously (Bartlett 2006). Case reports of serotonin syndrome in nursing and medical literature are noteworthy for highlighting how the diagnosis is often missed, leading to a cascade of symptoms that can be fatal (Attar-Herzberg et al. 2009; Dvir and Smallwood 2008; Inott 2009; Lee et al. 2009; Prator 2006). Onset of symptoms is rapid, within 6 hours of ingesting two serotonergic agents (Boyer and Shannon 2005). Given the increasing use of SSRIs and other serotonergic agents, the prevention of serotonin syndrome must be a priority among nurse prescribers and begins with a thorough analysis of multidrug regimens for potential drug-drug interactions (see Table 11–7).

The American Psychiatric Association (2010) practice guideline for the treatment of major depression states that patients who are being switched from a monoamine oxidase inhibitor (MAOI) to an SSRI with a short half-life must

TABLE 11–7. Medications associated with serotonin syndrome

Drug class	Examples
Antidepressants/mood stabilizers	
Selective serotonin reuptake inhibitors	Sertraline, fluoxetine, fluvoxamine, paroxetine, citalopram, escitalopram
Serotonin-norepinephrine reuptake inhibitors	Venlafaxine, duloxetine, desmethylvenlafaxine
$Serotonin_{2A}$ receptor blockers	Trazodone
Monoamine oxidase inhibitors	Phenelzine, moclobemide, clorgyline, isocarboxazid, tranylcypromine
Tricyclic antidepressants	Amitriptyline, nortriptyline, desipramine, doxepin, imipramine, protriptyline
Other	Lithium, buspirone, nefazodone, bupropion
Amphetamines	Dextroamphetamine, methamphetamine, sibutramine
Analgesics	Cyclobenzaprine, fentanyl, meperidine, tramadol, codeine, methadone
Antibiotics	Linezolid
Anticonvulsants	Valproate, carbamazepine
Antiemetics	Metoclopramide, ondansetron, granisetron
Antimigraine	Sumatriptan, ergot alkaloids
Antiretrovirals	Ritonavir
Bariatric	Sibutramine
Drugs of abuse	MDMA (ecstasy), lysergic acid diethylamide (LSD), Syrian rue
Herbal drugs and supplements	*Hypericum perforatum* (St. John's wort), *Panax ginseng* (ginseng), tryptophan
Over-the-counter medications	Dextromethorphan, chlorpheniramine

Note. MDMA=3,4-methylenedioxymethamphetamine.
Source. Ables and Nagubilli 2010; American Psychiatric Association 2010; Boyer and Shannon 2005.

have a waiting period of at least 2 weeks after the discontinuation of one medication and the initiation of the other. When a switch is being made from fluoxetine to an MAOI, a waiting period of at least 5 weeks is needed before the MAOI is started. Classes of medications with serotonergic properties that can interact with antidepressants include analgesics, antiemetic agents, antimigraine medications, and antibiotics; drugs of abuse; herbal supplements; and over-the-counter medications (Table 11–7). Aspirin, nonsteroidal anti-inflammatory drugs, and acetaminophen should be used for mild to moderate pain in patients taking medications with serotonergic properties (Martinez et al. 2008).

Mild symptoms of serotonin syndrome include tachycardia, diaphoresis, tremor, diarrhea, and hyperreflexia (Boyer and Shannon 2005). In moderate cases of serotonin syndrome, patients may exhibit horizontal ocular clonus, agitation, and hyperthermia. The condition may then rapidly escalate to delirium, severe hypertension, a core body temperature of greater than 41.1°C, muscle rigidity, renal failure, and shock (Boyer and Shannon 2005). Abnormal laboratory values that can assist in making the diagnosis include metabolic acidosis, rhabdomyolysis, elevated serum aminotransferase, and creatine (Boyer and Shannon 2005).

The American Academy of Family Physicians stated in its clinical practice guide that the Hunter Serotonin Toxicity Criteria should be used in screening for serotonin syndrome (Ables and Nagubilli 2010). These criteria are presented as a stepwise decision tree with high sensitivity (84%) and specificity (97%) in diagnosing serotonin syndrome (Dunkley et al. 2003). According to the Hunter model, a diagnosis of serotonin toxicity requires one of the following signs or clusters of symptoms: spontaneous clonus; inducible clonus with agitation or diaphoresis; ocular clonus with agitation or diaphoresis; tremor and hyperreflexia; hypertonia with hyperthermia >38°C; and ocular or inducible clonus (Ables and Nagubilli 2010).

Once patients diagnosed with serotonin syndrome are hospitalized, nursing care focuses on supportive measures to address hyperthermia, dehydration, hemodynamic instability, and agitation (Prator 2006). Patients with moderate symptoms should be placed on fall precautions. Because these patients have the potential for clonic seizures and muscle contractions, their agitation is best managed with benzodiazepines, and physical restraints should be avoided (Inott 2009). Hyperthermia is due to muscular activity, not an alteration in hypothalamic temperature, and nursing measures to lower body temperature (e.g., cooling blankets) are indicated (Prator 2006). In severe cases (hyperthermia of 41.1°C), paralysis should be induced, accompanied with intubation and ventilation (Boyer and Shannon 2005). Abatement of symptoms after discontinuing the offending serotonergic agents depends on the half-life; with extended-release preparations of SSRIs, residual symptoms may persist for weeks (Prator 2006).

Adverse Effects Associated With SSRIs

Hyponatremia

Hyponatremia is defined as having a serum sodium level <135 mmol/L (Draper and Berman 2008). SSRIs and serotonin-norepinephrine reuptake inhibitors (SNRIs) can induce hyponatremia by triggering the syndrome of inappropriate antidiuretic hormone secretion (Smith 2010). Hyponatremia can occur in any age group prescribed SSRIs or SNRIs, but it is seen primarily in older adults, with occurrence in almost one-third of patients over age 65 (Jacob and Spinler 2006). Factors that contribute to hyponatremia in older adults prescribed SSRIs or SNRIs include female gender, low body mass index, lower baseline sodium, and concomitant use of thiazide diuretics, carbamazepine, neuroleptics, narcotics, theophylline, or nicotine (Wright and Schroeter 2008). Comorbid medical conditions that contribute to sodium loss can also increase risk (Inott 2009).

Hyponatremia develops in the first 1–3 weeks of treatment with SSRIs or SNRIs and can initially manifest as symptoms similar to depression, such as confusion, fatigue, and sleep disturbance (Smith 2010). Other symptoms include muscle weakness, nausea, vomiting, and bradycardia; if serum sodium levels fall below 125 mmol/L, symptoms can progress to delirium, seizures, respiratory distress, and death (Draper and Berman 2008). Mild symptoms are treated with fluid restriction and a loop diuretic (Draper and Berman 2008). In cases with moderate symptoms, the SSRI must be discontinued and a switch made to another class of antidepressant medication, such as a TCA (Howland 2007). If indicated, patients may be prescribed medications to prevent hyponatremia, such as demeclocycline or fludrocortisone (Howland 2007). In severe cases, treatment may warrant intravenous potassium, anticonvulsants, and mechanical ventilation (Wright and Schroeter 2008).

No evidence-based guidelines exist for the nursing or medical management of hyponatremia from SSRIs or SNRIs (Wright and Schroeter 2008). Case reports suggest that patients should not be rechallenged or given a trial on an SNRI if the offending agent was an SSRI or vice versa (Howland 2007). Best practices for nursing care include obtaining baseline serum sodium levels prior to prescribing an SSRI or SNRI to patients at high risk and repeating serum sodium level tests each week for the first 2 weeks of treatment and monthly thereafter (Rottmann 2007; Wright and Schroeter 2008).

Bleeding

SSRIs can deplete serotonin in platelets, thus causing diminished coagulation (Looper 2007). Large case-control and cohort analyses have found that use of serotonergic antidepressants is associated with gastrointestinal and uterine bleeding and that the risk of hemorrhage is increased with the concomitant use of acetylsalicylic acid or nonsteroidal anti-inflammatory medications (Looper 2007). Patients taking SSRI antidepressants had twice the volume of blood loss during surgery and a higher risk (OR=3.7) of requiring blood transfusions during hospitalization compared with patients on other classes of antidepressants (Movig et al. 2003). The risk of bleeding is highest for patients taking SSRIs and other medications that have a high level of potency for the serotonin receptor, such as paroxetine, sertraline, fluoxetine, and clomipramine (Looper 2007).

Careful nursing assessments should be conducted prior to any surgical procedure to determine whether a patient is currently taking an SSRI medication and, if so, what time the last dose was taken; whether the patient is taking acetylsalicylic acid or nonsteroidal anti-inflammatory medications, supplements that can increase bleeding (e.g., fish oil or vitamin E), or anticoagulants; and whether the patient has a history of bleeding or bruising (Howland 2007; Reeves et al. 2007). Postoperatively, nurses should carefully evaluate the patient for signs of gastrointestinal bleeding, such as tarry stools, coffee-ground emesis, or blood in the urine; hypotension; and tachycardia (Inott 2009). In patients who are at risk for bleeding, APNs should consider prescribing antidepressants with low serotonergic potency, such as a serotonin agonist (nefazodone), norepinephrine-dopamine reuptake inhibitor (bupropion), or serotonin-norepinephrine disinhibitors (mirtazapine) (Looper 2007).

Adverse Effects Associated With MAOIs

The MAOI class of antidepressants interacts to potentiate the effect of tyramine in food within an hour after ingestion. Symptoms are characterized by hypertension, occipital headache, dilated pupils, palpitations, nausea, vomiting, chills, and diaphoresis. In severe reactions, patients exhibit delirium, hyperpyrexia, and cerebral hemorrhage triggered by a hypertensive crisis. Hypertensive crisis requires emergency treatment to lower blood pressure with intravenous administration of labetalol or sodium nitroprusside (American Psychiatric Association 2010). Nursing management of severe reactions is the same as in serotonin syndrome and includes the use of cooling blankets to lower core body temperature.

Nurses should educate patients taking MAOIs to avoid foods high in tyramine and to use caution when eating preparations such as gravies that can mask ingredients high in tyramine (Table 11–8). Patient education should include written material containing a list of foods high in tyramine that may be carried by the patient at all times. A medical alert bracelet indicating that the patient has been prescribed an MAOI should be worn in case of a medical

TABLE 11–8. Tyramine food restrictions for monoamine oxidase inhibitors

To be avoided	To be used in moderation
Cheese (except for cream cheese)	Coffee
Overripe (aged) fruit (e.g., banana peel)	Chocolate
Fava beans	Colas
Sausage, salami	Tea
Sherry, liqueurs	Soy sauce
Sauerkraut	Beer, other wines
Monosodium glutamate	
Pickled fish	
Brewer's yeast	
Beef and chicken liver	
Fermented products	
Red wine	

Source. Reprinted from Krishnan K: "Monoamine Oxidase Inhibitors," in *The American Psychiatric Publishing Textbook of Psychopharmacology,* 4th Edition. Edited by Schatzberg AF, Nemeroff CB. Washington, DC, American Psychiatric Publishing, 2009, pp. 389–401. Copyright © 2009 American Psychiatric Publishing. Used with permission.

emergency. Some clinicians advise patients to carry nifedipine for immediate use in the event of a hypertensive crisis (Krishnan 2009). The American Psychiatric Association (2010) cautions that this practice has not been approved by the FDA and can precipitate dangerously low hypotension.

Adherence to Antidepressant Treatment

Relapse prevention in major depression begins with promoting adherence to antidepressant treatment. Adherence consists of three behaviors: 1) acquiring the prescribed medication; 2) self-administering the medication at the proper time, dose, and route; and 3) taking the medication for as long as the medication is prescribed (Ruppar et al. 2008). At each step, environmental, treatment, and patient characteristics can moderate medication adherence.

Continuation of antidepressant treatment 4–6 months after an acute episode significantly decreases the risk for relapse; however, studies have found that medication adherence to antidepressant treatment steadily decreases over time to a range of between 44% and 66% at 6 months (Katon et al. 2001; McInnis 2007; Zivin et al. 2009). Concurrent psychotherapy significantly enhances adherence to antidepressant treatment, with 68% of patients in psychotherapy adhering to antidepressant treatment compared with 43.7% of patients not receiving psychotherapy (Olfson et al. 2006). This relationship between antidepressant treatment adherence and psychotherapy is noteworthy because while the rate of Americans receiving antidepressants has doubled from 13.3 to 27 million between 1996 and 2005, the percentage of Americans receiving psychotherapy has declined (from 31.5% to 19.87%) during this same period (Olfson and Marcus 2009).

Racial and ethnic health disparities continue to persist in depression treatment. Approximately half as many African Americans (4.5%) and Hispanics (5.2%) as Caucasians (10.1%) receive antidepressant treatment (Olfson and Marcus 2009). Rates of adherence to antidepressants have been found to be significantly lower among Hispanics (46.2% vs. 58.7% of non-Hispanics), patients with less than a high school education (52% vs. 64.8% of those with >12 years of education), patients without private health insurance (50.8% vs. 60.1% of those with insurance), and patients in lower socioeconomic groups (48.2% vs. 61.4% of those in middle- and upper-income families) (McInnis 2007; Olfson et al. 2006). Other patient characteristics associated with nonadherence to antidepressants include perceived social stigma, comorbid substance abuse and personality disorders, symptom remission or lack of remission, and side effects (Hardeman and Narasimhan 2010).

Primary adherence is defined as the rate at which patients fill new prescriptions and is a proxy for whether patients achieve the first step in the definition of adherence—acquiring the medication. Analysis of 195,930 e-prescriptions from 2003 to 2004 found that antidepressants were the fourth most prescribed class of medication and had a primary adherence rate of 78.6% compared with a rate of 76.5% for all classes of medication (OR=0.88; 95% CI=0.82–0.94) (Fischer et al. 2010). Similarly, a study of Veterans Affairs patients hospitalized for depressive disorders found a primary adherence rate with antidepressants of 79% at 3 months following discharge (Zivin et al. 2009). Studies of adherence and primary adherence suggest that approximately 20% of patients never fill prescriptions for antidepressant medications and an additional 10%–30% fail either to adhere to dosing schedules or to take antidepressants as long as indicated.

Children and Adolescents

Complex treatment regimens, side effects, the cost of medications, and family members' ambivalence about the value of treatment are a few of the factors that contribute to nonadherence across the life span. Risk factors for nonadherence in a pediatric population include individual, family, disease, and treatment factors that are specific for younger patients and their families (see

TABLE 11–9. Risk factors associated with pediatric treatment nonadherence

Correlates	Risk factors
Individual	History of poor adherence
	Adolescence
	History of behavioral difficulties
	Past emotional difficulties
	Presence of denial regarding illness
	Low self-esteem
	Internal locus of control
Family	Lack of parental supervision
	Parental conflict
	Parental psychopathology
	Poor family support
	Low socioeconomic status
	Lack of family cohesion
	Poor pattern of family communication
Disease	Long duration of illness
	Illnesses with few symptoms
	Feelings of pessimism regarding illness
Treatment	Complexity of the treatment regimen
	Unpleasant medication side effects
	Low level of perceived efficacy of treatment
	Treatment with high financial costs

Source. Reprinted from Shaw RJ, DeMaso DR: *Clinical Manual of Pediatric Psychosomatic Medicine: Mental Health Consultation With Physically Ill Children and Adolescents.* Washington, DC, American Psychiatric Publishing, 2006, p. 230. Copyright 2006, American Psychiatric Publishing. Used with permission.

Table 11–9). In an effort to improve pediatric treatment adherence, the American Academy of Child and Adolescent Psychiatry (2009) recommends health education for pediatric patients and their families, as well as developmentally appropriate behavioral interventions for younger patients. Table 11–10 lists treatment approaches for pediatric treatment adherence.

Collaborative care models stress the importance of close communication between primary care and mental health specialists. With children, the collab-

TABLE 11–10. Treatment approaches for pediatric treatment adherence

PRIMARY REASON FOR NONADHERENCE	TREATMENT MODALITY
Forgetfulness	Increased parental supervision Memory aids (e.g., pill boxes, pagers, telephone reminders)
Inadequate awareness of consequences of nonadherence	Reeducation of patient and family regarding medical issues
Lack of appropriate parental supervision of treatment Lack of awareness of need for parental supervision Logistical issues (e.g., working parents)	Education of the family regarding adolescent developmental need for supervision Establishment of effective system for supervision of treatment
Adolescent developmental issues Cognitive immaturity Acting out of separation conflicts Adolescent omnipotence/denial Peer group issues	Education of the family Increased parental supervision Behavioral interventions (i.e., incentives, behavior modification programs) Possible referral for individual and/or family therapy in refractory cases
Family psychopathology Parental conflict Poor communication Parental psychiatric illness (e.g., depression, substance abuse)	Family therapy Possible referral of parent for individual psychiatric treatment
Psychiatric illness Depression Attention-deficit/hyperactivity disorder Posttraumatic stress symptoms Oppositional defiant disorder	Individual psychotherapy Family therapy Possible use of psychiatric medications

Source. Reprinted from Shaw RJ, DeMaso DR: *Clinical Manual of Pediatric Psychosomatic Medicine: Mental Health Consultation With Physically Ill Children and Adolescents.* Washington, DC, American Psychiatric Publishing, 2006, pp. 235–236. Copyright 2006, American Psychiatric Publishing. Used with permission.

oration is broadened to include school health professionals, who may be integral to monitoring treatment efficacy. Antidepressants have surpassed psychostimulants used in the treatment of attention-deficit/hyperactivity disorder as the medication class of most concern to school nurses (Brock et al. 2005). Child psychiatric specialists should collaborate with school nurses to share perceptions about antidepressant treatment efficacy and management strategies for untoward effects that can affect patient adherence.

Knowledge about a family's beliefs and attitudes is vital to understanding a child's or adolescent's nonadherence with antidepressant treatment. Since the FDA issued a black box warning about suicidality and SSRI use in children and adolescents, a survey of parents' attitudes toward antidepressants found that parents perceived antidepressants as both beneficial and risky, with African American parents having the least favorable view (Stevens et al. 2009). Less favorable views by African American families toward mental health treatment have been associated with less familiarity with mental health services and less willingness to seek mental health care (Hines-Martin et al. 2004).

Parental concerns about the risks associated with antidepressant treatment can result in decreased contacts with clinicians to evaluate medication efficacy (Worley and McGuiness 2010). Providing families with a regular schedule of follow-up visits or phone contacts and the involvement of all health care professionals in monitoring target symptoms, especially signs of self-harm or suicidal ideation, are essential to allaying the fears of caregivers that antidepressant treatment may be more harmful than beneficial to their child.

Supervising adolescents' adherence to antidepressant treatment presents a unique challenge to parents and prescribers. Many parents want to support their adolescent's need for autonomy and may minimally supervise medication administration. Nurses must educate parents that adolescents need supervision and support to maintain treatment, especially at the initiation of treatment or after symptoms have remitted. Ultimately, parents are accountable for making sure that their child takes antidepressant medication as prescribed, and clinicians should make careful efforts to support caregivers in this role (Worley and McGuiness 2010). One helpful way to support parents is to keep the administration of medications as simple as possible to account for work or family schedules.

Adults

Clinical practice guidelines from the Institute for Clinical Systems Improvement (see "Web Resources" later in this chapter) recommend collaborative care models for depression treatment in primary care because these models have been demonstrated to result in improvements in treatment adherence and depression outcomes. A systematic review of randomized controlled trials that investigated the effectiveness of interventions to enhance adherence to antidepressant treatment found that educational interventions failed to improve adherence, whereas collaborative care interventions had a significant impact on adherence in both acute and continuation phases (Vergouwen et al. 2003). The positive impact of collaborative care models on patient outcomes is a result of interventions to enhance medication adherence and increased collaboration to support evidence-based prescribing practices (Vergouwen et al. 2003).

In collaborative care models, patients should receive written information personalized for their language preference or videotapes to enhance their understanding about depression treatment (Katon et al. 2001). The Institute of Clinical Systems Improvements guidelines for depression treatment (see "Web Resources" later in this chapter) state that the FDA requires that patients prescribed antidepressants must receive FDA-approved medication guides. Nurses should ensure that all education materials, including FDA medication guides, are consistent with a patient's language preference and literacy level.

In addition to providing health education, nurses engage patients with motivational interviewing or behavioral counseling techniques to manage side effects, address attitudes toward treatment, and provide suggestions or helpful reminders to take medication as ordered. Nurse contacts may be in person but more often are made using electronic media or phone calls that typically last less than 10 minutes and occur every other week for the first 3–7 months of treatment (Vergouwen et al. 2003). Nurses must be mindful that when patients have inadequate literacy skills, the odds that patients will inappropriately identify medication are increased 10–18 times compared with patients with adequate literacy skills (Kripalani et al. 2006). When language preference is different between nurses and patients, patients may give misleading nonverbal cues that they comprehend information. If there is doubt that patients understand any aspect of antidepressant treatment, nurses must enlist the assistance of a medical interpreter or, with the patient's permission, friends and family members to facilitate communication (Campinha-Bacote 2007).

Ethnic and racial disparities in accessing depression treatment and adhering to antidepressant medication reinforce the importance of developing models of collaborative care that are culturally sensitive. Motivational interviewing by nurses should incorporate language, beliefs, personal preferences, and social customs of minority populations (Interian et al. 2010). In one collaborative care model serving a Latino population, focus groups were conducted with members of a Latino community who had experience with antidepressant treatment. The purposes of the focus groups were to elicit information about positive and negative experiences with antidepressants and to provide members of the Latino community an opportunity to educate clinicians about values and beliefs that might impact medication adherence (Interian et al.

2010). Motivational interviewing addressed the key concerns identified in the focus groups, such as social stigma, fear of lifelong treatment, and *familismo* (familism—valuing family expectations over individual needs) (Interian et al. 2010).

Older Adults

Among older adults, the inability to afford insurance copayments and out-of-pocket costs associated with medication is the primary reason for medication nonadherence (Wilson et al. 2007). Most intervention studies to improve medication adherence with older adults fail to address the impact of cost on medication adherence (Ruppar et al. 2008). APNs should consider the inability to afford medication or lack of understanding about the medication regimen in evaluating medication adherence for all older adults (Zurakowski 2009). The HIGN clinical practice protocol for depression specifically recommends that nurses educate older adults about the importance of adhering to prescribed treatments and provide specific information about medication side effects (Kurolowicz and Harvath 2008) (see "Web Resources" later in this chapter).

Surveys of Medicare beneficiaries found that older adults also fail to fill prescriptions because they do not think the medication is necessary or they are afraid of the medication's side effects and contraindications (Kennedy et al. 2008). Evidence-based interventions to enhance medication adherence among older adults mirror many of the same educational and administrative interventions used in collaborative care models; these interventions include providing written information, health education, medication reminders, and monitoring (Ruppar et al. 2008). The HIGN clinical practice protocol "Reversing Adverse Drug Events" includes innovative recommendations that use information technology to help older adults evaluate contraindications with prescription and nonprescription medications, as well as alcohol (see Web Resources below) (Zwicker and Fulmer 2008).

Licensed health care professionals are required in some states to assess the ability of older adults in assisted living to safely self-administer medication (Mitty and Flores 2007). The Mini-Mental State Examination is commonly used to evaluate cognitive ability, and vision may be evaluated by an ophthalmologist. If mild changes are noted in vision or cognition, treatment adherence can be improved by lowering the number of daily doses, simplifying medication orders, or altering labeling and packaging (Ruppar et al. 2008).

A systematic review of 14 measurement instruments used to evaluate the ability of older adults to self-administer medications concluded that the Drug Regimen Unassisted Grading Scale (DRUGS) and the Medication Management Instrument for Deficiencies in the Elderly (MedMaIDE) were the only instruments with strong interrater and test-retest reliability (Elliott and Marriott 2009). MedMaIDE was also found to be a cost-effective method for evaluating factors associated with nonadherence in community-dwelling older adults when compared to electronic monitoring (Aspinall et al. 2007). MedMaIDE consists of three performance domains: 1) whether an older adult knows how to get his or her medication (e.g., resources to procure the medication and when to get refills); 2) what the patient knows about his or her medication (e.g., reason for medication, time, route, and dose); and 3) whether the patient knows how to take his or her medication (e.g., is able to open packaging and count correct number of pills). MedMaIDE is scored using a dichotomous yes-no scale (Orwig et al. 2006).

Similar to MedMaIDE, DRUGS is an assessment tool that scores a patient's ability to properly identify medication, open packaging, and describe the dosing schedule (Edelberg et al. 1999). DRUGS also includes a grid to role-play medication administration at different times of the day (Hutchison et al. 2006). The HIGN clinical practice protocol for "reducing adverse drug events" recommends that nurses evaluate medication self-management with the DRUGS tool at every transition of care for older adults (see "Web Resources" later in this chapter) (Zwicker and Fulmer 2008).

Conclusion

The scope of practice for APNs in the evidence-based use of antidepressants can be conceptualized with the ACE-ME model—assessment, collaboration, education, monitoring, and evaluation (Gould and Mitty 2010). In this chapter I reviewed evidence-based tools used by nurses in both community and hospital settings that have application to patients who are prescribed antidepressants. Expert panels of nurses in gerontology have devised practice protocols that can be used with depressed older adults to minimize adverse events associated with antidepressants and to improve treatment adherence and patient outcomes. On the advanced practice level, studies demonstrate that the prescribing practices of psychiatric nurse specialists are consistent with APA's evidence-based treatment algorithms (American Psychiatric Association 2010). Compelling scientific evidence suggests that when nurse specialists in psychiatry collaborate with their primary care colleagues, depressed patients are more likely to adhere to treatment and have better outcomes. Nurses have important contributions to make with their colleagues in medicine to advance the mutual goal of promoting evidence-based practice in the use of antidepressants and the care of depressed patients.

KEY CLINICAL CONCEPTS

- Advanced practice psychiatric nurses are more likely than nurse practitioners or physicians to prescribe antidepressants according to evidence-based guidelines in children, adults, and older adults.
- Collaborative care models, in which nurse specialists have a key role, are endorsed by the USPSTF for depression management in children and adults in primary care settings.
- Evidence-based measurement tools used by nurses in community and hospital settings have applications for patients prescribed antidepressants to minimize harms associated with side effects.
- Evidence-based protocols for use by nurses with children, adults, and older adults improve adherence to antidepressant treatment.

Suggested Readings

Bulat T: Clinical practice algorithms: medication management to reduce fall risk in the elderly—part 3, benzodiazepines, cardiovascular agents and antidepressants. J Am Acad Nurse Pract 20:55–62, 2008

Dunkley EJ, Isbister GK, Sibbritt D, et al: The Hunter Serotonin Toxicity Criteria: simple and accurate diagnostic decision rules for serotonin toxicity. QJM 96:635–642, 2003

Hendrich A: Predicting patient falls: using the Hendrich II Fall Risk Model in clinical practice. Am J Nurs 107:50–58, 2007

Kurlowicz L, Harvath TA: Depression, in Evidence-Based Geriatric Nursing Protocols for Best Practice, 3rd Edition. Edited by Capezuti E, Zwicker D, Mezey M, et al. New York, Springer, 2008, pp 57–82

Molony SL: Monitoring medication use in older adults: the Beers Criteria can be used in identifying medication-related risk. Am J Nurs 109:68–78, 2009

Trinite T, Loveland-Cherry C, Marion L: U.S. Preventive Services Task Force: an evidence-based prevention resource for nurse practitioners. J Am Acad Nurse Pract 21:301–306, 2009

Zwicker D, Fulmer T: Reducing adverse drug events, in Evidence-based Geriatric Nursing Protocols for Best Practice, 3rd Edition. Edited by Capezuti E, Zwicker D, Mezey M, et al. New York, Springer, 2008, pp 257–308

Web Resources

American Academy of Child and Adolescent Psychiatry: A Guide to Building Collaborative Mental Health Care Partnerships in Pediatric Primary Care. Washington, DC, American Academy of Child and Adolescent Psychiatry, June 2010. Available at: http://www.aacap.org/galleries/PracticeInformation/Collaboration_Guide__FINAL_approved_6-10.pdf. Accessed August 2, 2011.

American Academy of Child and Adolescent Psychiatry: When to seek referral or consultation with a child and adolescent psychiatrist: recommendations for pediatricians, family practitioners, psychiatrists, and non-physician mental health practitioners. Washington, DC, American Academy of Child and Adolescent Psychiatry, 2010. Available at: www.aacap.org/cs/root/physicians_and_allied_professionals/when_to_seek_referral_or_consultation_with_a_child_and_adolescent_psychiatrist. Accessed May 17, 2011.

Agency for Healthcare Research and Quality: National Guideline Clearinghouse

American Academy of Child and Adolescent Psychiatry: Practice parameter for the psychiatric assessment and management of physically ill children and adolescents. February, 2009. Available at: www.guideline.gov/content.aspx?id=15186. Accessed May 17, 2011.

American Association of Poison Control Centers: Selective serotonin reuptake inhibitor poisoning: an evidence-based consensus guideline for out-of-hospital management. May 1, 2009. Available at: www.guideline.gov/content.aspx?id=11293. Accessed May 17, 2011.

American Association of Poison Control Centers: Tricyclic antidepressant poisoning: an evidence-based consensus guideline for out-of-hospital management. May 1, 2009. Available at: www.guideline.gov/content.aspx?id=9906. Accessed May 17, 2011.

Hartford Institute for Geriatric Nursing: Depression, in Evidence-based geriatric nursing protocol for best practice. August 4, 2008. Available at: www.guideline.gov/content.aspx?id=12260. Accessed May 17, 2011.

Hartford Institute for Geriatric Nursing: Reducing adverse drug events: evidence-based geriatric nursing protocol for best practice. August 4, 2008. Available at: www.guideline.gov/content.aspx?id=12258. Accessed May 17, 2011.

Institute for Clinical Systems Improvement: Major depression in adults in primary care. December 2009. Available at: www.guideline.gov/content.aspx?id=14857. Accessed May 17, 2011.

Registered Nurses Association of Ontario: Prevention of falls and fall injury in the older adult. June 21, 2005. Available at: www.guideline.gov/content.aspx?id=7091. Accessed May 17, 2011.

U.S. Food and Drug Administration

Approved Medication Guides: Available at: www.fda.gov/Drugs/DrugSafety/ucm085729.htm. Accessed May 17, 2011.

U.S. Preventive Services Task Force

Trinite T, Loveland-Cherry C, Marion L: An evidence-based prevention resource for nurse practitioners. J Am Acad Nurse Pract 21:301–306, 2009. Available at: www.uspreventiveservicestaskforce.org/uspstf09/epbnursep/epbnursep.htm#refb4. Accessed May 17, 2011.

Major Depressive Disorder in Children and Adolescents. Release Date: March 2009. Available at: www.uspreventiveservicestaskforce.org/uspstf/uspschdepr.htm. Accessed May 17, 2011.

Screening for Depression in Adults. Release date: December 2009. Available at: www.uspreventiveservicestaskforce.org/uspstf/uspsaddepr.htm. Accessed May 17, 2011.

Substance Abuse and Mental Health Services Administration (SAMHSA) National Registry of Evidence-Based Programs and Practices

Partners in Care. Date of Review: November 2009. Available at: www.nrepp.samhsa.gov/ViewIntervention.aspx?id=126. Accessed May 17, 2011.

Telemedicine-Based Collaborative Care. Date of Review: January 2010. Available at: www.nrepp.samhsa.gov/ViewIntervention.aspx?id=127. Accessed May 17, 2011.

References

Ables AZ, Nagubilli R: Prevention, diagnosis, and management of serotonin syndrome. Am Fam Physician 81:1139–1142, 2010

American Academy of Child and Adolescent Psychiatry: Practice parameter on the use of psychotropic medication in children and adolescents. J Am Acad Child Adolesc Psychiatry 48:961–973, 2009

American Academy of Child and Adolescent Psychiatry: A Guide to Building Collaborative Mental Health Care Partnerships in Pediatric Primary Care. Washington, DC, American Academy of Child and Adolescent Psychiatry, June 2010. Available at: http://www.aacap.org/galleries/PracticeInformation/Collaboration_Guide__FINAL_approved_6-10.pdf. Accessed August 2, 2011.

American Academy of Pediatrics, Committee on Psychosocial Aspects of Child and Family Health and Task Force on Mental Health: Policy statement—the future of pediatrics: mental health competencies for pediatric primary care. Pediatrics 124:410–421, 2009

American College of Physicians: Nurse Practitioners in Primary Care, Policy Monograph. Philadelphia, PA, American College of Physicians, 2009

American College of Preventive Medicine: Screening adults for depression in primary care: a position statement of the American College of Preventive Medicine. J Fam Pract 58:535–538, 2009

American Psychiatric Association: APA clinical practice guideline for major depression, 3rd edition. Am J Psychiatry 167(suppl):1–152, 2010

Aspinall S, Sevick MA, Donohue J, et al: Medication errors in older adults: a review of recent publications. Am J Geriatr Pharmacother 5:75–84, 2007

Attar-Herzberg D, Apel A, Gang N, et al: The serotonin syndrome: initial misdiagnosis. Isr Med Assoc J 11:367–370, 2009

Bartlett D: Serotonin syndrome: a subtle toxicity. J Emerg Nurs 32:277–279, 2006

Bhatia SK, Rezac AJ, Vitiello B, et al: Antidepressant prescribing practices for the treatment of children and adolescents. J Child Adolesc Psychopharmacol 18:70–80, 2008

Boyer EW, Shannon M: The serotonin syndrome. N Engl J Med 352:1112–1120, 2005

Brock K, Nguyen B, Liu N, et al: The use of antidepressants in school-age children. J Sch Nurs 21:318–322, 2005

Bronstein AD, Spyker DA, Cantilena LR Jr, et al: 2008 Annual report of the American Association of Poison Control Centers' National Poison Data System (NPDS): 26th annual report. Clin Toxicol (Phila) 47:911–1084, 2009

Brown EL, Raue PJ , Schulberg H, et al: Clinical competencies: caring for late-life depression in home care patients. J Gerontol Nurs 9:10–14, 2006

Brown EL, Raue PJ, Roos BA, et al: Training nursing staff to recognize depression in home healthcare. J Am Geriatr Soc 58:122–128, 2010

Bulat T: Clinical practice algorithms: medication management to reduce fall risk in the elderly, part 3: benzodiazepines, cardiovascular agents and antidepressants. J Am Acad Nurse Pract 20:55–62, 2008

Callaham M, Kassel D: Epidemiology of fatal tricyclic antidepressant ingestion: implications for management. Ann Emerg Med 14:1–9, 1985

Campinha-Bacote J: Becoming culturally competent in ethnic psychopharmacology. J Psychosoc Nurs Ment Health Serv 45:27–33, 2007

Centers for Disease Control Task Force on Community Preventive Services: Guide to Community Preventive Services, Mental Health and Mental Illness. Atlanta, GA, Centers for Disease Control, 2009

Cipher DJ, Hooker RS, Guerra P: Prescribing trends by nurse practitioners and physician assistants in the United States. J Am Acad Nurse Pract 18: 291–296, 2006

Comer JS, Olfson M, Mojtabai R: National trends in child and adolescent psychotropic polypharmacy in office-based practice, 1996–2007. J Am Acad Child Adolesc Psychiatry 49:1001–1010, 2010

Darowski A, Chambers SA, Chambers DJ: Antidepressants and falls in the elderly. Drugs Aging 26:381–394, 2009

Delaney KR: Upcoming health care reforms: stepping up to the challenges. Arch Psychiatr Nurs 23:287–289, 2010

Draper B, Berman K: Tolerability of selective serotonin reuptake inhibitors: issues relevant to the elderly. Drugs Aging 25:501–519, 2008

Dunkley EJ, Isbister GK, Sibbritt D, et al: The Hunter Serotonin Toxicity Criteria: simple and accurate diagnostic decision rules for serotonin toxicity. QJM 96:635–642, 2003

Dvir Y, Smallwood P: Serotonin syndrome: a complex but easily avoidable condition. Gen Hosp Psychiatry 30:284–287, 2008

Dwyer LL: Polypharmacy in nursing home residents in the United States: results of the 2004 National Nursing Home Survey. Am J Geriatr Pharmacother 8:63–72, 2009

Edelberg HK, Shallenberger E, Wei JY: Medication management capacity in highly functioning community living older adults: detection of early deficits. J Am Geriatr Soc 47:592–596, 1999

Elliott RA, Marriot JL: Standardised assessment of patients' capacity to manage medications: a systematic review of published instruments. BMC Geriatr 9:27, 2009

Estrin I, Goetz R, Hellerstein DJ, et al: Predicting falls among psychiatric inpatients: a case-control study at a state psychiatric facility. Psychiatr Serv 60:1245–1250, 2009

Feldman S, Bachman J, Cuffel B, et al: Advanced practice psychiatric nurses as a treatment resource: survey and analysis. Adm Policy Ment Health 30:479–494, 2003

Fick DM, Cooper JW, Wade WE, et al: Updating the Beers Criteria for Potentially Inappropriate Medication Use in Older Adults: results of a U.S. consensus panel of experts. Arch Intern Med 163:2716–2724, 2003

Fick DM, Mion LC, Beers MH, et al: Health outcomes associated with potentially inappropriate medication use in older adults. Res Nurs Health 31:42–51, 2008

Fischer MA, Stedman MR, Lii J, et al: Primary medication non-adherence: analysis of 195,930 electronic prescriptions. J Gen Intern Med 25:284–290, 2010

Foy JM, Kelleher KJ, Laraque D: American Academy of Pediatrics Task Force on Mental Health: enhancing pediatric mental health care: strategies for preparing a primary care practice. Pediatrics 125:S87–S108, 2010

Gilbody S, Bower P, Fletcher J, et al: Collaborative care for depression: a cumulative meta-analysis and review of longer term outcomes. Arch Intern Med 166:2314–2321, 2006

Glod CA, Manchester A: Prescribing patterns of advance practice nurses: contrasting psychiatric mental health CNS and NP practice. Clin Excell Nurse Pract 4:22–29, 2000

Gould E, Mitty E: Medication adherence is a partnership, medication compliance is not. Geriatr Nurs 31:290–298, 2010

Hamrin V, Magorno M: Assessment of adolescents for depression in the pediatric primary care setting. Pediatr Nurs 36:103–111, 2010

Hanlon JT, Boudreau RM, Roumani YF, et al: Number and dosage of central nervous system medications on recurrent falls in community elders: the Health, Aging and Body Composition Study. J Gerontol A Biol Sci Med Sci 64:492–498, 2009

Hardeman SM, Narasimhan M: Adherence according to Mary Poppins: strategies to make the medicine go down. Perspect Psychiatr Care 46:3–13, 2010

Hendrich A: Predicting patient falls: using the Hendrich II Fall Risk Model in clinical practice. Am J Nurs 107:50–58, 2007

Henke RM, McGuire TG, Zaslavsky AM, et al: Clinician and organization level factors in the adoption of evidence-based care for depression in primary care. Health Care Manage Rev 33:289–299, 2008

Hines-Martin VP, Usui W, Kim S, et al: A comparison of influences on attitudes towards mental health service use in an African-American and White community. J Natl Black Nurses Assoc 15:17–22, 2004

Howland RH: Unusual and serious adverse effects of SSRIs: recognition and management. J Psychosoc Nurs Ment Health Serv 45:15–18, 2007

Howland RH: Prescribing psychotropic medications for elderly patients. J Psychosoc Nurs Ment Health Serv 47:17–20, 2009

Hutchison LC, Jones SK, West DS, et al: Assessment of medication management by community living elderly persons with two standardized assessment tools: a cross-sectional study. Am J Geriatr Pharmacother 4:144–153, 2006

Inott TJ: The dark side of SSRIs: learn how to recognize medical and surgical complications associated with these commonly used antidepressants. Nursing 8:31–33, 2009

Interian A, Martinez I, Rios LI, et al: Adaptation of a motivational interviewing intervention to improve antidepressant adherence among Latinos. Cultur Divers Ethnic Minor Psychol 16:215–225, 2010

Jacob S, Spinler SA: Hyponatremia associated with selective serotonin-reuptake inhibitors in older adults. Ann Pharmacother 40:1618–1622, 2006

Jacobs JT: Treatment of depressive disorders in split versus integrated therapy and comparisons of prescriptive practices of psychiatrists and advanced practice registered nurses. Arch Psychiatr Nurs 19:256–263, 2005

Joint Commission: Sentinel event statistics as of June 30, 2010. 2010. Available at: www.jointcommission.org/SentinelEvents/Statistics. Accessed May 18, 2011.

Katon W, Rutter C, Ludman EJ, et al: A randomized trial of relapse prevention of depression in primary care. Arch Gen Psychiatry 58:241–247, 2001

Kaye L, Warner LA, Lewandowski CA, et al: The role of nurse practitioners in meeting the need for child and adolescent psychiatric services: a statewide survey. J Psychosoc Nurs Ment Health Serv 47:34–40, 2009

Kennedy J, Tuleu I, Mackay K: Unfilled prescriptions of Medicare beneficiaries: prevalence, reasons and types of medicines prescribed. J Manag Care Pharm 14:553–560, 2008

Kerber CS, Dyck MJ, Culp KR, et al: Antidepressant treatment of depression in rural nursing home residents. Issues Mental Health Nurs 29:959–973, 2008

Kerse N, Flicker L, Pfaff JJ, et al: Falls, depression and antidepressants in later life: a large primary care appraisal. PLoS One 3:E2423, 2008

Kim EA, Mordiffi SZ, Bee WH, et al: Evaluation of three fall-risk assessment tools in an acute care setting. J Adv Nurs 60:427–435, 2007

Knight M, Coakley C: Fall risk in patients with acute psychosis. J Nurs Care Qual 25:208–215, 2010

Knight M, Houseman EA: A collaborative model for the treatment of depression in homebound elders. Issues Ment Health Nurs 29:974–991, 2008

Kurlowicz L, Harvath TA: Depression, in Evidence-Based Geriatric Nursing Protocols for Best Practice, 3rd Edition. Edited by Capezuti E, Zwicker D, Mezey M, et al. New York, Springer, 2008, pp 57–82

Kripalani S, Henderson LE, Chiu EY, et al: Predictors of medication self-management skill in a low-literacy population. J Gen Intern Med 21:852–856, 2006

Krishnan K: Monoamine oxidase inhibitors, in The American Psychiatric Publishing Textbook of Psychopharmacology, 4th Edition. Edited by Schatzberg AF, Nemeroff CB. Washington, DC, American Psychiatric Publishing, 2009, pp 389–401

Lee J, Franz L, Goforth HW: Serotonin syndrome in a chronic-pain patient receiving concurrent methadone, ciprofloxacin, and venlafaxine. Psychosomatics 50:638–639, 2009

Looper KJ: Potential medical and surgical complications of serotonergic antidepressant medications. Psychosomatics 48:1–9, 2007

Martinez M, Marangell LB, Martinez JM: Psychopharmacology, in The American Psychiatric Publishing Textbook of Psychiatry, 5th Edition. Edited by Hales RE, Yudofsky SC, Gabbard GO. Washington, DC, American Psychiatric Publishing, 2008, pp 1053–1131

McInnis M: Adherence to treatment regimens in major depression: perspectives, problems and progress. Psychiatric Times 24:17–22, 2007

Mitty E, Flores S: Assisted living nursing practice: medication management, Part 1: assessing the resident for self-medication ability. Geriatr Nurs 28:83–89, 2007

Mojtabai R, Olfson M: National trends in psychotropic medication polypharmacy in office-based psychiatry. Arch Gen Psychiatry 67:26–36, 2010

Molony SL: Beers Criteria for Potentially Inappropriate Medication Use in Older Adults part II: 2002 criteria considering diagnoses or conditions. Try This: Best Practices in Nursing Care to Older Adults—General Assessment Series. 2008. Available at: http://consultgerirn.org/uploads/File/trythis/try_this_16_2.pdf. Accessed May 18, 2011.

Molony SL: Monitoring medication use in older adults. Am J Nurs 109:68–78, 2009

Movig KL, Janssen MW, de Waal Malefiit J, et al: Relationship of serotonergic antidepressants and need for blood transfusion in orthopedic surgical patients. Arch Intern Med 163:2354–2358, 2003

Nelson LS, Erdman AR, Booze LL, et al: Selective serotonin reuptake inhibitor poisoning: an evidence-based consensus guideline for out-of-hospital management. Clin Toxicol (Phila) 45:315–332, 2007

Olfson M, Marcus SC: National patterns in antidepressant medication treatment. Arch Gen Psychiatry 66:848–856, 2009

Olfson M, Marcus SC, Tedeschi M, et al: Continuity of antidepressant treatment for adults with depression in the United States. Am J Psychiatry 163:101–108, 2006

Orwig D, Brandt N, Gruber-Baldini AL: Medication management assessment for older adults in the community. Gerontologist 46:661–666, 2006

Prator BC: Serotonin syndrome. J Neurosci Nurs 38:102–105, 2006

Qaseem A, Snow V, Denberg TD, et al: Using second-generation antidepressants to treat depressive disorders: a clinical practice guideline from the American College of Physicians. Ann Intern Med 149:725–733, 2008

Raphel S: New recommendations on screening and treatment for major depressive disorder in children and adolescents. J Child Adolesc Psychiatr Nurs 22:170–171, 2009

Razzi CC: Incorporating the Beers Criteria may reduce ED visits in elderly persons. J Emerg Nurs 35:453–454, 2009

Reeves RR, Wise PM, Cox SK: SSRIs and the risk of abnormal bleeding. J Psychosoc Nurs Ment Heal Serv 45:15–21, 2007

Registered Nurses Association of Ontario: Prevention of falls and fall injuries in the older adult. Nursing Best Practices Guideline. March 2005. Available at: www.rnao.org/Storage/12/617_BPG_Falls_rev05.pdf. Accessed May 18, 2011.

Richardson L, McCauley E, Katon W: Collaborative care for adolescent depression: a pilot study. Gen Hosp Psychiatry 31:36–45, 2009

Rottman CN: SSRIs and the syndrome of inappropriate antidiuretic hormone secretion. Am J Nurs 107:51–58, 2007

Ruppar TM, Conn VS, Russell CL: Medication adherence interventions for older adults: literature review. Res Theory Nurs Pract 22:114–147, 2008

Scudder L: Prescribing patterns of nurse practitioners. J Nurse Pract 2:98–106, 2006

Smith JM: Clinical implications of treating depressed older adults with SSRIs: possible risk of hyponatremia. J Gerontol Nurs 36(4):22–29, 2010

Sorock GS, Quigley PA, Rutledge MK, et al: Central nervous system medication changes and falls in nursing home residents. Geriatr Nurs 30:334–340, 2009

Stevens J, Wang W, Fan L, et al: Parental attitudes toward children's use of antidepressants and psychotherapy. J Child Adolesc Psychopharmacol 19:289–296, 2009

Trinite T, Loveland-Cherry C, Marion L: U.S. Preventive Services Task Force: an evidence-based prevention resource for nurse practitioners. J Am Acad Nurse Pract 21:301–306, 2009

Upshur C, Weinreb L: A survey of primary care provider attitudes and behaviors regarding treatment of adult depression: what changes after a collaborative care intervention? J Clin Psychiatry 10:182–186, 2008

U.S. Preventive Services Task Force: Screening for depression in adults: U.S. Preventive Services Task Force recommendation statement. Ann Intern Med 151:784–792, 2009a

U.S. Preventive Services Task Force: Screening and treatment for major depressive disorder in children and adolescents: U.S. Preventive Services Task Force recommendation statement. Pediatrics 123:1223–1228, 2009b

U.S. Preventive Services Task Force: About the USPSTF. August 2010. Available at: www.uspreventiveservicestaskforce.org/about.htm. Accessed May 18, 2011.

Van Leuven K: Psychotropic medications and falls in older adults. J Psychosoc Nurs Ment Health Serv 48:35–43, 2010

Vergouwen AC, Bakker A, Katon WJ, et al: Improving adherence to antidepressants: a systematic review of intervention. J Clinical Psychiatry 64:1415–1420, 2003

Williams SB, O'Connor EA, Eder M, et al: Screening for Child and Adolescent Depression in Primary Care Settings: A Systematic Evidence Review for the U.S. Preventive Services Task Force. Rockville, MD, Agency for Healthcare Research and Quality, 2009

Wilson I, Schoen K, Neuman P: Physician-patient communication about prescription medication nonadherence: a 50-state study of America's seniors. J Gen Intern Med 22:6–12, 2007

Wolfe BE, Talley SL, Smith AT: Psychopharmacologic first-line strategies in the treatment of major depression and psychosis: a survey of advanced practice nurses. J Am Psychiatr Nurses Assoc 14:144–151, 2008

Woolcott JC, Richardson KJ, Wiens MO, et al: Meta-analysis of the impact of 9 medication classes on falls in elderly persons. Arch Intern Med 169:1952–1960, 2009

Worley J, McGuiness TM: Promoting adherence to psychotropic medication for youth, part 1. J Psychosoc Nurs Ment Health Serv 48:19–22, 2010

Wright SK, Schroeter S: Hyponatremia as a complication of selective serotonin reuptake inhibitors. J Am Acad Nurse Pract 20:47–51, 2008

Zivin K, Ganoczy D, Pfeiffer PN, et al: Antidepressant adherence after psychiatric hospitalization among VA patients with depression. Adm Policy Ment Health 36:406–415, 2009

Zurakowski T: The practicalities and pitfalls of polypharmacy. Nurse Pract 34:36–41, 2009

Zwicker D, Fulmer T: Reducing adverse drug events, in Evidence-Based Geriatric Nursing Protocols for Best Practice, 3rd Edition. Edited by Capezuti E, Zwicker D, Mezey M, et al. New York, Springer, 2008, pp 257–308

Index

*Page numbers printed in **boldface** type refer to tables or figures.*